the new rules of menopause

A Mayo Clinic Guide
to Perimenopause
and Beyond

Stephanie S. Faubion, M.D., M.B.A.
Director of Mayo Clinic Women's Health

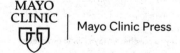
MAYO CLINIC | Mayo Clinic Press

MAYO CLINIC PRESS

Medical Editor Stephanie S. Faubion, M.D., M.B.A.

Publisher Daniel J. Harke

Editor in Chief Nina E. Wiener

Managing Editor Anna L. Cavallo

Art Director Stewart J. Koski

Production Design Amanda J. Knapp

Illustration and Photography Mayo Clinic Media Support Services, Mayo Clinic Medical Illustration and Animation

Editorial Research Librarians Anthony J. Cook, Edward (Eddy) S. Morrow Jr., Erika A. Riggin, Katherine (Katie) J. Warner

Copy Editors Miranda M. Attlesey, Alison K. Baker, Nancy J. Jacoby, Julie M. Maas

Contributors Paru S. David, M.D.; Julia A. Files, M.D.; Karen Grothe, Ph.D., L.P.; Laura M. Hamilton Waxman; Kejal Kantarci, M.D.; Ekta Kapoor, M.B.B.S.; Ann E. Kearns, M.D.; Juliana (Jewel) M. Kling, M.D., M.P.H.; Susan N. Kok, M.D.; Carol L.Kuhle, D.O., M.P.H.; Rachel Lehmann-Haupt; Robin M. Lloyd, M.D.; Denise M. Millstine, M.D.; Dawn M. Mussallem, D.O.; Hannah C. Nordhues, M.D.; John A. Occhino, M.D., M.S.; Chrisandra L. Shufelt, M.D.; Taryn L. Smith, M.D.; Richa Sood, M.D., M.S.; Jacqueline (Jackie) M. Thielen, M.D.; Suneela Vegunta, M.D.

Additional contributions from Kirkus Reviews and Rath Indexing

Image Credits All photographs and illustrations are copyright of MFMER, except the following: COVER: smartboy10 / DigitalVision Vectors via Getty Images | p. 277: bubaone / DigitalVision Vectors via Getty Images; ksana-gribakina / iStock /Getty Images via Getty Images; my vector illustration / iStock / Getty Images via Getty Images

To stay informed about Mayo Clinic Press, subscribe to our free e-newsletter at MCPress.MayoClinic.org or follow us on social media.

The information in this book is true and complete to the best of our knowledge. This book is intended only as an informative guide for those wishing to learn more about health issues. It is not intended to replace, countermand or conflict with advice given to you by your own physician. The ultimate decision concerning your care should be made between you and your doctor. Information in this book is offered with no guarantees. The authors and publisher disclaim all liability in connection with the use of this book.

For bulk sales to employers, member groups and health-related companies, contact Mayo Clinic, 200 First St. SW, Rochester, MN 55905, or email SpecialSalesMayoBooks@mayo.edu

ISBN 978-1-945564-11-6

Library of Congress Control Number: 2022942482

Printed in China

Big rocks analogy, page 245, is provided with permission by Franklin Covey Co.

Sections on gratitude and mindfulness, Chapters 14 and 15, are based on content from *The Mayo Clinic Guide to Stress-Free Living*, by Amit Sood, © 2013. Reprinted by permission of Da Capo Lifelong Books, a member of The Perseus Book Group.

When you purchase Mayo Clinic newsletters and books, proceeds are used to further medical education and research at Mayo Clinic. You not only get answers to your questions on health, you become part of the solution.

About the author

Stephanie S. Faubion, M.D., M.B.A., is the Penny and Bill George Director of Mayo Clinic's Center for Women's Health and is chair of the Department of Medicine at Mayo Clinic in Jacksonville, Florida. Dr. Faubion has practiced as a physician in the Women's Health Clinic at Mayo Clinic for over 18 years. She also serves as medical director for The North American Menopause Society. She has a broad interest in women's health and has evaluated and treated women with menopausal, hormonal and sexual health concerns. Her research encompasses sex and gender-based differences in disease, menopause, hormone therapy, healthy aging, and sexual health and dysfunction in women — addressing questions that come directly from the clinical dilemmas faced every day in medical practice. A leader in women's health, Dr. Faubion frequently lends her expertise to the *New York Times*, *Washington Post*, *Wall Street Journal*, CNN, NBC News and other national media.

Table of Contents

A note on terms

From Stephanie S. Faubion, M.D., M.B.A., and the editors

ALL GENDERS ARE WELCOME HERE

In this book, the term *woman* is frequently used to refer to the target audience. Gender-specific language may also be used to reflect the scientific publications that were referenced in gathering up-to-date research and information. However, this book is for all people. We recognize that not everyone experiencing menopause may identify as a woman or use the same pronouns. In addition, not all people who identify as midlife women will experience the typical biological and hormonal shifts of menopause.

Sex — a label of biological characteristics assigned at birth — is an important variable in your health. A better understanding of sex-based differences in health and disease is critical to truly individualizing medicine in the future. But gender identity — how you identify and express yourself — is not often considered separately from sex in research studies. As a result, it's not included as a factor in clinical practice guidelines and recommendations.

More study is needed on issues around gender as it relates to menopause. In these pages, we have tried to use an inclusive approach to the topic of menopause, acknowledging the gaps in knowledge that still exist.

For additional guidance on menopause and midlife health for transgender and nonbinary people, talk with a doctor or practitioner who is empathetic, knowledgeable and respectful of your needs. To find a doctor with transgender expertise, check the websites for the World Professional Association for Transgender Health (WPATH) or Health Professionals Advancing LGBTQ Equality (GLMA, previously known as the Gay & Lesbian Medical Association).

DOCTOR, HEALTH CARE PROVIDER, PRACTITIONER?

At the time of publication, *health care provider* may be the most common catchall term in the United States for the professional roles that provide medical care, including doctors, nurse practitioners, certified nurse midwives and physician assistants. Many other specialists also fit under this umbrella. However, we prefer other terms, such as *practitioner* or *clinician*, when a general term is needed. These words put less focus on the business transactions of health care and more focus on the professional credentials of the people providing care. In this book, you'll see *practitioner* used more frequently for that reason.

The term *doctor* is also used in these pages with some flexibility. The title of *doctor* is earned through specific academic degrees, and we want to respect that expertise. We also acknowledge that in conversation, *doctor* is often used more loosely to include other qualified professionals you might see for care, such as a nurse practitioner. In the interest of keeping this text reader friendly, we've allowed for some flexibility in how it's used here.

Menopause today: What's happening to my body?

In 2019 comedian Wanda Sykes performed a comedy routine about menopause that was part of her Netflix special *Not Normal.* "This is our plight, right?" she said emphatically. "When you're young, you're fertile; you're producing eggs. You're bringing life into the world ... And then you get older, no more eggs. You can't bring any more life into the world, so they just set you on fire!" This reference to hot flashes — the sudden feeling of warmth that's a common symptom of the menopause transition — resonated. The audience broke into the kind of laughter that gave the impression: Yeah, that sounds about right.

NOT YOUR MOTHER'S MENOPAUSE

In the past, conversations about perimenopause and menopause didn't often happen on celebrity stages. They tended to be private chats with your mom or among your sisters or girlfriends, or they didn't happen at all. For some, these conversations were tinged with cultural taboos and shame around aging. And let's face it, many people have traditionally not been very comfortable talking about their "lady parts." But this is fortunately changing.

In the generation now entering their post-fertility years, many people born with a uterus and ovaries have a distinctly different attitude. Women are not interested in suffering in silence. They are listening to podcasts, using apps, participating in online conversations and buying books because they want to know what to expect in the menopause transition, they want answers and they want effective solutions. More than ever before, in public spaces people are talking about this stage of life with humor and curiosity. They're talking about it as a normal part of life — because it is! Menopause is a universal experience for about half the world's population. By 2030, 1.2 billion people worldwide will be postmenopausal.

If you've seen Sykes' comedy set and haven't reached menopause yet, you might worry that it's about to hit you like a truck. But the reality is that the changes typically happen over a number of years. As you enter your 40s and early 50s, you may experience some of the symptoms of perimenopause (the transition period of several months to several years before menopause).

Menopause actually starts when you've had your last period — although it's not official until you haven't had a period for a full year. It can be a disorienting stage. At the same time that you're noticing these changes in your body and hormonal cycles, you may also be at the height of your confidence and career and finally feeling settled in your life. But suddenly, maybe you're finding yourself wide awake at 3 a.m., staring at your phone. Or you're finding it harder to focus on reading an email. But then again, that may be because your kid won't take a nap or won't stop whining at you or isn't home yet even though it's midnight. Maybe you've started to fear buttoning your favorite jeans or you've already jumped up a size.

And then, out of nowhere, every so often you feel like you've been set on fire, as hot flashes cause your neck and face to flush. That may create awkward moments in a video meeting or even a dinner date. Maybe you're starting to skip your period, and you haven't had one in more than a few months. In these moments, you hesitantly talk to a friend or your sister. You think, *What is happening to me?* Or if you suspect perimenopause, you think, *Really, now? It happened to my mom when I was going to college. I still have kids in school. I feel so much younger!*

Compared to women of previous generations, who more often got married and pregnant at a younger age, many of today's women nearing or entering the menopause transition are in a different phase of life. At 50, you may still be working as hard or harder than you did in your 30s. Maybe you're starting a new company. Perhaps you're falling in love for the first time, or the fourth. And if you were busy building a career in your prime fertility years, or it took you a bit longer to meet a parenting partner, maybe you're trying to start a family while many of your peers are talking about waking up drenched in sweat.

On the darker side, you could be wondering if you will face ageism at work, which can affect your self-esteem even if you know you're at the top of your game. You may be hearing more often about couples who are getting divorced. A few people in your social circles have been diagnosed with cancer, and you worry, *Could I be next?* Then you get a call from your aging mother, who doesn't remember that you already told her your son won his soccer game, and when you get annoyed about this, she questions whether you have a mood disorder, as if your irritability is related to some vague mental illness like the hysteria that women were labeled with in the 1950s.

The modern midlife sandwich of car pools and aging parents, often along with a demanding career, can easily be overwhelming, even apart from menopause. So it's completely understandable that starting to experience the physical and emotional symptoms of the menopause transition might push you to the brink. But knowledge is power. This book is full of empowering information, tips and stories to help you understand one of the most important rules of menopause: You don't have to suffer through it.

EMBRACING THE INEVITABLE

You may be one of the lucky ones. Not every woman will experience menopause symptoms; some will have a few symptoms, and some won't experience any. But all people with a uterus and ovaries will face the transition that leads to the end of menstruation, typically anywhere between their mid-40s to their mid-50s. For some, menopause may come prematurely and more suddenly and skip the typical lead-up. This may be due to medical interventions such as chemotherapy, pelvic radiation therapy or the surgical removal of your ovaries. For some people, menopause just comes early without any obvious reason.

The typical runway to the moment when your ovaries stop making estrogen and progesterone — the hormones responsible for the menstrual cycle and fertility — is a distinct stage of life known as perimenopause. It's a progression over the time when you're still releasing eggs but the number is getting low and quality is going downhill. The symptoms you may be experiencing in your body are directly related to living with less estrogen or experiencing significant swings in estrogen levels. These symptoms often include more-frequent headaches, irregular bleeding, night sweats, joint aches and hot flashes. It's not uncommon to have a general feeling of irritability, along with worsening depression and other mental health issues. For the majority of women who experience natural menopause, these symptoms increase during the transition to menopause, and they tend to be most common in the first few years after your final menstrual period.

Along with physical and mental symptoms, menopause can have social and societal effects. For example, if you're stressed about managing hot flashes at work, or you've been passed over for a promotion for someone younger, you're not alone. It's true that there is often a bias against peri- and postmenopausal women. It's a combination of sexism and a culture that puts youth on a pedestal.

For comparison, consider that men also experience age-related changes in midlife. For decades, pharmaceutical companies and advertisements have catered to middle-aged men with erectile dysfunction, while menopause symptoms still go underrecognized, undertreated and, worse, disparaged. This double standard and bias may be especially frustrating in a time when women in midlife are driving the global economy with their economic power and wisdom.

It's true: Many of the symptoms of the menopause transition ... well, they bite. What's most important is to focus on healthy conversations about aging and your body's natural transitions. While comedy routines are entertaining and good for bringing the conversation into the mainstream, women's changing bodies should not just be the punchlines of jokes — or worse, completely ignored.

Here's some good news: You're in great company. Millions of women around the world are going through the transition to menopause — and finally talking about it. The rules of your body are changing, but more than ever before, you can read the rule book. When symptoms cause suffering, you can seek the help you deserve. With the right tools to advocate for yourself, including some comedian-inspired attitude, you can turn menopause into a time to embrace the new rules of your body in the next phase of life.

Maybe just keep your fan handy.

A HISTORY OF MENOPAUSE

Looking into the history of menopause can offer some clues on both why the menopause transition has been stigmatized and why so many women have internalized menopause as the end of their relevance. History also explains why this change has been viewed as both a physical and mental disease.

But let's start with the positive side of what ancient culture can teach us about this time of life and why the menopause transition is also a time to celebrate. Anthropologists believe that menopausal women offer an advantage that has helped drive evolution. The "grandmother hypothesis" holds that women who could no longer biologically conceive children lived on to ensure the survival of their children's children, supporting them with their freed-up time. Studies have found that in hunter-gatherer societies, foraging grandmothers supplied food and child care. And in ancient Greece, as communities evolved from 700 to 480 B.C., postmenopausal women were viewed as renewed virgins and appointed as priestesses.

"Disease of deficiency"
As modern medicine has evolved, the views on menopausal women have been less flattering. In the 1700s and early 1800s, many still

thought menstrual blood contained toxic components. When periods stopped and those impurities weren't regularly flushed out, it was thought to cause a range of problems in the body. In another school of thought, the freedom from menstruation ultimately left women stronger, but the transition to this phase of life was a rocky time of internal disorder. By the 19th century, physicians in the United States widely viewed menopause as a "physiological crisis," according to Susan E. Bell, a professor of anthropology and sociology. This crisis was thought to lead to either "tranquility or disease, depending on a woman's prior behavior and her 'predisposition to malignancy.'"

These early views contributed to the practice of treating menopause as a disease or disorder, like diabetes or depression — the medicalization of menopause. In some ways, this approach helped doctors take menopause symptoms more seriously and work to find methods to resolve them. Women were no longer expected to suffer through their symptoms in silence.

Yet the medicalization of menopause also solidified the message that menopause is a health problem needing treatment, rather than a natural transformation that can be managed based on an individual's experience and preferences. It's a subtle difference in perspective that can make a big difference in a person's understanding of their body. Your body is not broken; it's just changing, and as with all change, it can sometimes be rocky.

In the 1930s and 1940s, this view became further entrenched because of the medical vocabulary that defined menopause as a "deficiency disease" in a series of papers written by a small, elite segment of medical professionals. These professionals were influential in medical policy and education, and many of their views have remained as the common wisdom. Furthermore, their ideas were based in a 19th century philosophical concept known as "the eternal feminine." This principle idealized the essence of a virtuous woman as modest, graceful, pure, delicate and polite.

This same group of doctors who considered menopause a deficiency disease also recommended estrogen as a treatment to help its symptoms. That helped convince the U.S. Food and Drug Administration (FDA) to approve estrogen therapy as a treatment. If a lack of estrogen caused the physiological symptoms, they thought, then the treatment was to replace the estrogen. As they wrote, this would "let her down more gently and gradually" and "remove temporarily the immediate cause of the symptoms."

One could argue that the idea was to restore the eternal feminine and to make men's lives easier. This diagnosis also allowed doctors to standardize therapeutics, which often neglected variation among individual women around doses needed, biologically different health profiles, and subjective experiences. It also led to books like *Forever Feminine*, published in 1966 by Dr. Robert A. Wilson. In it, he maintained that estrogen therapy could cure the "natural plague" of menopause.

Over the following decades, hormone therapy (HT) became the standard of care to ease the symptoms of menopause. It was used also to help stave off the risk of coronary heart disease, as observational data showed a preventive benefit. Then in 1985, the Framingham Heart Study reported a two-fold increase in heart disease associated with estrogen use over an eight-year period, and many in the medical community became more skeptical about HT. Around the same time, however, the Nurses' Health Study and several others reported a 50% lower risk of heart disease in those who used estrogen therapy. The contradiction created even more confusion. Ultimately, more evidence seemed to show the benefit of estrogen therapy for reducing heart disease risk. In 1992, a position paper from the American College of Physicians recommended that all postmenopausal women be offered estrogen therapy to help prevent heart disease.

Then in 2002, a landmark study stunned the medical community. The Women's Health Initiative (WHI) trials had been launched in the early 1990s to study several leading health concerns in women. It was one of the largest preventive health studies in U.S. history, involving more than 160,000 postmenopausal women ages 50 to 79. But part of the study was stopped early when it found that the combination of a particular type of estrogen (conjugated equine estrogens) and a progestin (medroxyprogesterone acetate) increased the risk of heart disease, stroke, blood clots and breast cancer. These risks outweighed other health benefits. The study, however, didn't distinguish among the broad age range of women studied. Many of the women in their 60s and 70s were well past the age range in which women are likely to seek treatment for menopause symptoms. In addition, the trial had looked at just one type of hormone therapy — conjugated equine estrogens plus medroxyprogesterone acetate.

Still, the media hype around these results caused most clinicians to stop prescribing HT for relief from menopause symptoms. By 2010, use of HT dropped to about 5% of women in their 50s and 60s. Robust debates broke out about the best approaches to managing menopause. Clinicians — and their patients — were left with a void in medical advice and treatment for the millions who were suffering from menopause symptoms.

Moving toward more inclusive medicine

For many years, the medical field looked at women's health by narrowly focusing on issues related to women's breasts and genitals instead of looking at the body and mind as a whole. Significant advances in research have moved women's health beyond the realm of outdated "bikini medicine." Sex-based biological differences in health and disease are now a more prominent focus of interest by the National Institutes of Health (NIH) Office of Research on Women's Health in the design and analysis of research and the reporting of study results. There are essential reasons to understand the impact of sex differences in the study of medications, interventions, and diagnostic tests, and to look at every woman as an individual patient.

Research has shown that women are 50% more likely than men to experience adverse drug reactions. And medicines may also have different effects in men and women. In 2013, for example, researchers found that zolpidem (Ambien), one of the bestselling prescription sleep aids, resulted in much higher blood levels of the drug in females. This led the FDA, for the first time, to reduce the standard dose for women to half of what was recommended for men. A growing body of research shows the need to pay closer attention to sex- and gender-based differences in health and disease across the board.

In addition, there is a large gap in the literature on the menopause experience in racial minorities and transgender individuals. In the late 1990s, a group of scientists published initial results from the Study of Women's Health Across the Nation (SWAN). This 23-year study looked at the menopause transition among an ethnically and racially diverse (Black, Chinese, Hispanic, Japanese and white) group of midlife women in the United States. Among many conclusions, the study found that Black women have a higher tendency toward early and more-frequent hot flashes. We know that women who experience hot flashes early often have an increased risk for heart disease and that Black women also have a higher risk, compared to other groups of women. But more research is needed to better understand what the differences in menopause symptoms mean for people in minority racial groups. How are symptoms, racial and cultural identities, and health outcomes related? By current statistics, 1 in 3 women will die of cardiovascular disease. A better, more inclusive understanding of risk factors is critical to make real improvements in women's health for all.

New standard of care

Since the results of the WHI trial first came out, more analysis has helped give a clearer picture of its takeaways. In 2015, an article in the *New England Journal of Medicine* addressed the fact that HT was largely abandoned in the years following the WHI. The article discussed the flawed interpretations of the WHI study — in particular, that the results from a largely older group of women have been applied to health care decisions for people in their 40s and 50s.

Meanwhile, later analyses of the WHI trial as well as other studies have confirmed that the benefits of HT outweigh the risks for most healthy younger women experiencing menopause symptoms. If clinicians use an individualized approach to symptom management, hormone therapy can be an incredibly effective, low-risk treatment. Indeed, for those who are appropriate candidates, it can dramatically improve symptoms and quality of life.

The North American Menopause Society and other leading women's health organizations now recommend the use of HT as a safe and effective treatment option for most symptomatic women who are within 10 years of menopause onset and under the age of 60 years. HT has also been shown to prevent bone loss and fracture.

It's important to note that other treatments can help with symptoms in perimenopause too. Hot flashes, headaches, irregular bleeding, mood changes and other symptoms are common during this transition. Hormonal treatments in perimenopause may be different — stronger

— than the type prescribed after periods have completely stopped. Menopausal HT wouldn't be strong enough to override the hormonal fluctuation during perimenopause, when the ovaries are still working. In other words, it wouldn't control bleeding, prevent pregnancy or stop the falls in estrogen that cause migraines and mood issues. Treatment in perimenopause depends on which symptoms someone is experiencing. Options might include low-dose birth control pills, antidepressants, an IUD containing a progestin, or a nonsteroidal anti-inflammatory medication, which can control excessive bleeding.

Menopause management vacuum

More than 20 years after the publication of the WHI trial results, HT still gets a bad rap. Because the widely publicized initial results showed greater risks than benefits, without distinguishing among age groups or other nuances of the trials, there is still a great deal of confusion around treatment with HT in menopause. Many women who would be eligible for HT to improve symptoms are still skeptical because they haven't received updated information about the relative safety of HT from their health care providers. Many clinicians are still practicing under the older concept that HT is dangerous. Efforts to communicate the favorable balance of risks and benefits of HT in younger, healthier postmenopausal women have not improved prescription rates. These low prescription rates even extend to the use of low-dose vaginal estrogen for management of genitourinary symptoms in postmenopausal women and particularly among those who are cancer survivors.

The challenge goes deeper than the remaining skepticism related to the WHI trials. Many clinicians simply aren't well equipped to address menopause symptoms with their patients because medical training programs don't properly equip them for menopause management. A recent survey of residents in U.S. obstetrics and gynecology, internal medicine and family medicine training programs showed that most trainees received no more than an hour or two of instruction on menopause and generally felt unprepared to manage women with menopause symptoms. This dearth of postgraduate training means women now live in a menopause management vacuum, which has created a market opportunity, for better and for worse.

THE NEW FRONTIER OF WOMEN'S HEALTH

Women entering the menopause transition years now represent a significant segment of a $28 trillion worldwide female economy. Many of these women are experiencing symptoms that significantly disrupt their quality of life. And they're not holding back. Their curiosity and attitude are driving what is now estimated to be a $600 billion market for menopause management.

In response to this demand, startup companies are mushrooming in every area of menopause management from over-the-counter hair and skin care products to alternative natural supplements that tout nonhormonal hot flash remedies and weight-loss probiotics. There are energy bars dubbed "power food for the pause" (so you can approach menopause "like a boss!") and FDA-approved off-label prescriptions. And the technology industry, finally focused on women's health, is racing to fill the gaps in the menopause market with apps, devices, digital therapeutics, virtual clinics and more.

This broad spectrum of choices will undoubtedly overwhelm you as you immediately see that many of the products don't have scientific backing or offer ways for women to further explore the risks versus benefits. Some products come attached with claims from doctors, but unfortunately that's not automatically a sign that the product does everything it claims to do. On the one hand, this market sheds much-needed attention on women's health and this treatment gap. On the other hand, it means that women seeking treatment need to become savvy health consumers.

It's important to keep a high degree of skepticism regarding health claims about menopause management solutions that seem too good to be true and often lack high-quality evidence to back them up. It's essential to understand how to tell a helpful and scientifically sound approach from snake oil, especially when either may come with a celebrity doctor's endorsement. The first rule of thumb is to be a wary consumer. If it looks too good to be true, it probably is. If someone is promising you a cure to menopause or the fountain of youth and anti-aging solutions, remember: There is no miracle cure for menopause (or aging)! Let this be your mantra: *It's not a disease. It's a natural process with symptoms that can be alleviated.*

So, what if your clinician seems to have no idea what you're talking about when you try to discuss perimenopause and the menopause transition, or worse, suggests you just tough it out? If possible, find a more knowledgeable provider. If you're worried that your clinician is touting treatments that are not evidence based — or you're simply not getting the expert support you need to manage symptoms — it's time to call in reinforcements. Look to reputable sources such as Mayo Clinic or the North American Menopause Society. These organizations can help point you to reliable, accessible menopause providers and certified practitioners in menopause management.

A NEW RULE BOOK

This book is designed to give you the information you need to take charge and be your own advocate in the transition to menopause. It's organized into three parts.

In Part One, you'll learn how and why your body's rules are changing as you go through perimenopause and menopause. Chapters focus on defining and explaining the phases of the menopause transition, specific challenges and solutions in perimenopause, and changes throughout the body. You'll also find discussions of early menopause and the many different experiences of menopause depending on your identity, background and surroundings. If your daily refrain in midlife has been, "What's going on?" Part One is a solid place to start.

Part Two gets at why you're probably reading this book: managing menopause symptoms. With chapters focusing on the latest expertise in medication therapy, holistic therapies and strategies targeted to each symptom, this section will empower you to find the most effective solutions for your symptoms and your life with your own health care provider. With recent discoveries and advances, there are more options than ever before that can be tailored to fit your individual story.

In Part Three, chapters look further down the road. The average 55-year-old woman can expect to live another 30 or more years after reaching menopause — that's one-third of your life! And while you'll be free from the risk of unintended pregnancy, staying on top of other health risks that come along with aging can help you get the most out of this season of life. These chapters hold important information about screenings, preventive care and lifestyle tips for a healthy heart, strong bones, sound mental health and much more.

Whether you immediately dive into Chapter 1 or jump ahead in search of more specific answers, this book can help you gain some perspective on menopause and understand your body's transition. This may ultimately help you feel stronger, have a better sense of control and own the process.

The transition to menopause is your unique experience. It's a natural progression. You don't have to suffer through it. And you get to help write your own rules!

1

Understanding it

1

What is menopause?

On the topic of new rules: It may seem like the rules of your body are changing and no one told you. You turned 45 and weight started creeping on, even though you're staying active. Suddenly you're feeling an occasional hot flash, and more than ever, you can't remember where you left your phone. Then your period gets a little wonky.

It's not just in your head — your body is changing. As you approach and enter menopause, your chemistry and physiology are shifting to a new set of rules and a new normal.

THE BASICS

Put simply, you've reached menopause when you've had your last period and your menstrual cycle has stopped. But for most women, you won't know for sure that you've hit this landmark (and a health care provider won't diagnose it) until a full year after your last period.

The years before and after, as you near menopause and transition through it, bring big changes in the body. This is a normal life stage that happens to everyone born with a uterus and ovaries. But it can feel anything but normal!

Menopause occurs when your ovaries stop making estrogen and progesterone — female hormones that are key for menstrual cycles and fertility. In most women, menopause happens naturally, somewhere around age 52. Menopause can also be the result of a medical procedure, such as chemotherapy, pelvic radiation therapy or the surgical removal of the ovaries.

Most women will notice changes in their bodies in the years before menopause (perimenopause) and after menopause (postmenopause). These changes, like menopause itself, are different for everyone. Some women experience many symptoms of menopause, including hot flashes and drenching night sweats, which can be hugely disruptive to daily life and last for years. Others notice hardly any disruptions.

Each person's experience is unique. And while some of the changes you encounter may be surprising or unpleasant — or both! — keep in mind that what you're going through is a natural part of life. And, even more importantly, know that there are ways to treat or help manage these symptoms. You don't have to suffer.

Don't worry — you've got this!

HORMONAL CHANGES DURING YOUR LIFETIME

Throughout your life, hormones play a vital role in your health and development. Hormones are chemical substances that influence other cells in your body, kind of like little chemical messengers. When you were young, low levels of the female hormone estrogen influenced the growth of your bones and muscles, as well as your brain, heart and blood vessels. As you neared puberty, estrogen production increased and you got your first period.

During your reproductive years, hormone levels rise and fall monthly. In fact, it's this consistent fluctuation that controls your menstrual cycle. At the beginning of each month's cycle, estrogen and progesterone levels are low. They start to rise, thickening the lining of

HORMONE PRIMER

Your hormones change throughout your life, playing important roles in reproductive health. Here's a look at the key ones.

Estrogen This female hormone is released by the ovaries. It helps regulate the menstrual cycle during the reproductive years. Estrogen levels rise and fall during your menstrual cycle, and they significantly decrease by menopause. Prior to menopause, estradiol (ess-truh-DIE-ahl), also called E2, is the primary estrogen in your body. After menopause, estrone (ESS-trohn), or E1, becomes the dominant form.

Progesterone This female hormone, also released by the ovaries, stimulates the uterus to prepare for pregnancy and helps maintain a pregnancy. Progesterone levels drop after menopause.

Follicle-stimulating hormone (FSH) This hormone, secreted by the pituitary gland, stimulates the ovaries to produce eggs. (In men, FSH stimulates the production of sperm.) FSH levels go up and down during your menstrual cycle and rise at menopause.

Luteinizing (LOO-tin-ize-ing) hormone (LH) This hormone, also secreted by the pituitary gland, triggers ovulation. Levels of LH also rise at menopause.

Testosterone This hormone, which is more dominant in men, belongs to a class of hormones called *androgens*. It is also produced in small amounts in women, by the ovaries and adrenal glands. Testosterone plays a role in sexual function. Testosterone levels go down gradually with age and do not decline specifically because of menopause.

Anti-mullerian (anti-muh-LEER-ee-en) hormone (AMH) This ovarian hormone is thought to regulate the number of follicles that develop with each menstrual cycle. Levels of AMH are linked to the number of eggs in reserve and can be measured to predict fertility. Researchers are still exploring whether AMH testing, alone or with other factors, also might be used to estimate how close you are to menopause.

HOW HORMONE LEVELS FLUCTUATE

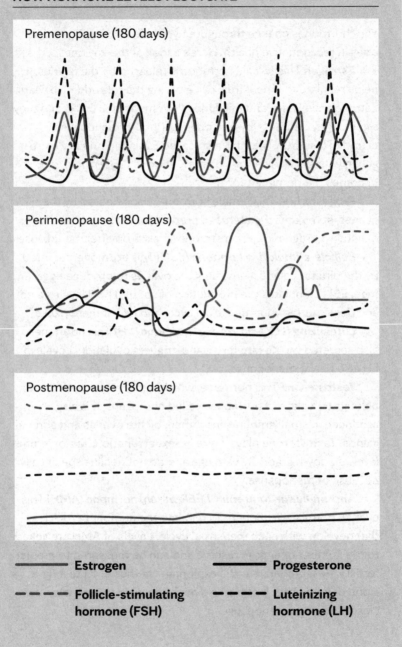

Premenopause (180 days)

Perimenopause (180 days)

Postmenopause (180 days)

——— Estrogen

——— Progesterone

– – – – Follicle-stimulating hormone (FSH)

– – – – Luteinizing hormone (LH)

your uterus as it gets ready for an egg (oocyte). About 14 days into the cycle, hormone levels rise again as you ovulate — which is when the egg leaves your ovary and travels down the fallopian tube to your uterus. If you don't become pregnant at this point (because the egg is not fertilized by a sperm), hormone levels start to fall, and your uterine lining is shed as you have your period. This happens over and over again, month after month, throughout your reproductive years.

As you age, however, and near the end of your reproductive years — typically around your mid-40s — the consistent rise and fall of hormones starts to change. The rate at which your ovaries make estrogen and progesterone becomes less predictable.

These hormonal changes mark the beginning of perimenopause. They can cause irregular menstrual cycles and other symptoms, such as hot flashes and vaginal dryness. These fluctuations and changes may last several years before you experience your last menstrual cycle.

Eventually, the production of reproductive hormones slows so much — and the number of eggs stored in the ovaries diminishes enough — that your periods stop altogether. When this happens, and you haven't had your period for at least 12 months, you'll know you've reached menopause.

STAGES OF MENOPAUSE

Menopause may be marked by your last period, but this life change doesn't happen overnight. The menopause transition typically has three stages: perimenopause, menopause and postmenopause.

Perimenopause
Many of the symptoms that most women think of with menopause — from hot flashes to irregular periods — actually start in perimenopause.

Perimenopause, which means *around menopause,* is the time leading up to menopause (or your last period). Women typically start perimenopause in their mid-40s (47 is average). But it's normal for it to start anywhere from the early 40s to early 50s.

Perimenopause is prompted by fluctuations in your estrogen and progesterone levels. Changes in your menstrual cycle are often the

WHAT IS PREMATURE MENOPAUSE?

Premature menopause is when menopause happens before the age of 40. It can happen naturally, or it may be caused by medical interventions such as surgery or cancer treatment. Just as in menopause at an average age, women who go through premature menopause quit having their periods and are unable to get pregnant without reproductive assistance. It's estimated that about 1% of women experience premature menopause.

If you have stopped having your period before age 40 and don't know why, see your health care provider for further evaluation. Women who go through menopause early are likely to benefit from hormone therapy to prevent some potential health risks down the road. Premature menopause is covered in detail in Chapter 4.

first sign. Initially, you may notice a longer time between periods, or notice that you are bleeding for more or fewer days than usual. Your menstrual blood may have more clots, or it may change color slightly. Hot flashes and night sweats are also common. Later in perimenopause, periods may change again. They might occur even further apart or closer together again for a time, and other symptoms may be added to the mix.

Perimenopause feels different for every woman who experiences it. A few lucky women will breeze through both perimenopause and menopause without any symptoms that disrupt their daily routines. Some will experience the signs and symptoms for just a year or two, while others will be in perimenopause for nearly 10 years before reaching menopause. Most often, women will remain in the perimenopause stage for 4 to 8 years.

While every person's experience is unique, research has identified some patterns. For example, the Study of Women's Health Across the Nation (SWAN) found that the perimenopause stage tends to be longer

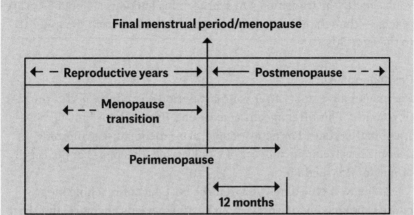

MENOPAUSE TIMELINE

Adapted from World Health Organization. Research on the Menopause in the 1990s: Report of WHO scientific group. WHO Technical Series 866; 1996.

for women who begin it earlier. In addition, Black women in the study were in perimenopause longer than white, Chinese and Japanese women. More research is needed to fully understand these patterns.

Because symptoms aren't always clear — and they can change over time — it can be hard to know exactly when you start perimenopause. If you're experiencing menstrual changes and other perimenopausal signs and symptoms, it's a good idea to talk to your health care provider. Together, you can make sure there isn't another reason for these changes.

For more in-depth discussion of perimenopause, turn to Chapter 3.

Menopause

Menopause is a milestone you don't know you've reached until an entire year has gone by. That's because menopause is considered official only when you haven't had a period for 12 full months.

Why wait a year to make the call? Because some people will think they've gone through menopause after going a few months without a period, only to be surprised by several more cycles. However, once you've gone a full year without a period, you can be pretty sure that you've made the transition. On average, this happens at about 52 years of age — though there is a wide range of "normal," from the mid-40s to the later 50s.

Postmenopause

Postmenopause starts after your last period and continues for the rest of your life. This often means at least one-third of your life will be spent in this stage. For many people, after menopause symptoms become less frequent and less of a daily issue, this phase of life is full of newfound freedom.

Many women will tell you that the best part of reaching menopause is not having to worry about getting periods anymore. But there are other benefits too. For instance, you also don't have to worry about getting pregnant. And many of the uncomfortable or disruptive symptoms you might have experienced in perimenopause — such as breast pain or mood swings — usually go away as well. Your hormones should settle into steady, low levels instead of fluctuating like they did during your reproductive life.

Some of the symptoms of perimenopause may continue into postmenopause. Hot flashes often stick around for a few years or more, and vaginal dryness may stay for good or even worsen with time. Other body changes often crop up over time as well, thanks to lower levels of estrogen and other natural aging processes. Fortunately, many of these conditions can be managed with treatments and lifestyle changes to help you stay comfortable and active.

CHANGES TO THE MENSTRUAL CYCLE

Often, one of the first signs of perimenopause is a change in the menstrual cycle. This is primarily due to natural changes in ovulation (including changes in the frequency of ovulation) and hormone levels, including those of estradiol, the primary estrogen made by the ovaries. No matter how regular (or irregular) your periods have been historically, these changes can disrupt your menstrual cycle.

CHANGES IN FERTILITY

Your ability to get pregnant is at its peak in your 20s, and then pregnancy becomes less likely with age. This decline in fertility typically starts after age 35 and continues through menopause.

Once you start perimenopause, conceiving is more difficult, but still possible. In fact, you can still get pregnant even if you haven't had a period in several months. It's only when you're postmenopausal that you can no longer conceive naturally.

For some women, reaching this stage of life can be an adjustment and it might feel like a loss. Even if they had not planned to have more (or any) children, they may mourn the loss of their fertility as a part of their identity. For others, the loss of fertility is a time of relief — a time to relax and enjoy sex without worrying about birth control or the risk of pregnancy.

Just be careful not to discard your contraception too soon. It's worth repeating: Women do get pregnant in the years and months leading to menopause. In fact, the changing menstrual cycles common during perimenopause can cause unpredictable ovulation — making it difficult to know when you are most likely to get pregnant.

Of course, this unpredictability can also make it frustrating if you are trying to get pregnant as you enter perimenopause. In Chapters 3 and 4, you'll find more information on options to help improve your chances and other ways to grow your family.

For some, the changes are subtle. For others, the changes are obvious — and disconcerting. Your period may come more often or less often. It may last several more days than usual, or it might be surprisingly short. If you've had years of an unpredictable period, it may suddenly run like clockwork. It may be lighter, resulting only in brief spotting, or heavier than ever, bleeding through pads or even your clothing.

One of the most frustrating facts for many women is that all the above may be true. One month, your period may arrive a week late and be lighter. Then your next one comes a week early and seems alarmingly heavy.

For some, heavy or prolonged bleeding can affect social lives, sexual relationships or stress levels. Less frequently, unusually heavy menstrual cycles may cause fatigue, headaches or anemia. It's important to contact your health care provider if you have any abnormal bleeding.

It may be reassuring to know that you're not alone — and that this roller coaster won't last forever. Nearly all women (about 90%) who go through natural menopause will experience changes to their menstrual cycles before their last period. For most people, these changes will resolve in an average of 4 to 8 years. For some, symptoms can last longer.

RED FLAGS: MENOPAUSE, OR SOMETHING MORE?

Changes to your menstrual cycle are usually a normal part of perimenopause. But in some cases, abnormal bleeding may require further evaluation to rule out a more serious condition. Talk to your health care provider if you experience any of the following:

- You stop having periods before age 45.
- Your periods become so heavy that you have to change tampons or pads every hour or two for two or more hours.
- Your periods last longer than seven days, or several days longer than usual.
- You are bleeding or spotting between periods.
- Your periods are becoming closer together, regularly occurring fewer than 21 days apart.

Your health care provider can help you decide whether these changes are a normal part of your perimenopause experience or if they might indicate another condition.

WHAT CHANGES YOU MIGHT EXPECT

Many changes happen to women as they enter midlife. Some of these are positive. For instance, many women in their 40s and 50s find themselves feeling more confident, self-assured and decisive than ever before. Some of these changes, on the other hand — such as those happening to your body and its systems — may seem much less positive.

If you're nearing menopause, you've probably heard the stories. You've at least overheard talk about hot flashes and weight gain, about mood swings and libido changes. You may worry about what's going to happen when you hit menopause — because it can be so different for every person.

Physically, some women may notice only a few minor changes — some breast tenderness, perhaps, or the occasional hot flash — in the years before menopause. Others may feel like their world has turned upside down.

Read on to learn more about the changes you might experience during the menopause transition, including:
- Hot flashes and night sweats
- Sleep problems
- Weight gain
- Mood changes
- Breast pain
- Vaginal problems
- Urinary problems
- Headaches
- Cognition and memory challenges
- Joint pain
- Changes to your hair, skin and eyes
- Hearing changes
- Dental concerns
- Bone changes
- Cardiovascular issues

If that list seems depressing, don't close the book yet. Yes, some of the changes to your body can be challenging. But it's not hopeless. Keep

" Menopause took me completely by surprise. Especially growing up in a Black family where women's health issues were never discussed — from puberty through menopause — I had not heard women talking about menopause. While I was happy that my very heavy periods were getting lighter and less frequent in my late 40s, I was shocked by my inability to focus and my emotional volatility. I also became more sensitive to temperature, including getting very hot at times when others were comfortable. Perhaps most upsetting was the fact that I could no longer sleep through the night.

A family camping trip helped me finally connect these symptoms with menopause. With so much time together, it became clear that my daughter (who was just starting to cycle) and I were both emotionally volatile. There was a lot of crying and shouting, and we frequently couldn't even recall why afterward. As an aside, I'm proud of my husband for suggesting I might want to discuss my mood swings with my doctor, without saying that I was becoming unhinged.

When I visited my primary care provider, she was clearly hesitant to prescribe anything and terrified of breast cancer as an outcome of

reading. Part 2 is full of expertise on the most effective ways to treat or manage menopause symptoms. In addition, personal stories like the one above are featured throughout the book, giving voice to a wide variety of experiences from real people.

Making it through

Menopause is a natural part of life — not an illness. You may encounter none of the symptoms outlined in that lengthy list, or you may experience several of them. Whatever your experience is, know that more resources than ever before are available to help you understand and manage it. By working with a knowledgeable, trusted health care

taking estrogen. I understood that risk, but I have no family history, and my menopause symptoms were having a big impact on my life. She eventually put me on hormone therapy at a low dose.

The result was that while my symptoms improved somewhat, I had heavy spotting. All the time. For a year. I essentially had my period for a year. But I did not want to return to that doctor, and I kept hoping it would clear up.

I finally found a doctor who specialized in women's health and menopause care. Seeing that doctor was fantastic. I'm now on both progesterone and estrogen, which together control the symptoms and the spotting. My brain fog and volatility have resolved, and I am so much happier. I still sometimes find myself awake at night, but it's no longer every night. My relationships and my career are both moving forward.

In addition, it has been helpful to join an online community to hear about others' symptoms. I also try to talk about my experience so that others are not in the dark. Finding a doctor who can partner with you to tackle perimenopause and menopause is essential. You matter!

provider, and gathering other tools of your choice, you have what you need to manage any of the symptoms you encounter and make it to the other side of menopause while living an active, vibrant and healthy life.

2

Body changes from head to toe

You are not imagining things. Your eyes are drier. Your skin is itchier. You're getting hairs in new places. And the shape of your body is shifting — even if you're eating less and moving more than you used to. These signs and symptoms are real, and they're part of the natural transition that your body goes through as your periods come to an end.

You were expecting hot flashes, right? Not joint pain and dry eyes? You're definitely not alone.

Many women don't even think about menopause when odd symptoms first appear. After all, many symptoms of the transition start when your periods are still fairly regular, and many have no obvious connection to hormones. It's common to worry that something is wrong with your health, instead of recognizing changes as part of a natural process.

Researchers are still learning about all the symptoms associated with menopause. But this is clear: The gradual loss of estrogen in your bloodstream is responsible for a wide range of changes throughout your body — not just in your reproductive system.

This chapter lays out the physical changes you may experience. Once you understand all the things that may be happening to your body, you can decide how to manage them. Of course, you don't have to treat every symptom. In some cases, it's helpful just to have the reassurance that what you're feeling is perfectly normal.

EVERY PERSON'S SYMPTOMS ARE DIFFERENT

There is no timeline or blueprint for the transition to menopause. Every person born with ovaries goes through it differently. So it's impossible to predict exactly which symptoms you may experience or when they may creep up.

Perimenopause typically begins years before your final menstrual period. (See page 31.) Physical symptoms related to hormone changes often begin then — not the day your periods permanently stop. Women in all phases of perimenopause and menopause report a wide range of body changes. For some, the physical symptoms that emerge completely disrupt their daily routine. Others barely seem to notice anything different. And some are somewhere in between.

Wherever you fit on that spectrum, it's important to be aware of and informed about what's happening.

WHAT'S CAUSING THESE CHANGES?

The short answer is hormones.

As you approach your late 30s, your ovaries start making less estrogen and progesterone — the hormones that regulate menstruation — and your fertility declines. In the years before menopause, your hormone levels may rise and fall unevenly, dramatically and unpredictably. This often causes your menstrual periods to become longer or shorter, heavier or lighter, and more or less frequent, until eventually you have no more periods. (Fun fact: You may have any or all of those variations before your period stops!)

These fluctuations affect more than your menstrual supplies and whether you can get pregnant. Changes in your hormone production can set off a cascade of physical changes throughout your body.

Estrogen is a powerhouse. It's made mainly in the ovaries and released into your bloodstream, where it travels to cells all around your body — including your reproductive organs, brain, heart, blood vessels and bones. It helps to regulate many bodily functions. When estrogen dips, you may feel it from head to toe.

At the same time, you may experience symptoms that aren't directly related to a decline in estrogen. In other words, you can't blame your hormones for everything. Some changes in your body are simply due to growing older.

Your options for treating menopausal symptoms may be different from your options for treating symptoms that have nothing to do with hormones. Your doctor or practitioner can help you separate out your symptoms and manage them appropriately.

SYMPTOM SPECIFICS

The rest of this chapter gives a closer look at the various body changes associated with the menopause years. If this list seems overwhelming — well, you're not wrong. Symptoms can affect nearly your whole body, and some are unpleasant. But they are a natural part of major shifts within your body's systems.

Remember: You probably won't experience every symptom on this list severely. But knowing what's going on (and why) can empower you to talk about these changes, normalize them, and seek out solutions when needed. In Part Two, you'll find much more on how to manage or treat any symptoms that are throwing you off.

HOT FLASHES

As estrogen production decreases significantly around menopause, most women experience temperature dysregulation to some degree, most often in the form of hot flashes. Hot flashes, hot flushes and night sweats are all the same thing. The only difference is that night sweats happen at night. The medical term for all of these is *vasomotor symptoms*. They are the most common symptom of the transition to menopause.

A hot flash is a sudden feeling of warmth or heat that spreads over your body. It's usually most intense around the face, neck and chest. During a hot flash, your skin gets flushed, red or blotchy, as if you're blushing. You might start sweating — sometimes profusely. Your heart may beat faster too. Once the heat passes, you may develop chills.

Sometimes, flashes are mild, causing just a slight feeling of warmth. Others may leave you looking like you just left hot yoga. Night sweats come in the same range. Some can be strong enough to jolt you from sleep, needing to change your pajamas.

A hot flash typically lasts one to five minutes. It can repeat several times an hour, a few times a day or just once or twice a month. This varies widely from person to person. But you'll likely have your own consistent patterns. In general, flashes become more frequent as your periods wind down. Hot flashes typically peak in the two years after your last period. Then, they decline with time.

Hypothalamus changes

For a long time, we haven't known exactly what causes hot flashes. But researchers are finally beginning to gain a better understanding.

A part of the brain called the *hypothalamus* produces hormones that regulate a number of functions in your body, including hunger and thirst. One of the main jobs of the hypothalamus is to keep your body temperature not too hot and not too cold.

But in the transition to menopause, as estrogen levels fluctuate and fall, this temperature regulation can be thrown out of whack. That's because estrogen circulating in the brain helps control chemical signaling from neurons that release kisspeptin, neurokinin B and dynorphin, known as KNDy (pronounced "candy") neurons. As estrogen levels fluctuate, this signaling goes unchecked.

As a result, your hypothalamus may overreact to any small rise in your core body temperature — such as when you sit in a sunny room or drink a hot coffee. The hypothalamus senses this extra warmth and mistakenly believes that you're too hot. It starts a chain of events to cool you down, which includes opening blood vessels near the surface of your skin to increase blood flow and release heat. Ironically, this attempt results in sudden warmth, flushing and sweating.

Triggers

Hot flashes may seem unpredictable and erratic. But for many people, there are predictable triggers.

Hot flashes may happen when your body has a faulty reaction to a minor boost in your temperature. So it's no surprise that many common triggers of hot flashes cause your body temperature to spike temporarily. This can happen even if these triggers were no problem in the past. Here are some common culprits:

- **Spicy foods.** When your tongue is on fire, it can spark a hot flash. Even if you like your food highly spiced, your body may sense a rise in temperature and feel the need to cool down.
- **Certain beverages.** Many researchers have looked at the connection between caffeine and hot flashes with mixed results. One study from Mayo Clinic found that postmenopausal women who drank caffeinated beverages — such as coffee, tea or soda — experienced more bothersome hot flashes and night sweats than postmenopausal women who didn't use caffeine. Alcoholic beverages can also be a problem.
- **Smoking.** If you need another reason to quit smoking cigarettes, this is it. Current smoking and a history of smoking have both been linked to an increased risk of hot flashes. If you smoke, your hot flash risk may increase with the number of cigarettes or packs that you smoke. The exact relationship among smoking, nicotine and hot flashes isn't fully understood. It's possible that smoking affects the way your body metabolizes estrogen. Whatever the connection, it's clear that smoking worsens hot flashes.
- **A warm environment.** As estrogen declines and your body thermostat becomes more sensitive, you may find that you're comfortable in only a small temperature range. Any environment that's too warm can trigger a hot flash. Hot, constrictive clothing, warm bedding or other things in your environment may push you out of your comfort zone.
- **Stress.** It's tough to stay cool under fire — particularly during menopause. A stressful situation such as a contentious meeting or traffic jam may be enough to trigger a hot flash. If you experience ongoing stress, you may also be more likely to have more-frequent hot flashes.

MOOD CHANGES AND BRAIN FOG

Midlife changes in the brain can throw off your memory, mental processing abilities and mental health. Mood swings, depression and what's often called brain fog are some of the most common symptoms in perimenopause and menopause.

Some of these effects are clearly the result of hormone levels fluctuating and shifting. Others may result from a complex combination of menopause and natural aging in the brain. Here's a look at what may be going on.

Mood

Ever since you were a teenager, hormones have been affecting your moods. This is because hormones in your blood affect the chemicals in your brain that control mood.

Over the years, you may have noticed mood fluctuations around your menstrual cycles. If you've been pregnant or had a baby, your shifting hormones throughout gestation and postpartum might've sent you on a roller coaster of emotions as you cried — either happy or sad tears — over the tiniest thing.

As you head into menopause, your changing hormones may, once again, affect your moods. The level of estrogen in your body rises and falls unevenly during perimenopause. Then, after your final period, your estrogen level drops and stabilizes at a lower level.

Estrogens have a positive effect on neurotransmitters involved in mood regulation. In addition, research has linked fluctuating estrogens with mood disorders. So it's not surprising that mood swings and the risk of depression tend to increase during the transition to menopause and the first few years after reaching menopause. In fact, research suggests that some anxiety symptoms, such as nervousness and worry, occur more frequently during perimenopause than at any time before it. These mood swings may be frequent or occasional. They may seem cyclical, like those during your reproductive years, or they may just leave you feeling generally more emotional or irritable.

However, mood changes may also be caused by what's happening in your life. Managing work, raising kids, caring for aging parents and other responsibilities in midlife can feel like a high-stress juggling act.

Your relationship with your partner may be changing as kids grow and your priorities and goals evolve. Your network of friends may be morphing because of career- or family-oriented moves. You may also have complex emotions around the transition to a new phase of your life without periods. All together, these factors can easily lead to anxiety, irritability or a depressed mood.

Of course, other menopause symptoms can contribute to emotions that feel out of control too. Sleep problems, hot flashes and menopause-related fatigue can affect your mood.

Depression

While mood swings can involve lows that last hours or even days, depression is different. Depression is a serious mood disorder that interferes with your daily life. It may appear as severe sadness or no longer enjoying your usual activities. You may not feel like eating, going to work or even getting out of bed. Depression can affect your relationships, your job and your physical health.

It's not clear exactly what role hormones play in developing depression. However, research does suggest that menopause-aged women — and, specifically, women in the perimenopause stage — are at an increased risk of depression. This may be, in part, because of the amount of hormone changes happening in your body as it begins the transition to menopause. On the bright side, once you go through menopause and are considered postmenopausal, the risk of depression goes down.

Other factors that may contribute to your risk include poor sleep, anxiety, a history of depression, stressful life events and weight gain or a higher body mass index. Menopause at a younger age or menopause caused by removal of the ovaries can also increase the risk of depression.

Brain fog

No, you're not crazy if you feel like you're struggling more to concentrate or remember where you left your phone. Perimenopause really may affect your memory and processing. Research from several cognitive studies suggests that complaints of brain fog are valid. Among the different mental tasks studied, verbal memory and learning appear to be some of the most common areas of complaint during perimenopause. But despite these common complaints, women still typically have a normal range of function. Studies show that only around 12% of women in perimenopause have cognitive impairment that's clinically significant.

Brain fog during this time is likely due to a complex combination of factors, including menopause changes and other natural aging in the brain. Fluctuating hormone levels may contribute to trouble concentrating or recalling information, because estrogen and progesterone receptors in the brain are involved in cognitive function. Add in poor sleep, depression or hot flashes — or all of those — and it's no wonder if you feel like you can't think straight. For most people, though, brain fog seems to resolve after the transition to menopause.

HAIR GONE WILD

As you approach menopause — and postmenopause — it's common to find too much hair in some spots and too little in others. In fact, some studies show that about 70% of women who have been through menopause and didn't take hormone therapy during the transition develop more hair on their faces while losing hair on their heads and in the pubic region. It's common for these changes to happen during perimenopause too.

Here are some of the hairy signs that you may notice:

Hair loss

If you or your stylist has noticed that your hair is suddenly shedding or gradually thinning, that's very typical around menopause. It may be time for a new hairstyle to work with the changes to your mane. Hair thinning during menopause can affect the top of your scalp, or you may develop a receding hairline along the top of your forehead.

That's because hormones influence hair growth. The exact mechanism isn't well understood, but estrogen receptors are found on hair follicles. Estrogen seems to influence hair follicles in some way that relates to hair density. If your hair grew thick and fast during pregnancy — and maybe even changed texture — this connection may sound familiar. Unfortunately, on the flip side of hormone changes, you'll see the opposite of those full locks you may have had during pregnancy.

Hair loss may also affect the eyebrows and pubic hair. In rare cases, women can develop patches of hair loss or near or total baldness.

Facial hair

Hirsutism (HUR-soot-iz-um) is the medical term for excessive hair growth in women. It results in hair on body parts such as the face, chest and back, where men typically grow hair. Many women experience facial hirsutism during menopause — especially on the chin, upper lip and cheeks.

For some women, this manifests as fine hairs or peach fuzz, which can appear on larger areas of the face. Others have lone, dark, quick-growing rogue hairs that curl out of the chin or cheeks. In some cases, facial hair may grow to resemble a faint mustache.

The reason, again, may be related to a change in hormones. At puberty, your ovaries begin to produce a mix of female and male sex hormones. This is what causes hair to grow in your armpits and pubic area. Hirsutism can occur if the mix becomes unbalanced with a high proportion of male sex hormones (androgens). This commonly happens during menopause, as the ratio between estrogen and androgens shifts. Some hair changes may also be part of the natural process of growing older or related to family history and not related to hormones.

Hair changes can be mild or severe, inconvenient, or anxiety inducing. Your health care provider can talk through options for managing your concerns. If hair changes are affecting your body image and self-esteem, it's worth doing something about them.

EYE CHANGES

Sex hormone receptors have been found in many of the tissues of the eyes. This includes the colored part of your eye (iris), the clear elliptical structure behind the iris (lens), the protective dome of clear tissue at the front of your eye that helps your eye focus (cornea), and the transparent tissue that covers the white part of your eye (conjunctiva). These hormone receptors are also in the lubricating glands in the eyelids.

Researchers haven't figured out the exact role of the estrogen and androgen receptors found in those areas. However, it seems that sex hormones are involved in maintaining a state of equilibrium in your eyes in different ways. As a result, you may notice various changes to your eyes as hormones fluctuate throughout your life — during your menstrual cycle, during pregnancy and at the time of menopause.

Women report a host of eye complaints that occur with menopause. These include:

- Blurred vision
- Swollen and reddened eyes
- Tired eyes
- Trouble with contact lenses
- Vision changes

Think about your own eyesight. Do you find yourself holding books or your phone at arm's length to read them? You might be experiencing presbyopia (prez-bee-OH-pee-uh) — the gradual loss of your eyes' ability to focus on nearby objects. It's a natural part of aging. However, your ability to see may also be altered by changes or swelling in your corneas or other parts of your eyes as your hormones change. Many women find that they need reading glasses just before menopause.

Dry eyes

One of the most common eye problems around the time of menopause is dry eye syndrome. Dry eyes occur when you can't produce enough tears or the tears aren't lubricating well enough (think: aren't oily enough) to provide enough moisture for your eyes. The medical term for this condition is *keratoconjunctivitis sicca* (ker-uh-toe-kun-junk-tih-VY-tis SIK-uh). Tear production tends to fall off as you get older. But women tend to report worse dry eyes and more severe effects than men. This may be due in part to hormonal changes.

Dry eyes can be uncomfortable and distracting. Your eyes may sting or burn. Dry eyes can also cause scratchiness or an odd sensation that feels as if you have something stuck in your eye. A lack of tears can also make you very sensitive to light (photophobia) so that it's difficult to drive or be outside without sunglasses. Environmental factors, such as wind and low humidity, can exacerbate the problem and make symptoms worse, so you may be more affected in certain seasons or in different climates. Some medications and conditions, such as rheumatoid arthritis and Sjogren's syndrome, can also worsen the problem.

Glaucoma

Recent research has shown a clear link between menopause hormone changes and glaucoma. Glaucoma is a group of eye conditions that damage the optic nerve. This damage is often caused by an abnormally high pressure in the eye (intraocular pressure). Signs might include patchy blind spots in your vision or, in a more advanced case, tunnel vision.

Compared with women of the same age who haven't reached menopause yet, menopausal women tend to have higher pressure in the eye. The mechanism behind this isn't fully understood, although research has linked certain estrogen receptors in women with a higher risk of glaucoma. In addition, estrogen therapy has been shown to reduce eye pressure in postmenopausal women, and in one study, it reduced the risk of glaucoma in Black women.

Altogether, evidence suggests that going through menopause is a significant risk factor for developing glaucoma. It's important to have regular eye exams that include measurements of your eye pressure so a diagnosis can be made in its early stages and treated appropriately. If glaucoma is recognized early, vision loss can be slowed or prevented.

HEARING CHANGES

Do you have a hard time hearing the conversation in a crowded room? Do you find yourself reaching for the remote to turn up the TV? Do you ask friends and family to repeat themselves, especially when talking on the phone?

Maybe you haven't noticed any changes in your hearing yet, especially if you're still in perimenopause or early menopause. But as you age, it's common to experience gradual hearing loss. The medical term for this type of hearing loss is *presbycusis* (prez-bih-KYU-sis). About one-third of people in the United States age 65 and older have some degree of hearing loss. Even among people ages 55 to 64, about 1 in 12 have hearing loss.

In addition, there is some evidence of a relationship among menopause, estrogen and hearing. Some researchers have found that estrogen may protect and preserve your hearing as you age. When you lose estrogen, you may lose some of your ability to hear right along with it. In addition, women who use hormone therapy to replace estrogen may have slightly better hearing than those who don't.

If you notice changes in your hearing, you may need to see your health care provider or an audiologist. Various tests may be used to quantify your hearing ability and look for evidence of hearing loss.

MOUTH AND DENTAL CHANGES

Dryness is a recurring theme. The drying effects of menopause can be prominent in your mouth as well.

The mucous membrane that lines the inside of your mouth (oral mucosa) contains estrogen receptors. So do the glands that produce your saliva (salivary glands). Estrogen seems to support the health of these structures in your mouth, helping to keep your saliva flowing. As a result, saliva production may decrease with estrogen production.

Is less spit in your mouth really a bad thing? Well, yes. Saliva washes away food particles, enhances your ability to taste and helps with digestion. A low flow of saliva may lead to the following oral conditions and problems:

Dry mouth
Xerostomia (zeer-o-STOE-me-uh) refers to any condition in which your mouth is unusually dry. In addition to a parched, dehydrated feeling in your mouth or throat, you may notice bad breath, a changed sense of taste or lipstick sticking to your teeth. Dry mouth can affect the health of your teeth, as well as your appetite and your enjoyment of food.

Burning mouth syndrome
This is the medical term for ongoing or recurrent burning in your mouth without an obvious cause. The discomfort can affect the

tongue, gums, lips, insides of your cheeks, roof of your mouth or widespread areas of your whole mouth. Symptoms may vary from mild discomfort to intense pain, as if you scalded your mouth. This condition is more frequent in postmenopausal women.

Cavities

As noted above, saliva helps wash away food particles. It also helps prevent tooth decay by neutralizing the acids produced by bacteria in your mouth. As estrogen and saliva drop, some women dread trips to the dentist's office because they count more cavities than ever before. Tooth decay can also cause tooth pain, tooth sensitivity or pain while eating or drinking.

Gum infections

Changes in your hormones may change the balance of healthy bacteria in your mouth. This can leave your gums susceptible to plaque and make it more difficult to fight off infection. Gum infections, such as gingivitis and periodontitis, are both common in postmenopausal women.

Gingivitis is a common, mild form of gum disease that causes irritation, redness and swelling (inflammation) of your gums. Because it's mild, you may not be aware that you have this condition. In contrast, periodontitis (per-e-o-don-TIE-tis) is a serious gum infection that damages the soft tissue and destroys the bone that supports your teeth. Periodontitis can lead to tooth loss, if left untreated.

If you're experiencing uncomfortable changes in your mouth or teeth, make an appointment with a dentist. The sooner you seek care, the better your chances of finding cavities, gum disease and other dental conditions before they lead to more-serious problems.

SKIN PROBLEMS

You're probably well aware that you may develop wrinkles, creases and sagging skin as you age. A lot of magazine pages, commercials and beauty products are dedicated to the idea of keeping your skin young and fighting these effects with anti-aging solutions. However, you may not be aware of all the skin changes you may experience as your hormones shift around menopause.

The truth is that hormones play a very important role in the health of your skin. The estrogen and androgens produced by your ovaries since puberty have nourished your skin for decades. Your androgen hormones help control oil production in your skin. At the same time, young skin is rich in estrogen receptors in the two outer layers — the dermis and epidermis — and it's clear that estrogen helps with some important jobs there. One of those jobs is metabolizing collagen — a fibrous type of protein that makes up your body's connective tissues and keeps your skin supple and pliable. As estrogen decreases, it greatly affects the amount of collagen in your skin, leaving skin thinner and wrinkled. Declining estrogen has other effects on the skin too.

As your hormone levels change, you may notice a pronounced effect on your skin, from your face to your ankles. If you think back, you may remember changes in the appearance of your skin at other times in your life when your hormone levels made a major shift. Remember how your skin changed during puberty? Or during pregnancy? Or after you delivered a baby? Or when you tried a new birth control pill? Or even during your monthly menstrual cycle?

Here are some of the common skin changes that you might find during the menopause transition:

Acne

It may seem completely unfair that you're growing older and reverting to your teenage skin all at once. Is it really possible to have wrinkles and pimples at the same time?

Unfortunately, yes. Pimples pop up when hair follicles become plugged with oil and dead skin cells. When your body produces an excess amount of oil (sebum) and dead skin cells, the two can build up on hair follicles. They form a soft plug, creating an environment where bacteria can thrive. If the clogged pore becomes infected with bacteria, it gets inflamed. The plugged pore may cause the follicle wall to bulge and produce a whitehead. Or the plug may be open to the surface and may darken, causing a blackhead. If blockages and inflammation develop deep inside hair follicles, cystlike lumps can form beneath the surface of your skin.

It's very common for women who had pimples in their teen years to experience an encore in midlife. This time around, lumps may be tender and appear deep beneath the surface of the skin.

The problem is androgen circulating throughout your body. As your estrogen levels drop, the ratio of androgen to estrogen in your body can shift. This can cause adult acne, particularly on the chin, jaw line and neck.

This problem can be distressing and frustrating. Be assured that effective treatments are available. They may just take a little time. You may need to work with a dermatologist to find a treatment that works for you.

Bruising

In addition to keeping skin supple, collagen provides a protective layer between the surface of your skin and your blood vessels. As estrogen decreases and the amount of collagen in your skin changes, your skin may become thinner. As a result, slight injuries may be more likely to cause bruising as you age. You may notice more cuts, bruises and other marks on your skin. It may also take longer for these wounds to heal.

Dry skin

Dry eyes, dry mouth, dry skin — you see the pattern. For some women, menopause feels like a drought.

Dryness is a common condition in aging skin. The medical term is *xerosis* (zer-OH-sis). For women, though, flaking and itching is very common around the time of menopause, as the production of skin-smoothing collagen drops. The changing ratios of hormones can also affect the water content in your skin and oil production in your body, which can contribute to the problem. In addition, if the transition to menopause has you sweating a lot — such as soaking your sheets as a result of night sweats — your skin may be feeling the effects of all that loss of liquid and moisture.

You may notice parched, dry skin on your back, ankles, elbows, face or torso. It can cause significant itching and discomfort. It can also be aggravated by the climate or season. You may be the itchiest in winter or if you live in or visit dry climates.

Wrinkles

Frown lines. Crow's-feet. Forehead lines. All sorts of wrinkles and creases can appear — or deepen — as estrogen declines. This is partly due to decreased collagen in the deep layers of your skin, causing it to lose its elasticity and tone. In addition, decreased production of natural oils dries your skin and makes it appear more wrinkled. You may notice more-pronounced lines around your eyes and mouth and on your neck. Some wrinkles can become deep crevices or furrows.

You can't do much to reverse the hormone changes that contribute to wrinkles. But there are other factors that you can control. These include ultraviolet light, smoking and constant squinting. Avoid all of these things as much as you can. If the lines and creases on your face bother you, you'll find information about treatments in Chapter 21.

Other problems

There are other skin changes and conditions associated with menopause. You may notice thickening of the skin on your palms and heels. Some women also develop rosacea (roe-ZAY-she-uh) at this time. This common skin condition causes persistent redness in the face and often produces small, red pus-filled bumps. Signs and symptoms may flare up for a period of weeks to months and then diminish again before once again appearing. Rosacea can be mistaken for acne, an allergic reaction or other skin problems. Talk to your health care provider if you're concerned about other changes to your skin.

JOINT CONCERNS

Joint pain is discomfort that arises from any joint — the point where two or more of your bones meet. Joint pain is sometimes called *arthralgia* or — particularly if inflammation or joint changes are involved — *arthritis*. The joint can feel stiff and achy. You also may feel some soreness each time you move the affected joint.

Joint pain and arthritis are common with age and are caused by wear-and-tear damage to your joint's cartilage — the hard, slick coating on the ends of your bones. This wear and tear can happen over many years or it can be hastened by an infection or injury in the joint.

FIBROMYALGIA OR MENOPAUSE?

Sleep disturbance, joint aches, and fatigue are common symptoms of perimenopause and menopause. They're also some of the main symptoms of fibromyalgia, a disorder characterized by widespread muscle and bone pain. Fibromyalgia pain is accompanied by fatigue, sleep, memory and mood issues. Experts believe that this disorder amplifies painful sensations by affecting the way your brain and spinal cord process painful and nonpainful signals.

Fibromyalgia is 2 to 3 times more common in women than in men. And as it happens, it most often starts in midlife. For those who are already diagnosed, symptoms may also worsen with menopause. A link to hormone changes in menopause has been suggested, but the connection isn't well understood. Based on limited data, hormone therapy has not proven to help with fibromyalgia symptoms, but more study is needed.

If you have fatigue and recent pain in multiple spots around your body that's severe enough to interfere with your daily life, talk with your health care practitioner. A clinician can help figure out what may be causing your symptoms and discuss possible treatments. In any case, you deserve help to feel better.

But many women notice joint pain for the first time during perimenopause. And, in fact, recent research has shown a connection between joint pain and the loss of estrogen. As it turns out, this joint pain — separate from arthritis — is another common symptom of menopause.

Some studies indicate that women with joint pain or stiffness may get some relief with hormone therapy. It's important to note hormone therapy isn't prescribed to treat joint pain in menopause — but this may be a side benefit. The relationship between joints and estrogen isn't fully understood, and more research is needed in this area.

If your knee feels stiff or you're having trouble getting your rings over your swollen finger joints, you can be reassured that these symptoms are common. At the same time, don't be too quick to shrug off new pain without investigating its cause, especially if pain is severe.

There are many reasons for pain in or around your joints. It's possible that your pain is actually radiating from the bone, ligament, tendon or the small sacs of fluid (bursae) that reduce friction between moving parts in your joint. Pain also may be traced to an injury or mechanical problem.

Arthritis — true joint damage — is more common after you've reached menopause, so it's important to get joint pain checked out early on. Your health care practitioner can help you sort out the cause of your pain and the best treatment. If the cause is an injury, focusing on hormones won't be the right solution.

GENITAL AND URINARY CHANGES

Your vagina is a muscular canal that extends from the neck of your uterus (cervix) to your vulva — the outside of the female genital area. The vulva is the area of skin that surrounds the urethra and vagina, including the clitoris and labia. The health of your entire female genital area — inside and outside — is an important part of your overall health.

Problems here can affect your desire for sex, your ability to reach orgasm, your relationship and your self-confidence. So it's important to recognize changes in this area due to menopause. For some women, these changes are all too obvious as shifting hormones can have a major impact on the vagina and vulva.

The following vaginal conditions are common during the transition to menopause:

Vaginal dryness

Remember the dryness theme of menopause? In the early stages of perimenopause, you may begin to notice a slight decrease in the amount of vaginal lubrication you feel with sexual arousal and during sexual activity. This is often one of the first signs that estrogen is declining. As time goes on, you may notice a whopping dip in the amount of lubrication that you feel during sex. You may also notice vaginal dryness during daily activities, not just during sexual activities. Dryness may lead to discomfort and itchiness too. All of these sensations are very common and are a result of declining estrogen and decreased blood flow to your vagina.

Genitourinary syndrome of menopause (GSM)

This term is a medical name for the combination of vulvar, vaginal and urinary tract changes related to the loss of estrogen. The vaginal walls may appear thin, smooth, pale and dry during a pelvic exam. This is a change from the way the vagina looks before menopause, when it's well stocked with estrogen and the lining is thick and full of folds, allowing it to stretch during intercourse and childbirth. Vaginal dryness can be a symptom of GSM. Women with moderate to severe GSM may also feel vaginal burning, scratchiness or discomfort.

Most women experience some loss of fullness and thinning of the vagina during menopause. In some cases, it can be progressive and severe. As walls thin, the vagina becomes less flexible, more fragile and more susceptible to bleeding, spotting, tearing or pain during sexual activities or even during a pelvic exam. It can make sex very painful or even impossible. Changes to the vaginal tissues can lead to infections and irritation, redness, vaginal burning and discharge. Similar changes can happen with the urethra, leading to painful urination, frequent urination or leaking urine.

All these symptoms are the result of the decrease in estrogen production. As hormones shift, you may lose collagen under the skin near your vagina and urinary tract in the same way that you lose collagen elsewhere in your skin. As a result, the tissues of the vulva and the lining of the vagina can become thinner and less elastic or flexible. All these vaginal conditions can understandably alter your desire for sex or enjoyment of sex.

Other factors can contribute to this problem too. Smoking cigarettes or taking certain medications, such as antihistamines and antidepressants, can make things worse. So can a lack of sexual activity. In use it or lose it fashion, regular, *painless* sexual activity helps maintain vaginal health.

Estrogen also helps protect the health of your bladder and urethra — the tube that carries urine from the bladder. So changes in this area can cause bladder infections and urination problems such as incontinence. These problems may result from a combination of menopause, reproductive factors, and other body changes with age. They are covered in detail in Chapters 12 and 13.

WEIGHT GAIN

It's common for women in early menopause to report that their eating habits and exercise routines haven't changed but their waistline has. Sometimes, they're eating a healthier diet and working out harder than ever and still gaining in pant sizes. What gives?

When it comes to your weight and menopause, your body may seem to be following a new set of rules. The eating habits and exercise routines that used to work for you may suddenly seem like they're not enough. Or you may feel as if you just can't cheat on healthy habits anymore — you can't skip a few days of exercise or stuff yourself on a special occasion without seeing the effects on your bathroom scale.

These observations aren't off. Your weight and body shape may be changing in different ways all at once in midlife. First, hormone changes with the menopause transition can result in changes in your body composition, including an increase in the fat accumulation around the center of your abdomen. During and after menopause, women tend to gain weight in more of an apple shape rather than in the pear shape that is more common before menopause. In practical terms, you may gain weight in your stomach area instead of your thighs and hips. It may not budge easily.

It's important to note that this fat redistribution — gaining more fat around the belly — contributes to the risk of cardiovascular disease. Recent research has clarified that even for women with a normal body mass index (BMI), having a thicker waistline seems to increase the risk of heart disease and heart failure. For more explanation of BMI, turn to Chapter 16.

Second, many women also gain overall weight during this time — about 1.5 pounds per year, on average, during the menopause transition. However, it's unclear whether menopause is directly responsible for any extra pounds. Midlife weight gain may be triggered by loss of muscle that's part of natural aging, and by lifestyle changes that happen at this time, rather than hormonal changes. For example, sleep deprivation is often associated with weight gain. As a result, women who struggle to sleep well during menopause may pack on unwanted pounds, even though hormones aren't directly to blame.

Similarly, life events that happen around menopause might change your diet or exercise habits and contribute to menopausal weight gain. For example, if you become an empty nester or undergo a divorce at this time, it may change how much you cook and how much you eat out. It may also have a significant effect on your weekly calendar and activity level. You may inadvertently be eating more calories or a less nutritious diet — and burning off less — without really realizing it.

Genetic factors might also play a role in menopause weight gain. If your parents or other close relatives carry extra weight around the belly, you're likely to do the same. Aging plays a role too. As you age, muscle mass typically diminishes, while fat increases. When muscle mass decreases, it can decrease the rate at which your body uses calories and make it more challenging to maintain a healthy weight. If you continue to eat as you always have and don't increase your physical activity, you're likely to gain weight.

When you add up all of these factors, the math is clear: You will probably need to work harder to maintain your weight during perimenopause and menopause. Even if you're able to maintain your weight, you may carry it differently, and your clothes may not fit the same.

That's OK. There's no good reason to drive yourself mad trying to maintain a flat stomach for the rest of your life. On the flip side, there's no reason to give up and resign yourself to an extra 10 or 20 pounds. Extra weight is associated with some health risks, including heart disease. So it's important to keep a focus on healthy lifestyle choices even more than your BMI as you age. You'll learn more about healthy lifestyle changes that can keep you feeling great as you age in Part 3.

TAKE ACTION

For some women, understanding all the changes that are happening to the body during menopause is a relief. It's a much-needed validation

TRACK YOUR SYMPTOMS

The changes laid out in this chapter make it clear why perimenopause and menopause can be such a bewildering time in your body. There's a lot going on, even if your symptoms are mild.

It can be hard to keep track of all your symptoms over time, but taking notes can be good for your health. When you talk with your health care provider, it's helpful if you can report on the timing, severity and range of menopause symptoms you've experienced. That can be valuable information as you discuss treatment options. It may also help your practitioner find any symptoms that don't fit with the rest of your personal menopause puzzle.

Many symptom-tracking apps for smartphones or tablets are available to make quick work of organizing your data. Some track a range of symptoms beyond hot flashes, including sleep, mood, sexual function and weight, to give a broader picture. Talk to your health care provider and your friends for a recommendation (or to kick off team research). You may also want to consider how much detail you want to track, other app features such as community boards, and — as a savvy digital consumer — the longevity of an app and the company that created it. A handwritten list can also work, if you prefer low tech. With each symptom, you may want to note the date, severity, any potential triggers and solutions you tried. Write down any questions for your practitioner too.

that what they're seeing and feeling is real. For others, this extensive list of menopause symptoms is daunting.

However you feel, as you notice the symptoms of menopause, talk with your doctor. Even though the symptoms discussed in this chapter are normal and natural, you don't have to suffer through them. Your health care practitioner can help you figure out a plan to deal with any uncomfortable or embarrassing symptoms. More than ever before, as the transition to menopause is better researched and understood, you have options for managing symptoms. These include lifestyle changes, hormone therapy and other medications, as well as holistic and integrative therapies, such as meditation and more. Don't be afraid to advocate for your needs and seek treatment.

If you're among the lucky ones who aren't thrown off by any symptoms of menopause, that's great. This is a good time to check in with your practitioner and talk about a plan to keep it that way.

Before your appointment, keep track of any menopause-related symptoms that you've noticed. However you log your information, take it with you when you visit your health care provider, and use it to talk through your symptoms and concerns. Then you can work together to develop an informed, thoughtful plan for helping you feel your best.

Finally, a word of caution: Take new symptoms seriously, and don't chalk everything up to hormones or natural aging. Although the transition to menopause can be responsible for a wide range of body changes and sensations, other serious conditions can cause some of the same signs and symptoms — mouth pain, vision changes, bruising or joint pain, for example. It's important to rule out other causes of new signs and symptoms, particularly if they come on suddenly or are particularly severe.

Pay attention to your body, and keep in touch with your health care provider as things change. Menopause-related changes are just one part of your overall health. It's also important to consider your unique personal medical history, your family history, your health habits and other factors as you evaluate changes in your body. Menopause is only one piece of the puzzle.

3

Perimenopause (or, Are we there yet?)

Around your early 40s to early 50s, you might start experiencing signs that your hormones are shifting. Perhaps you're moodier, having bigger reactions to what should be small conflicts. Maybe you're starting to get massive headaches. You may wonder if there's something wrong with you, even though nothing in your life is technically wrong. The cycles of your period are starting to get shorter, and your period could be lighter — or it could be heavier.

Welcome to perimenopause.

In this stage, your body is getting ready to shift from the hormonal cycles that support fertility to new levels in menopause. This transition often lasts 4 to 8 years before your final period, and wild swings in your hormone levels can kick off a range of symptoms.

As with menopause symptoms, everyone experiences perimenopause differently. This is in part because a person's psychosocial experience influences the reaction to symptoms. So a woman's perimenopause is influenced by everything from her quality of life, levels of stress, social stigmas and mental health, including a history of depression, anxiety, post-traumatic stress disorder, or mood disorders.

Racial and ethnic differences also affect perimenopause experiences. The Study of Women's Health Across the Nation (SWAN), for example, found that African American women in the transition to menopause may experience more frequent vasomotor symptoms such as hot flashes and night sweats, compared with other racial groups. They also reported more discomfort with symptoms. Experts don't yet fully understand these racial differences.

Bottom line: While certain changes are common in perimenopause, your experience will be your own. But with a solid understanding of what's going on, you'll be well equipped to advocate for your needs, adjust what you can in your lifestyle, and manage the transition smoothly.

CHANGING HORMONAL PATTERNS

If you're feeling thrown off-kilter by perimenopause, there's good reason. Most likely, you've been going through the hormonal patterns of the reproductive cycle since you were a teenager. Each month, your ovaries have been getting a signal of follicle-stimulating hormone (FSH) from your pituitary gland, which tells the immature eggs in your ovarian follicles to start to grow. As the follicles and eggs mature, they produce more estrogen and progesterone. Then the hormone inhibin B sends a "turnoff" signal to stop the pituitary from making more FSH. At that point, one of your ovaries releases a mature egg, and if there is sperm to meet it, there's a chance of conceiving a baby. If not, then your progesterone levels drop, leading to your period.

In perimenopause, those patterns change. The pituitary gland still dishes out FSH to stimulate your ovaries to make more estrogen. Your ovaries are still releasing eggs — but not every month, and their quality and supply is lower. Because of this, your body is making less inhibin B. So FSH levels continue to rise, signaling to the ovaries to produce more estrogen. But with a lower egg supply, your estrogen levels respond less to the FSH signal and become more erratic.

Inevitably, your body is reacting in new ways to these changing signals. Your brain circuits and your body's systems are used to functioning with a certain pattern of estrogen levels, and then those levels starts to fluctuate wildly. It's no wonder if you're experiencing symptoms from this transition. Think of when Han Solo hits the controls to take his spaceship to hyperspace in *Star Wars*. At first, the ride is a little bumpy.

A cascade of symptoms

The wild cycles of high and low estrogen during perimenopause can be very unsettling physically and emotionally. These fluctuations of estrogen can be more erratic, meaning higher highs and lower lows, than during a typical menstrual cycle. This is what's behind hot flashes and night sweats, middle-of-the-night awakenings, and the moodiness, anxiety, and foggy thinking that are common in perimenopause.

These hormonal shifts are also why your periods are becoming more irregular and unpredictable. As you approach menopause, this abnormality is entirely, well, normal. If you have a persistent change of seven days or more in the length of your menstrual cycle, you may be in early perimenopause. If you have a space of 60 days or more between periods, you're likely in late perimenopause.

Other common symptoms of perimenopause include migraine headaches that last up to 1 to 2 days right before your period, joint pain, and increased irritability or anxiety, especially right before your period.

Some studies have found that women who tend to be more sensitive to premenstrual syndrome (PMS) also have stronger reactions to the hormonal changes of perimenopause. Let your health care practitioner know about any symptoms or changes, as some health changes that seem unconnected may indeed be related to your hormones. Also, it's important to note that early-onset hot flashes in perimenopause — which start before you're noticing big fluctuations in your period — may be a predictor of future heart disease risk. So it's worth paying attention to anything that seems out of the ordinary and talking with your practitioner.

MANAGING THE TRANSITION

To help you manage this stage, it's important to see a doctor or other clinician who understands the menopause transition — even if you're not currently experiencing symptoms. Choose someone with whom you feel comfortable so that you can keep an open line of communication about any symptoms that do crop up, including emotional changes such as anxiety and depression. As your hormones shift over time, your health care team can help you find treatments and self-care tips to manage a variety of symptoms.

Some hallmarks of perimenopause, such as hot flashes, night sweats and mood changes, may continue long after your final period. Even so, health care practitioners approach the two stages in different ways and with separate treatments because of the difference in hormonal patterns at each stage. After the wild fluctuations in estro-

RED FLAGS: WHEN TO SEE A DOCTOR

Your period will become more irregular as you enter perimenopause — that's almost a given. This can mean bleeding that's lighter or heavier than in the past, more days of bleeding or fewer, and longer or shorter cycle lengths. When estrogen levels are higher in comparison to progesterone, it often results in heavier bleeding during your period as the lining of the uterus is shed. A skipped period can also cause the lining to build up, leading to heavier bleeding over the next few months.

But some symptoms may point to underlying problems with your reproductive system. Call your doctor right away if you're experiencing any of the following:

- Bleeding that's heavy enough that you need to change your tampons or pads every hour or two. This can be a sign of fibroids, infection, a sexually transmitted disease, a thyroid problem, endometrial polyps or, in very rare cases, cancer.
- Bleeding that lasts longer than seven days.
- Bleeding that occurs between periods.
- Periods that regularly occur less than 21 days apart.
- Bleeding with intercourse.

gen levels during perimenopause, in the years after your final period, estrogen falls to a more consistent, low level.

In addition, preventing pregnancy is still a concern until you're certain you've had your last period. This is why a low-dose birth control is a common hormone treatment for perimenopause. The hormone therapy offered in menopause, in contrast, doesn't contain high enough doses of hormones to override the perimenopausal swings of hormones and prevent ovulation.

How your doctor can help

If the following symptoms are disrupting your life, it's important to reach out to your health care practitioner. Treatments are available and can help you feel like yourself again.

Heavy/irregular bleeding If you're experiencing heavier periods or breakthrough bleeding in between your periods, your health care practitioner may recommend a low-dose birth control pill or an IUD with progestin. If you're looking for a nonhormonal option, nonsteroidal anti-inflammatory drugs (NSAIDs) or tranexamic acid (Lysteda) may offer some relief. These can reduce prostaglandin levels, which are elevated in women with excessive menstrual bleeding.

With heavy or irregular bleeding, a pelvic ultrasound may be recommended to check for polyps, fibroids or other causes.

Hot flashes A low-dose birth control pill can offer relief if hot flashes are frequent or severe (or both frequent and severe) and difficult to manage in your daily life. An IUD along with an estrogen patch, which could also improve your mood, may be another option.

Mood or mental health changes If you're experiencing new anxiety or depression in perimenopause, tell your health care practitioner right away. A low-dose antidepressant in the last two weeks of your cycle may help you get back to normal. For some women, a low-dose hormonal contraceptive can improve mood symptoms.

Headaches New or worse menstrual-related migraines are a common symptom of the unstable hormones in perimenopause. If headaches are a problem, continuous low-dose birth control can help.

What you can do

Some symptoms of perimenopause are best tackled through changes you make to your daily routine and habits. What's more, they can set you up for better health in menopause and beyond. While these aren't flashy solutions, they can make a real difference in your health and happiness — now and in the long run.

Minimize weight gain Extra pounds often start to creep on during this stage, even if you're eating and exercising like you always have. Unfortunately, increasing activity alone usually won't combat these midlife body changes.

Some shifts in your metabolism and body shape are related to aging rather than hormones. Both men and women tend to lose muscle mass and gain weight starting in midlife. But some changes, particularly in body composition, are likely related to the loss of estrogen. For instance, even if your weight doesn't change overall in perimenopause, some weight tends to be redistributed to fat around the middle. This is not only annoying for buttoning your jeans — it may affect your health. An increase in belly fat can raise your cardiovascular risk and risk of diabetes, even if your weight overall is in a healthy range.

The good news is that making some adjustments to your habits in this stage can have a lasting impact. A 2022 study published in the journal *Menopause* suggested that the perimenopause transition may be the most opportune time to focus on daily habits to improve your metabolism and minimize the changes to your body composition. In particular, researchers suggested it may help to focus on preserving muscle mass in the menopause transition, through a diet higher in protein and lower in carbohydrates and activity such as resistance training. (As a bonus, activity that builds muscle helps protect against the loss of bone density during the menopause transition too.) In addition, moderate to high-intensity exercise also may help you fight the drop in metabolism that's common in midlife. But more study is needed to know exactly how to fight these effects.

Limit alcohol While you might enjoy a glass of wine to relax with friends or unwind at night, cutting back on alcohol can actually help your body deal with perimenopause symptoms. Alcohol increases anxiety and can disrupt sleep. In addition, some research has found that drinking alcohol can trigger and intensify hot flashes. And even if you have healthy eating habits overall, drinking the same amount that you used to may lead to weight gain.

FERTILITY: WANT IT OR NOT?

A few generations back, women tended to have children younger. Because advanced degrees and careers are now viable options for so many women, many are having children later, when fertility can start to decline. More women are thinking about having a child after the age of 35, and often in their early 40s, so it's increasingly common for women to be both in early perimenopause and trying to get pregnant.

Your experience may be very different from your friends' during the perimenopause transition. Some will have kids going into high school and really want to avoid a happy — or not so happy — accident. Others will just be starting to try to get pregnant. Some women get pregnant as soon as they stop using birth control methods. For others, it can be more challenging.

No matter where you are in your life, it's important to talk to a health care provider about the effects of pregnancy on your lifestyle and health. Your desire to become pregnant or your feelings about the risk of getting pregnant will help you make a choice about the benefits of birth control or the use of advanced reproductive technology.

If you're trying to get pregnant in perimenopause, the most significant change is decreased fertility. Your chance of becoming pregnant every month declines because your ovulation is becoming less regular, you have fewer eggs, and the quality of eggs is not what it was in your 20s and 30s. But that doesn't mean you can't get pregnant. As long as you have periods, natural pregnancy is still possible.

If you don't want to get pregnant in perimenopause, your health care provider may prescribe a low-dose birth control pill. This can prevent pregnancy and also improve some of the symptoms of perimenopause, such as abnormal bleeding, hot flashes and mood fluctuation. Another option may be an IUD that dispenses a low dose of a progestin. This provides contraception and protects the uterine lining from overgrowth and prevents heavy bleeding. An estrogen patch can be used in addition to the IUD to help relieve hot flashes and sleep disturbances.

Preserving fertility
Historically, the birth control pill has allowed women to prevent

pregnancy, and thus enjoy sexual freedom and gain economic power. Today, that economic power enables women to freeze their eggs and then access their fertility further down the road. In 2012 the American Society for Reproductive Medicine (ASRM) removed the "experimental" label from the egg freezing procedure, called oocyte cryopreserva-

FERTILITY AFTER 40

The number of women having babies later in life has dramatically increased in recent years. About 9% of first births in the United States are now to women over age 35, which is a 23% increase from 20 years ago. More than 100,000 U.S. women a year give birth over the age of 40.

While it becomes harder to get pregnant over 35, and definitely over 40, when it does happen, there are upsides. An observational study of mothers over 40 found better health and development in their children up to 5 years of age. In this study, the children of older parents got hurt less and had higher rates of immunization and better social and language development. In addition, older parents tended to have more patience and give their children more attention. They also had more emotional and financial stability.

The main challenge of fertility after 40 is that it's harder to get pregnant naturally and even through reproductive medicine. When a girl is born, her ovaries hold 6-7 million eggs. In puberty, she has 300,000 to 500,000, and that number goes down to 25,000 by the time she turns 37. By the time a woman enters menopause, she has only 1,000 eggs. And it's not only an issue of quantity but also quality. Older eggs tend to have more genetic mutations. When an egg is fertilized, these changes can affect whether it develops into a healthy embryo and fetus. Because of this, miscarriage is a much bigger risk.

After about age 37, the ecosystem of your reproductive system changes. Lower egg quality, along with changes in the composition of reproductive hormones such as FSH, anti-mullerian hormone (AMH) and inhibin B, makes it more difficult to get and stay pregnant.

tion. Egg retrieval and freezing is now offered by a growing number of fertility clinics and doctors.

However, this process is expensive. Most health insurance plans don't cover it, or if they do, they cover only part of the cost. So this option remains out of reach for many people. And, of course, there are

Diseases like leiomyomas, tubal disease and endometriosis also become more prevalent as you age. In addition, a history of ovarian surgery, chemotherapy, pelvic infection, or smoking, or a family history of early menopause, may affect the size of the ovarian follicles that hold and release eggs. This could impact fertility too.

And let's not forget: It's not just about women. As men age, their sperm decline in numbers, start swimming slower and develop more genetic abnormalities. Research has shown that babies born to older fathers experience increased rates of many diseases, including neurodevelopmental disorders on the autism spectrum.

Reproductive technology can help a lot, and its use is growing. A recent demographic study predicted that by the year 2100, 400 million people worldwide could be conceived with assisted reproductive technologies. But these methods are not foolproof, and age is still a factor. In women under 35 with fertility obstacles, a little over 40% of IVF cycles lead to bringing home a baby. That percentage goes down to 12% in women ages 41 to 42 years, 5% in women ages 43 to 44 years, and 1% for women older than 44 years. Women over 40 may have the option of using donor eggs from younger women, and more than half those cycles result in a child.

If you're over 40 and hoping to get pregnant, talk to your doctor about your options before you start trying. Working with your health care team and understanding your own body, as well as the statistics and risks, is essential to help you make smart decisions and achieve a healthy pregnancy and birth before you reach menopause.

still many uncertainties around the success and long-term effects of preserving fertility through this method or others. If you're interested in exploring this route to fertility, talk with your doctor.

PREDICTING THE FUTURE

If you haven't frozen your eggs, then working with a reproductive endocrinologist may help you assess the state of your fertility by measuring your FSH and anti-mullerian hormone (AMH) levels. Studies suggest that FSH, estradiol and inhibin B are only poor to fair measures of a woman's ability to conceive or how her ovaries will respond to stimulation. However, increasing research is showing that measuring AMH levels in combination with age may help predict your ability to conceive each month. Studies of this testing are ongoing, and with growing evidence it may be a helpful predictive tool that's available more widely. If your AMH levels are indeed low, then IVF with either your own eggs or donor eggs could be the next step to pregnancy.

NAVIGATING THE ROAD AHEAD

As you enter the transition to menopause, no matter your age, the key to navigating your changing body is awareness and education. The information throughout this book can help you understand the wide range of what's typical and the solutions that are available. Use it as a jumping-off point for discussing your specific situation with your doctor and advocating for yourself.

If you're experiencing new physical or mental symptoms, talk with a health care practitioner who's well versed in perimenopause and menopause. A trusted clinician can help you manage your symptoms, flag other health issues, and advise you on the best path to either achieving or avoiding pregnancy as you near your final period.

PERSONAL STORY: SARAH | AGE 43

" I still have my period. And, given my age, statistics say that I may have it for several years to come. But I'm definitely feeling the signs of changing hormones.

I was 40 when I first started getting symptoms, and at first, I didn't realize what was happening. Menopause wasn't on my radar. So when I started noticing more facial hair, mood swings and weight gain (after maintaining the same weight for two decades), I just figured that aging and a busy lifestyle were the culprits. I'd never even heard of perimenopause.

In fact, when I started experiencing breast tenderness at 41, I thought, to my great surprise, that I was pregnant. After all, breast pain had been my first indicator of pregnancy with my sons 10 and 13 years earlier. I was so sure. When a pregnancy test came back negative, I was both relieved and confused.

Within a year, my periods became irregular. While they still arrived about every four weeks, they became more unpredictable. One month I'd have a light period that lasted only a few days. The next month, my period would last a full week and be so heavy that changing tampons and pads felt like a full-time job.

I told my health care provider about my symptoms. I worried that something might be wrong with me. But after an evaluation, she said that I'd started perimenopause. I was surprised — but also relieved that my symptoms weren't a sign of something more serious.

Now, irregular periods and my other perimenopausal symptoms (like that cyclical breast tenderness) have become my norm. And while I can't say I necessarily enjoy the process, it's just another part of my day, like attending meetings or driving my kids to activities. That said, I am looking forward to completing this cycle and going through menopause. Now that I'm on my way, I'm ready for the next phase.

4

Premature menopause

By their late 40s or early 50s, most women have started noticing the symptoms of perimenopause. They are watching for the signs of their final period — often with open arms.

For some, though, menopause comes much earlier. They stop having their periods in their 20s, 30s or early 40s. Women who go into menopause before age 40 are said to have premature menopause. This condition affects about 1% to 3% of women. Around 5% to 10% of women go through menopause between the ages of 40 and 45, which is considered early menopause.

There are many reasons your ovaries might stop working early. Regardless of the reason, premature menopause is a manageable condition. This chapter will help you understand it and walk you through the actions you can take to protect your health — and, if it's important to you, your dreams of building a family.

PREMATURE MENOPAUSE: WHY IT HAPPENS

Thanks to medical research, more diseases and conditions than ever can be treated or cured. Unfortunately, some of the treatments that can save your life can also damage your ovaries. If you go through menopause because of medical treatments, such as surgery, chemotherapy or radiation, it's called *induced premature menopause*. If you experience menopause on your own before age 40 — as a result of health conditions, some genetic conditions or even unknown reasons — it's known as *premature ovarian insufficiency (POI)*. *Primary ovarian insufficiency* is another common term for it.

Menopause due to removal of the ovaries

For various reasons, sometimes the ovaries need to be surgically removed during the childbearing years. This procedure is called an *oophorectomy* (oh-uh-fuh-REK-tuh-me). Depending on the procedure, this may bring on different levels of menopause symptoms.

If you have an operation to remove both ovaries (bilateral oophorectomy), for instance, you'll stop getting your monthly period immediately, your hormones will drop quickly and you will enter menopause.

If, instead, you have surgery to remove your uterus (hysterectomy), but you keep your ovaries, you will immediately stop getting your period and will be unable to become pregnant. You will not be in menopause, though, because your ovaries will still continue to make the hormones estrogen and progesterone. This means you also aren't likely to experience menopause symptoms. However, women who have a hysterectomy may experience menopause a few years earlier than average.

Sometimes one ovary is removed in surgery (unilateral oophorectomy). In this case, your body may continue to use the other ovary to produce hormones. For example, you may have a hysterectomy with unilateral oophorectomy. Still, this is linked to experiencing earlier menopause than those who have a hysterectomy alone.

If you do undergo premature menopause related to the removal of both ovaries, your menopause symptoms may be stronger than they would have been if you had reached menopause naturally. This is because in natural menopause, you experience a slow decline in estrogen and progesterone over time. But when your ovaries are surgically removed, you experience a sudden and immediate stop to your hormone production, including a portion of your testosterone production.

In this situation, symptoms such as hot flashes may begin as soon as the day after surgery. Fortunately, there are effective options for managing these symptoms. Before surgery, talk to your health care provider about your treatment options.

Other causes of premature ovarian insufficiency

When something's not quite right in your body, it's natural to want answers. You may want to know what caused it, how it happened and how you can fix it. Unfortunately, for 75% to 90% of people who experience premature ovarian insuffiency (POI), health care providers simply don't know the cause.

Some factors that may contribute to POI are:

Genetic disorders Certain chromosomal problems — such as those involved in your reproductive hormones or ovarian development — can cause POI. For instance, in a condition called *Turner syndrome*, women are born without all or part of one X chromosome, and as a result, their ovaries may be underdeveloped. Turner syndrome is one of the most common causes of primary ovarian insufficiency.

There is also evidence that women who carry the FMR1 gene — which is linked to a condition called *fragile X syndrome* — are at an increased risk of POI. These women may initially have regular menstrual cycles, but their hormone levels more closely match those of aged ovaries. Many other genetic syndromes are also associated with primary ovarian insufficiency. However, most are extremely rare.

Autoimmune diseases When you have an autoimmune condition, your body's immune system mistakes your own cells as invaders and attacks them. In some cases, such as in thyroid disease, lupus or rheumatoid arthritis, your immune system may attack your ovaries, preventing them from making hormones. This can ultimately lead to POI.

Metabolic disorders Certain metabolic disorders, such a galactosemia, may contribute to POI. For instance, people with galactosemia are unable to break down galactose — a sugar found in milk. Research shows that the defects in galactose metabolism may influence ovarian function.

Infectious causes Mumps and HIV, among other infections, may contribute to POI by damaging ovarian tissue.

Family history If you have a family history of early menopause or POI, you are more likely to have early menopause yourself.

Chemotherapy-induced menopause

Chemotherapy is medicine that's designed to attack and kill cancer cells. Unfortunately, as it attacks fast-dividing cells, it may also damage your ovaries.

Not all chemotherapy drugs affect the reproductive system. Some may have no effect on your ovaries, while others can cause either a temporary or a permanent stop to your periods. Your risk of going into menopause depends on many factors, including your age, the kind of chemotherapy drugs you'll take and the amount of chemotherapy used.

Typically, any damage done is to the follicles — the fluid-filled sacs that hold your eggs. Women who've received chemotherapy may have decreased numbers of maturing follicles. While some women aren't affected, others may experience menopause after a single dose.

Even if you do experience ovarian insufficiency due to chemotherapy, the condition may be temporary. Some women — especially those under 40 — may find that their fertility returns months or even years after they complete treatment.

Radiation-induced menopause

Like chemotherapy, radiation therapy can be a highly effective method of fighting cancer. When this radiation is centered on your pelvic area, though, it can damage your ovaries. In fact, radiation therapy is typically more damaging to your ovaries than chemotherapy is.

The effect of radiation on your fertility depends on your age and the dose you receive. Radiation-induced ovarian insufficiency may sometimes be temporary, especially in younger women and in those who receive lower doses. These women may find that their periods return 6 to 18 months after treatment. Sometimes a procedure to move the ovaries outside the field of radiation (oophoropexy) may be done.

ADDRESSING YOUR PHYSICAL HEALTH

When you experience POI or premature menopause, your hormone levels drop significantly. The premature or early loss of estrogen can impact your health in a number of ways. It may affect:

Cardiovascular health Research suggests that premature meno-

CONSIDERING OOPHORECTOMY

In some situations, such as treating ovarian cancer, removing the ovaries (oophorectomy) may be a necessity. But you may also consider removing the ovaries as a preventive health measure. This is known as *prophylactic oophorectomy*. If you want to reduce your high risk of developing breast or ovarian cancer, for example, this may be one option.

Oophorectomy is not a decision to be made lightly. It carries significant risks. In particular, removing both ovaries will cause immediate menopause. Common signs and symptoms of menopause, such as hot flashes and vaginal dryness, are likely to occur and are often more severe than in women who go through menopause naturally. Oophorectomy may also increase your risk of depression or anxiety, heart disease, osteoporosis and premature death.

In addition, the procedure may take an emotional toll. If you want to have children (or more children), the loss of your fertility may be crushing. Some women also struggle with their sense of femininity.

On the other hand, if your cancer risk is high, removing the ovaries reduces that risk significantly. If you're premenopausal and you have changes to the BRCA genes, which make proteins to help repair DNA, this procedure can reduce your breast cancer risk by up to 50% and your ovarian cancer risk by 80% to 90%. The trade-offs may be well worth it.

If your risk of breast cancer or ovarian cancer is high, you can talk with your health care practitioner about whether to preventively

pause may be associated with an increased risk of heart disease and stroke. This may be because of estrogen's effect on endothelial function, the health of the cells that line your blood vessels. For more on cardiovascular problems after menopause, see Chapter 19.

Bone health Estrogen plays a key role in the strength of your bones. As a result, when you go through premature menopause, you have an

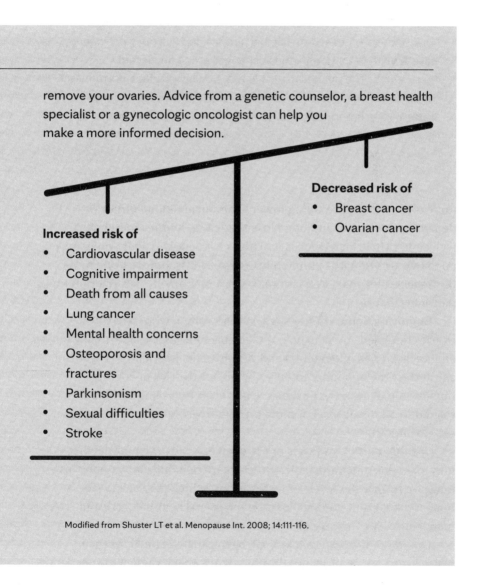

remove your ovaries. Advice from a genetic counselor, a breast health specialist or a gynecologic oncologist can help you make a more informed decision.

Decreased risk of
- Breast cancer
- Ovarian cancer

Increased risk of
- Cardiovascular disease
- Cognitive impairment
- Death from all causes
- Lung cancer
- Mental health concerns
- Osteoporosis and fractures
- Parkinsonism
- Sexual difficulties
- Stroke

Modified from Shuster LT et al. Menopause Int. 2008; 14:111-116.

UNDERSTANDING PREMATURE OVARIAN INSUFFICIENCY

Premature ovarian insufficiency (POI) might seem like a technical term for premature menopause. But the two aren't exactly the same thing.

POI describes what's happening in the ovaries when they're not releasing eggs regularly. POI involves many of the changes of menopause — ceased menstrual periods and a drop in estrogen levels. With POI, though, these changes aren't necessarily permanent. The ovaries may still occasionally produce hormones and release eggs. Some women may even have an occasional return of their periods, and 5% to 10% are able to conceive.

increased risk of developing lower than normal bone mineral density (osteopenia) and bone loss that causes bones to become weak and brittle (osteoporosis). This is especially true if you experience POI or premature menopause in your 20s, before bone mass has reached its peak. You can read more on bone health after menopause in Chapter 18.

Cognition Some studies suggest that women who have their ovaries removed and who do not take hormone (estrogen) therapy have an increased risk of dementia and cognitive decline. The younger the age at the time of oophorectomy, the higher the risk of cognitive impairment. However, the data are less clear for women with POI related to other causes. For more on cognitive issues and menopause, see Chapter 20.

Sexual health Low levels of estrogen can cause symptoms that may make sex uncomfortable. Women experiencing early menopause may also have lower levels of testosterone, which may negatively impact sexual functioning. For more on sexual health during and after menopause, see Chapter 12.

Quality of life Low levels of estrogen can be blamed for menopause symptoms such as hot flashes, night sweats, vaginal dryness and mood changes. Read more about menopause symptoms in Chapter 2, and see Chapters 6 through 13 for how to manage them.

HELP FROM HORMONES

Everyone who goes through menopause may benefit from hormone therapy. The primary goal may be managing symptoms such as hot flashes or mood swings. In women with premature or early menopause, adding ovarian hormones back into the body also may help prevent heart disease, protect cognition and minimize vaginal dryness. And hormone therapy is vital for preventing bone loss after premature menopause.

In people experiencing premature or early menopause, higher doses of estrogen may be needed, compared with the doses for women going through natural menopause. Higher doses are often given to mimic the estrogen production in reproductive aged women, not only to treat symptoms, but also to lower the health risks from the loss of estrogen in younger women. Most health care providers recommend that women with early or premature menopause take hormone therapy until at least the age of natural menopause — about 52 years old.

STEM CELL THERAPY FOR POI

Stem cells are the body's raw materials — the source of all other cells with specialized functions. In a lab, stem cells can be grown and guided into becoming specific cells that can regenerate and repair damaged or diseased tissues. This technology may be a game changer for many medical conditions, including POI.

So far, studies of stem cell use in other animals have shown some potential in regaining ovarian function. Transplanting stem cells could help restore hormone levels and even activate follicles. For now, more research is still needed to know if this treatment is safe and effective in people before it's ready for primetime.

But hormone therapy isn't a cure-all. While it can reduce or remove many of the negative health consequences of POI or premature menopause, it does not remove them all. Mood changes and sexual function, in particular, may not be entirely managed with hormone therapy. To learn more about hormone therapy, see Chapter 6.

What about the risks?
Much has been written about the risks of hormone therapy. If you have POI or premature menopause, you may worry especially about taking hormone therapy at a young age or for a longer time.

Don't let this concern you. The medical trials that revealed the risks of hormone therapy were conducted with older, postmenopausal

COULD YOU BE EXPERIENCING POI?

Women who are experiencing POI often don't realize it. That is because the signs aren't always clear.

Someone in the early stages of POI may stop having periods altogether, or she may initially just skip one or two. She may have some of the symptoms of menopause — such as hot flashes or vaginal dryness — or she may not have any, yet. This is because even if someone has POI, the ovaries may still occasionally release estrogen and eggs.

So how do you know if your symptoms are early signs of POI or a separate health problem?

Your best bet is to talk to your health care practitioner. If your periods change significantly (become noticeably longer or shorter, or vary markedly from your usual schedule) or stop altogether for three cycles before age 40, make an appointment.

It's important to get checked out, since missing periods could be a sign of another health concern. Plus, if you're experiencing POI, you're at a higher risk of developing health conditions such as osteo-

women — not women in premature or early menopause. The results simply cannot be applied to younger women. In fact, we know that the risks of not taking hormone therapy can be devastating for this group.

The bottom line: If you have premature menopause and you do not take estrogen, you have a much higher risk of dementia, Parkinson's disease, cardiovascular disease, osteoporosis, sexual dysfunction, depression, anxiety and death.

COPING WITH PREMATURE MENOPAUSE

Going through menopause can be an emotional time at any age. You may struggle through daily symptoms and feel anxious about your body

porosis and heart disease. Diagnosis can be a powerful tool, allowing you to take steps to make sure you stay as healthy as possible.

To help find the cause of your symptoms or skipped periods, your health care provider may:

- Ask about any menopause symptoms you've been having.
- Conduct a pregnancy test. This will make sure that any missed periods aren't due to pregnancy.
- Test your hormone levels. Blood tests can evaluate your level of follicle-stimulating hormone (FSH) to determine if it is in the menopausal range.
- Check for medical conditions that may be affecting your period. Blood tests may measure thyroid-stimulating hormone (TSH), fasting glucose, serum calcium or phosphorus levels, to name a few.
- Check your ovarian reserve. An anti-mullerian hormone (AMH) level is a test that can estimate your ovarian reserve. A pelvic ultrasound can be used to check the quantity of eggs in your ovaries.

and your identity in the months or years ahead. If you go through early or premature menopause, these feelings may be even more intense.

You may feel shocked at the diagnosis, certain that you're too young to go through this. You may feel confused or unsure what steps to take next. If you'd hoped to have children in the future — or even if you hadn't really decided yet — you may feel devastated over the loss of your fertility.

You may feel angry about the changes premature menopause makes in your daily life, like the symptoms you might have or the hormones or other medication you may have to take. Experiencing hot flashes or vaginal dryness in your 20s or 30s may make you feel like you're growing old overnight — and aging beyond your friends. Premature or early menopause can be traumatic and isolating. It may lead to feelings of depression and anxiety.

The good news is that you don't have to go through this alone. There are many resources available to help you get the answers you deserve and make sense of your circumstances. Take care of your emotional and mental health with this advice:

Gain perspective. Going through menopause in your 20s or 30s might not have been part of your life plan. But that doesn't mean you

WHAT ABOUT TESTOSTERONE?

Estrogen and progesterone aren't the only hormones that are depleted during menopause. When you experience premature menopause, particularly if your ovaries are removed, you'll also have a decrease in ovarian androgens. Androgens are the male sex hormones, such as testosterone. For some women, a decrease in testosterone isn't a concern. For others, the loss of testosterone may contribute to problems with sexual dysfunction. This is because testosterone plays a role in sexual desire and arousal. As a result, some women may benefit from testosterone therapy.

can't still realize your dreams. Many women experience POI or premature menopause and go on to have healthy, productive lives with symptoms under control — and even families of their own.

Get accurate information. Educate yourself about what's happening with your body. No question is a dumb question. Your health care provider is there to help you get answers. When looking for information online, make sure to stick to reputable websites, especially those aligned with established medical institutions, such as *www.MayoClinic.org* or those ending with .gov.

Seek emotional support. Ask your health care provider to recommend a counselor and support group. Support groups are made up of people who understand what you're going through because they're going through it too. They can offer the compassion and encouragement that others might not. If a local group isn't an option, an online group, such as through Mayo Clinic Connect or the Daisy Network, may be a helpful community offering support and real-life tips. In

CONCEIVING NATURALLY WITH PREMATURE OVARIAN INSUFFICIENCY: IS IT POSSIBLE?

You've heard the stories. Women who were told they would never conceive — who had maybe even struggled with infertility due to premature ovarian insufficiency for years — suddenly become pregnant. Could it happen for you?

The answer is a cautious maybe — but the odds are low. Research tells us that about 5% to 10% of women who experience POI are able to become pregnant. So while there's hope, it's not a strong method of family planning. If your goal is to have children, your best bet is to consider the options in this chapter and talk with your health care practitioner. You may want to ask about ovarian reserve testing, which can help assess whether pregnancy with your own eggs might still be an option.

addition, talking with a counselor who specializes in premature menopause or fertility issues can help you gain a sense of control over your diagnosis.

Give yourself some time. Sometimes the greatest gift you can give yourself is time to come to terms with your diagnosis. It won't happen

PERSONAL STORY: SUSAN | AGE 43

" When I was 36 years old, I stopped menstruating. I also began experiencing hot flashes, night sweats, vaginal dryness/burning, increased anxiety and irritability, lack of concentration, insomnia, abdominal weight gain despite no change to my diet or exercise plan, and generalized body stiffness. I knew something was wrong.

I reached out to my primary care provider (PCP), and we monitored the symptoms for a couple months. Nothing changed. Then, lab work was drawn — with abnormal results. My PCP was concerned about infertility. I won't ever forget that appointment. My "plan" was to try to get pregnant after a much anticipated work trip that I had worked years towards attaining. There went my plan. I felt crushed.

After my work trip, I followed up with the Reproductive Endocrinology and Infertility Clinic regarding fertility options. Then I followed up with the Women's Health Clinic. There, I was diagnosed with Primary Ovarian Insufficiency (POI). In other words – early menopause. This was a turning point. I'd been focused on my infertility, but what I didn't know were the health risks associated with low estrogen levels at such an early age.

I was started on an estrogen patch, along with progesterone to promote a monthly uterine shedding and prevent endometrial thickening or cancer. The estrogen therapy significantly improved my symptoms. However, progesterone side effects are no joke — fatigue, stiffness (myalgia), depression, weight gain, nightmares and constipation. For me, synthetic progestin has had less severe side effects. When I'm on this medication for 12 days each month, I have found a few tricks that are helpful to reduce the side effects. To reduce fatigue, myalgia and

overnight. Allow yourself the space to come to accept it. You'll get there.

Allow — and talk about — your feelings of grief. It's natural to mourn your vision of how you'd build a family. It's normal to struggle with this shift in your identity. Have open communication as you

depression, I keep on an exercise routine including yoga and self-care activities. To reduce weight gain and constipation, I eat an extra well-balanced diet, drink lots of water, and minimize alcohol consumption. I've found that even one glass of alcohol increases fatigue and insomnia.

Seven years later, my symptoms are pretty well managed and I have learned more about my body than I ever imagined. As I age, I am more prone to vaginal irritation and yeast infections — which affects our sex life. Changing to a lubricant with no parabens/glycerin (such as Good Clean Love) has helped significantly. It also helps to "air the vagina" by avoiding tight fitting pants and going without underwear when I can. Drinking lots of water and reducing my sugar intake helps too.

The most challenging part of my POI journey has been the psychological and psychosocial hurdles. When I was diagnosed with POI, it was life changing. I had been ready to start a family. I found many people minimized the implications of this diagnosis, simply because they cannot relate. It's not terminal. It's not visibly debilitating. My favorite comment was, "at least it isn't cancer." It has changed my approach with other people facing life-altering diagnoses.

In addition, I live in a very family-oriented community. You learn to navigate through conversations. We have learned to focus on the many blessings in our life and that life can be fulfilling whether you have children or not.

That's my story. Though many of my friends have not gone through menopause yet, one day, when they reach that stage in their life, I will have years of advice to share with them.

manage your feelings. And allow yourself to envision a different version of your dreams.

CAN YOU STILL HAVE A FAMILY?

If you had hoped to have children in the future, facing premature or early menopause — or even the possibility of it — may feel like a punch to the gut. But you don't have to give up hope. Many women who experience POI or premature menopause go on to become parents.

Options that involve your own ovaries

There are several options that make use of or protect the ovarian function you currently have. If you're facing a medical condition or treatment that may compromise your fertility and you hope to have children in the future, ask your health care provider to refer you to a fertility specialist. A fertility specialist can help you decide on your best options for building a family, which may include:

Freezing your embryos (embryo cryopreservation) Embryo cryopreservation is when a specialist harvests your eggs, creates embryos with your partner's (or a donor's) sperm and then freezes and stores them for future in vitro fertilization. Embryos can be stored for many years before use — giving you the chance to regain your health or wait for the time to be right. And when it is right, embryos can be thawed and implanted in your (or a gestational carrier's) uterus. Embryo cryopreservation can have high success rates, but it can be expensive.

Freezing your eggs (oocyte cryopreservation) Oocyte cryopreservation is when your healthy eggs are harvested, then frozen for future in vitro fertilization. In order for you to use these eggs in the future, a partner or a donor will have to provide sperm. This can be a successful approach to preserving your fertility — but there are a couple of caveats. The procedure can be expensive. And just as in trying to get pregnant naturally, there are no guarantees.

Oophoropexy Radiation can be an effective method of treating cancer. But if you're undergoing radiation in your pelvic area, it can damage your ovaries and their ability to produce eggs. An oophoropexy can help minimize your risk of this damage. During an oophoropexy,

" As mom to a 12-year-old girl, I've had a lot of conversations with my daughter about how her body works, including what it means to have a period and why I don't have one anymore. I was surgically induced into menopause at age 33 due to ovarian cancer.

When I was growing up, I truly don't remember anyone telling me about "the change" and how challenging it would be.

In 2004, menopause information and treatment options were not what they are today. I learned more about the anticipated side effects from chemo and radiation than about what would happen after a full hysterectomy and oophorectomy. I was told I might have some hot flashes and night sweats, but no other info was shared.

Over the next decade, my patience began to wane. I experienced insomnia, increased urination (particularly at night), anxiety, depression, and rising blood pressure. When I heard Dr. Faubion speak at a cancer conference, I was shocked to learn that all my symptoms were related to menopause! I had no idea how a woman's body changes when it no longer has the protective effects of estrogen. I also didn't realize symptoms could last for years.

Today, while I still wake up half a dozen times a night (to pee), my blood pressure is under control, and I have a team of women's health experts helping me navigate my post-menopause quality of life. Due to my cancer, I am not a candidate for hormone therapy, but I have found other options that help me manage the ongoing challenges.

While I can't change the past, I do talk about it in hopes of raising awareness around menopause and the issues that younger women may face. And despite the grimaces from my daughter when I share nuggets of information, I know she will be more prepared whenever she reaches this milestone.

your health care provider moves your ovaries out of the area to be radiated. This is done before any radiation treatment, through a minimally invasive procedure.

PERSONAL STORY: LILI | AGE 24

" I was 22 years old when I was diagnosed with primary ovarian insufficiency. I'd never heard of it before. The doctor gave me a pamphlet and then referred me to an endocrinologist. It would be the first in a series of referrals, as I tried to get my symptoms under control: chronic insomnia, tachycardia, osteopenia, brain fog, loss of libido, depression and anxiety. You name it, and I probably experienced it. There was nothing to prepare me for it, and it was shocking. I never learned about menopause at school, and older women seemed to avoid the topic as if there were a veil of shame around it.

It's been an endless struggle to feel normal ever since my diagnosis. I've spent time both on and off hormone therapy, experimenting with diets such as carnivore and keto, and practicing yoga. I often feel like I have to intensely micromanage my life just to feel somewhat normal or healthy. This creates a feeling of isolation from my peers. In addition, I still struggle with symptom management and it affects my performance at work. Seeing a therapist has been helpful in teaching me to advocate for myself, both with doctors and with employers.

I wish medical providers knew that primary ovarian insufficiency affects more than just fertility. Primary ovarian insufficiency is a complex metabolic disease that can result in severe symptoms. I've met quite a few women in support groups that were facing disability since their initial diagnosis. These are young women. I'm concerned for those who lack health insurance and can't even afford treatment. In the future, I hope women's health will take more of a precedence in scientific research.

Freezing ovary tissue (ovarian cryopreservation) A promising new option involves freezing healthy ovarian tissue to protect it from chemotherapy or radiation damage during cancer treatment. After treatment is done, the tissue can be reimplanted. While this process is still experimental, it has proven to restore hormone production and fertility in some people.

Other avenues
If you were surprised by a diagnosis of POI and didn't have the opportunity to take preservation measures, there are still ways you can have a family.

In vitro fertilization (IVF) with donor eggs Even if you aren't able to produce eggs of your own (and even if you no longer have your ovaries), you may still be able to become pregnant via in vitro fertilization with donor eggs. In this procedure, eggs are collected from a donor, then fertilized with your partner's or a donor's sperm and implanted in your uterus.

IVF with donor eggs has high success rates in women who have experienced POI. In some cases, however, IVF isn't recommended. For instance, pregnancy can be dangerous for women with Turner syndrome. (See page 76.)

Gestational carrier You might consider using a gestational carrier — a woman who will carry a baby for you. In this situation, an embryo is created through IVF and is transferred to a gestational carrier's uterus. No genes from the gestational carrier are passed on to the child. Because laws for using another person (third-party) for pregnancy may vary depending on where you live, it's wise to contact a lawyer familiar with donor issues in your area for legal advice if you're considering this option.

Adoption Many who are unable to conceive a biological child turn to adoption to complete their families. Adoption can be a rewarding and fulfilling way to realize your dream of parenthood. In fact, many parents who pursued adoption say they now couldn't imagine building their families any other way.

5

Diverse experiences of menopause

Hot flashes, mood swings, sleepless nights. How many of us have turned to a mother, auntie or friend and asked, "Am I the only one?" If you've been reading this book, you know the answer is a resounding no. The menopause transition affects us all to one degree or another. But those effects vary widely. The question is: Why? Why do some women experience menopause like an 18-wheeler driving straight for them while others seem to skate right through it?

Genetics may be one part of the puzzle. But the picture is a lot more complicated than that. Emerging research points to a multitude of factors that may shape how you experience menopause. Some of these things relate to lifestyle — behaviors we may be able to change to improve our symptoms.

Other factors — like our bodies, background, exposure to adversity (including racism) and other experiences are simply part of who we are. These aspects of our unique life stories may extend beyond the personal, reflecting broader issues within society. No single person or

CORRELATION VS. CAUSATION

This book — and especially this chapter — pulls together findings from many research studies. It's important to keep in mind that frequently, when research finds that two things are associated, it doesn't mean one causes the other. Or, at least, the study didn't prove that one causes the other — it just showed a relationship. (This depends on how the study was done.) In other words, correlation is not the same as causation.

For example, we know that people who have chronic stress tend to experience earlier menopause and worse menopause-related symptoms. When that link is shown repeatedly in research, we can be pretty confident there's a connection. But often, we still don't know exactly why the two parts are linked — how one leads to another or if there's a separate factor that's involved in both.

book can solve these larger problems alone, but this chapter doesn't shy away from them either. The hope is that by arming you with scientifically and medically based knowledge, you'll feel empowered to seek out and ask for the health care you need and deserve.

YOUR LIFESTYLE

What you eat, how active you are, your sleeping, dietary or smoking habits — these are some of the behaviors that can affect the way you experience menopause. The good news? You have some control over these factors. In many cases, simple changes may improve bothersome symptoms and boost your overall health.

What you eat
A diet low in nutrition may make menopausal symptoms worse. One particularly sneaky culprit is ultraprocessed foods. Think snack cakes,

chicken nuggets, soda, chips, frozen dinners ... you get the idea. Convenient and tasty? Yes. Nutritious? Not so much.

One recent study looked at the diets of nearly 300 postmenopausal women. The women with higher amounts of ultraprocessed foods in their diets reported having more severe menopausal symptoms, including hot flashes and night sweats, sexual difficulties and issues with memory and concentration. In contrast, a plant-based diet is linked to reduced hot flashes, night sweats and sexual problems in menopausal women. If possible, aim for a diet that includes a variety of fruits, vegetables and whole grains. Limit saturated fats, oils, sugars and processed food. It just might make a difference in how you feel.

How much you move

You know exercise is good for your health, but did you know it may improve your menopause symptoms too? Some studies suggest that regular aerobic exercise may lessen hot flashes and night sweats, improve how well you sleep and boost your mood in the menopause years. But more research is needed to understand how — and how much — physical activity helps to reduce these symptoms.

The recommendation for most healthy adults is to get at least 150 minutes of moderate aerobic activity or 75 minutes of vigorous aerobic activity a week, or a combination of the two. A good rule of thumb is 30 minutes of moderate physical activity every day, such as brisk walking, biking, swimming or mowing the lawn. If you want to maximize your time, turn it up a notch with vigorous exercises like running, heavy yardwork and aerobic dancing. Just be sure to check with a doctor or other clinician first if you've been inactive for a while. And keep in mind that any amount of physical activity is good for your health. There's no shame in starting small.

How well you sleep

Like it or not, sleep is another factor that may affect how you experience menopause. It's unclear whether poor sleep contributes to symptoms like hot flashes or simply affects how you perceive and manage those symptoms. Hormonal shifts in menopause are known to cause night sweats and insomnia. So it's more likely that hot flashes lead to poor sleep, not the other way around. But at the very least, poor sleep may increase the risk of depression in women experiencing severe and frequent hot flashes. If you're regularly waking up exhausted, you won't have as much energy to face life's challenges — including the ups and downs of menopause.

But all is far from lost. There are effective options out there for treating sleep difficulties. Turn to Chapter 11 to read all about them.

If (and how much) you smoke
Research shows a strong link between smoking and the timing of menopause. Compared to people who have never smoked, those who currently smoke or did so in the past are at greater risk of entering menopause before the age of 45. The risk increases the longer someone has been smoking and the more cigarettes that person smokes in a typical week. Quitting can make a difference. The earlier someone quits smoking, the lower the risk of experiencing early menopause.

People who currently smoke heavily are more than two times as likely to have severe and frequent hot flashes. People who began smoking at age 15 or younger may also have a higher risk of these symptoms. But quitting before age 40 or quitting for more than five years can bring your risk down to nearly the same level as someone who's never smoked.

KICKING THE HABIT

If you've tried quitting without much success or want to quit but don't know where to begin, never fear — there are some great resources out there. Two trustworthy places to start are the American Cancer Society and the Centers for Disease Control and Prevention (CDC). Both these agencies offer a wealth of information and advice about quitting tobacco use on their websites. The CDC also provides free coaching in English at 1-800-QUIT-NOW (1-800-784-8669), in Spanish (1-855-335-3569), in Mandarin and Cantonese (1-800-838-8917), in Korean (1-800-556-5564) and in Vietnamese (1-800-778-8440).

YOUR BODY

A number of factors related to your body may impact your experience of the menopause transition. Here are several common ones.

Body mass index

Your body mass index (BMI) is a measurement based on your height and weight. It's not a perfect measure, but in general, a higher BMI indicates a higher percentage of total body fat. A BMI of 30 or higher is considered in the obese range. Having a BMI in that range may increase the risk of having worse and more-frequent hot flashes. A higher BMI is associated with higher levels of estrogen, but the link between weight and hot flashes is complex.

Your BMI may also play a role in the timing of menopause. Women with a BMI of 25 or higher may be more likely to enter menopause after the age of 51. In contrast, having a BMI of less than 18.5, which is considered underweight, may increase the chances of hitting menopause at age 45 or earlier.

Number of childbirths

Believe it or not, giving birth may affect when you enter menopause. This may be related to the interruption in ovulation during pregnancy. A recent study of more than 300,000 women found that the age of menopause increased with an increase in the number of a woman's childbirths. So, for instance, a woman who gives birth twice might enter menopause later than she would've if she had given birth once. But there is a limit — the effects of this phenomenon appear to be capped at three births. Another interesting factoid about having children? Women who are mothers may be more likely to view the end of menstruation with relief rather than regret.

YOUR LIVED EXPERIENCE

When you think about the many factors that affect your health, you might focus on the kind of stuff you've read about so far: your genetics, habits, physical makeup and medical history. What you may not consider is that the way you exist in the world, and the way the world treats you, can also impact your health. Maybe you already have a sense of that. Or maybe this is a new idea for you. Either way, this section will touch on some of the hidden issues that may affect your experience of menopause.

Socioeconomic status

The term *socioeconomic status* refers to aspects in someone's life such as educational background, income and occupation. And, yeah, it can have an impact on menopause. Research shows that women with higher levels of education, income and employment are more likely to have fewer or less-severe menopausal symptoms. A lower socioeconomic status is linked to earlier menopause, more-frequent hot flashes and more sleep problems during the menopause transition. Being homeless or uninsured are also risk factors for developing more severe symptoms.

Community attitudes and norms

How do you view the aging process in midlife? Do you bemoan each new wrinkle, fretting that you're going downhill? Or do you see growing older as a natural phase of life, maybe even something to honor and celebrate? The way you answer that question may have a lot to do with the culture or community you identify with.

Menopause-related concerns, including hot flashes, depression and negative body image, have been linked to a culture's attitudes about menopause. The status of women in a community may be another factor. In one study, women who lived in cultural communities where men held dominant family positions had worse menopausal symptoms. In contrast, women in communities that valued women-led families or shared decision-making between men and women had less-intense menopause symptoms. Women who identify with cultures that prize tightknit families and communities may also have a lower risk of severe menopause-related symptoms.

Sexual orientation may also play a role. A recent study examined the attitudes of women who identified as heterosexual, bisexual or lesbian. It found that heterosexual women tend to have the most negative views about menopause and experience more regret about the end of menstruation. The study found that bisexual and lesbian women typically view menopause in a more positive light. On the whole, they have fewer concerns about how the aging process in midlife will affect their sense of self.

Stressful circumstances

We all experience stress sometimes. Stress can be a healthy reaction to the demands of life. A small amount of stress can motivate us to confront challenges and do what needs to be done to overcome them. But if your stress switch is always turned on, it can wreak havoc on your mind and body. Chronic stress can increase your risk of a host of health problems, including anxiety and depression, tummy troubles, high blood pressure and heart disease. Chronic stress is also linked to earlier menopause and worse menopause-related symptoms.

Serious and stressful events, including violence, serious injury or sexual harassment, abuse or assault may also affect the experience of menopause. Previous trauma may increase the chances of an earlier menopause and more-frequent menopause-related symptoms. Even trauma that happened in childhood has been linked with worse menopause symptoms and may impact health and well-being in many ways later in life.

Racism and implicit bias

Let's be real: Our society has a long way to go to end racism and implicit racial bias — unconscious attitudes and stereotypes about minority racial groups. Those issues are reflected in everyday interactions and show up in laws, policies and institutions, including the health care industry.

It may come as no surprise, then, that members of minority groups are underrepresented in medical research about menopause. There's still a lot to explore and uncover, but emerging data points to the role that race — and racism — may play. For example, Black women are significantly more likely to experience frequent hot flashes and night sweats than are white women, and on average their symptoms last more than three years longer. Part of the reason may be due to structural racism — Black women are more likely to experience the socioeconomic factors linked to earlier menopause and more severe symptoms.

Everyday exposure to racism has also been linked to health problems during the transition into menopause. Repeated experiences or perceptions of discrimination are linked to higher blood pressure, increased rates of diabetes and risk factors that can lead to cardiovascular disease. It's thought that the wear and tear of these stressful encounters takes a toll on the body.

Adding to this picture is research on how people of color are treated for menopausal symptoms like hot flashes. One recent study of nearly 300,000 women veterans in midlife showed that non-Hispanic Black women and Hispanic women were less likely to receive prescriptions for hormone therapy compared to non-Hispanic white women — even if they experienced the same symptoms.

Gender identity

For people who identify as transgender or nonbinary, this part of their identity may impact their menopause experience.

As part of gender-affirming care, transgender people may be prescribed hormone therapy — including testosterone for trans men, and estrogen, often with an androgen blocker or synthetic gonadotropin-

GENDER TERMINOLOGY

Gender identity refers to your internal sense of your gender. The term *transgender* refers to a person whose gender identity doesn't match their assigned sex. A person whose gender identity and sex assigned at birth do match is considered cisgender. Someone who is gender nonconforming or gender fluid may not conform to societal expectations of what's consistent for any specific gender. Meanwhile, the terms *nonbinary* and *gender queer* refer to people who consider their gender to be outside of the categories of male or female. In addition, some people are born with differences of sexual development (DSD) — chromosomes or anatomy that differ from what's typical for either sex. *Intersex* is an older term for DSD.

releasing hormone (GnRH), for trans women. In addition, many undergo some form of surgery as part of their transition. How do these treatments affect menopause hormone shifts and symptoms? That answer is different for everyone. To manage any version of a midlife transition, it's key to work with a trusted health care practitioner, ideally one with knowledge of transgender health.

However, seeking and receiving care is often more difficult for those in the transgender community. In a national U.S. transgender survey, many reported avoiding seeing a doctor out of fear of anti-transgender bias. Among those who did seek care, 1 in 3 reported negative experiences such as being refused appropriate treatment or having to teach the clinician about transgender issues. Transgender people of color are especially likely to encounter discrimination in health care settings.

Insurance is another common problem, with limited coverage for care related to gender affirmation. Furthermore, gender-specific care such as menopause management or certain preventive screenings may

PERSONAL STORY: Linde | Age 79

" I experienced menopause as an intersex person. I was born with features of both sexes, and a recent genetic analysis determined that I have 46,XY sex reversal syndrome. Growing up, I was raised as a boy. But puberty never really hit me, so I didn't develop very masculine features.

As an adult, I was not very manly looking. But I lived well as a man, and I went on to get married and earn a PhD in biomedical sciences.

For 36 years, I was happily married to a woman. Then around age 55, things changed. I hit menopause, and I lost all the male attributes I'd had. In addition, suddenly my wife and I were always at each other's throats. She was going through menopause too, and we both experienced anger and listlessness. It was almost like a personality shift, and the marriage eventually ended.

not be covered for transgender people.

Given these factors, among others, it follows that people who are transgender and nonbinary also experience high levels of stress. And stress, in turn, can impact menopause symptoms as well (see page 98).

Experiences with health care

Regardless of gender identity, a knowledgeable medical expert who listens to you and whom you trust can have a positive effect on your health and well-being. But what if your doctor squirms or goes blank when you bring up menopause? What if you can't afford to see a doctor at all?

More than 1 out of 10 women in the United States between the ages of 18 and 64 are uninsured. Those numbers are even higher among women with lower incomes, women of color and women who are undocumented immigrants. In one study, uninsured women were more likely to say they experienced bothersome menopause symptoms compared to women who were insured.

As my body was feminizing after menopause, I began living as a woman, and later I had my testicles and micropenis removed. Now, my body matches how I feel. And for several years, I've been taking hormone therapy — estrogen, progesterone and testosterone. I think I live now the way I should have lived my whole life. I plan to stay on hormones for the long run, in consult with my endocrinologist.

If menopause irritability can happen to me, it can happen to anyone. I'd suggest reaching out for hormone therapy or other treatment at the first signs. In my experience, many family practitioners have no idea about hormone therapy.

I'm often treated as a stupid old woman — very different from my experience as a man. I have to "train in" each doctor. My medical education helps me advocate for myself. Part of my mission is to show that intersex people are normal people, just with slightly different bodies.

Another barrier to supportive health care is a lack of practitioners who are trained to discuss menopause and treat its symptoms. Research indicates that few medical residents feel prepared to talk about and manage menopause symptoms. A doctor who is uncomfortable with the topic — or worse, dismissive — may leave you feeling discouraged, confused and more anxious about what's happening with your body.

Immigration experiences

Each year millions of people leave or are displaced from their homelands. They arrive in a new country, seeking opportunities for a better education, career or way of life. Some have been uprooted as a result of difficult circumstances, such as war, poverty, political strife or environmental crises.

If you or someone close to you has immigrated to a new country, you know how hard it can be to pull up roots and slowly regrow them in a new place. Immigrants may experience a deep sense of loss, missing friends and family back home. They may have to learn a new language, adapt to unfamiliar cultural expectations and adjust to a different way of life. Many global migrants and refugees experience discrimination and struggle to find stable housing, work and access to health care. All of this can affect a person's mental and physical health.

Studies of women who have immigrated to the United States suggest that these experiences may affect the menopausal years too. The research shows a relationship between the length of time a person has lived as an immigrant in the United States and the severity of symptoms such as depression, sleep difficulties and problems with concentration or forgetfulness.

Even so, one study found that women who emigrated from outside the United States had on average less severe symptoms of menopause than women born in the United States. One possibility is that close family and cultural connections, which are more common in immigrant communities, may have health benefits that help protect women from more severe symptoms of menopause.

Another issue is that health care practitioners may be hesitant to educate immigrant women about menopause, feeling unprepared to discuss the topic in a way that's culturally appropriate.

Language barriers

The old adage "knowledge is power" is repeated for a reason. Being educated about health-related topics such as menopause can empower you to make better decisions. Research shows having access to reliable sources of health information may even improve your symptoms. Health care practitioners understand this, which is why they share medical knowledge in the form of health brochures, online sources, videos, apps and other guides.

But what happens if someone can't access that information because of a language barrier? Or what if the information doesn't reflect the reader's cultural values or experiences?

In the United States, finding reliable menopause information that is culturally sensitive and written in languages other than English can be a challenge. In desperation, people may turn to less trustworthy sources, such as social media or group chats, leading them down a rabbit hole of misinformation. This shortchanges someone who might benefit from an accurate understanding of their symptoms and how to manage them.

Exposure to pollution

The median age at which women reach menopause varies by region and by race and ethnicity. And among many factors, pollution may play a role. *Particulate matter* (PM) is the term for the tiny particles of dust, smoke and other chemicals in the air. Most of this air pollution comes from automobiles, industry and power plants, though it also comes from dirt roads, construction sites and fires.

Recent evidence suggests that living in areas of greater air pollution and more traffic is linked to a slightly earlier onset of menopause. In a large study of women across the United States, those living in areas with high PM levels in midlife reached menopause about half a month earlier than women in areas with the lowest PM levels.

GETTING THE MOST OUT OF YOUR HEALTH CARE

Your life experiences and identity may affect your journey through menopause, but they shouldn't affect the quality of your health care. If you've been let down by a medical encounter in the past, consider trying again. The urge to avoid the doctor's office is understandable if you've felt ignored or belittled or discriminated against, but you deserve to find a practitioner who sees, hears, respects and understands you.

The first step is to search for a clinician who is knowledgeable, experienced and reputable. The North American Menopause Society is a good place to start. Their website (www.menopause.org) has a search tool that allows you to locate menopause practitioners by U.S. ZIP code or by country.

And if you have trusted local friends, especially if they have already experienced perimenopause or menopause symptoms, don't be shy about asking them for a personal recommendation. That may

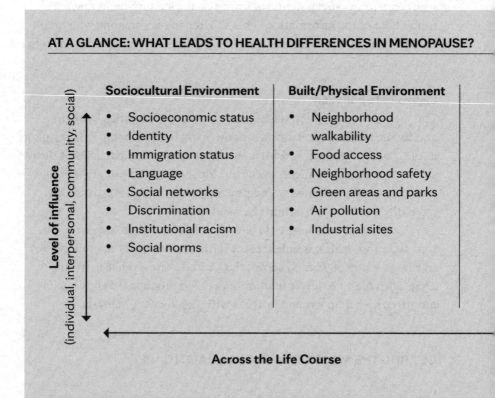

AT A GLANCE: WHAT LEADS TO HEALTH DIFFERENCES IN MENOPAUSE?

Level of influence (individual, interpersonal, community, social)

Sociocultural Environment	Built/Physical Environment
• Socioeconomic status	• Neighborhood walkability
• Identity	• Food access
• Immigration status	• Neighborhood safety
• Language	• Green areas and parks
• Social networks	• Air pollution
• Discrimination	• Industrial sites
• Institutional racism	
• Social norms	

Across the Life Course

help you find a practitioner who seems like a good fit.

The next step is to trust your gut. Does your practitioner understand where you're coming from and take your concerns seriously? Do you feel that they care about you and have your best interests at heart? Do you have confidence in their expertise and view them as trustworthy? These are the kinds of qualities that promote a strong doctor-patient relationship. And a strong relationship with a health care provider can have a positive effect on your health.

If a doctor or other clinician doesn't possess the qualities you're looking for — or if you perceive subtle (or not-so-subtle) forms of discrimination — move on and look for a better fit. You deserve a trusted ally who can be a source of comfort and guidance as you surf the sometimes wild waves of menopause.

Behavioral

- Diet
- Physical activity
- Sleep
- Stress management
- Coping strategies

Biological

- Sex hormones
- Allostatic load
- Telomere length
- Inflammatory markers
- Vasculature

Health Care System

- Health literacy
- Insurance coverage
- Access to care
- Patient-clinical relationship
- Treatment preferences
- Quality of care
- Health care policies

Conceptual Framework of Factors Driving Menopause Health Inequities (adapted from the NIMHD Minority Health and Health Disparities Research Framework)

2

Managing it

6

Hormone therapies

Did you flip right to this chapter? If you did, odds are your symptoms are interfering with your life and you want to get them under control *now*. You've heard how effective hormone therapy can be. However, maybe you're also concerned about the potential risks of taking these medications. There's a lot of conflicting information out there. How do you sift through it to know what might be the best choice for you?

This chapter will help you understand the different hormonal prescription therapies available for treating menopause symptoms — and their benefits and risks. Keep in mind that there's no magic bullet when it comes to treating menopause symptoms. But after reading this chapter, you'll be better prepared to have an informed discussion with your health care provider about what treatment may be the most safe and effective for you.

There are several factors that you and your health care provider will need to consider, including:
• What symptoms you're experiencing and their severity

- Your age
- How long it's been since menopause began or — if you're in perimenopause — whether you still need contraception
- Whether or not you have a uterus
- Whether you reached menopause naturally or as a result of surgery
- Whether you're experiencing menopause earlier than average
- Your personal history of cancer, especially breast, endometrial and ovarian cancers
- Your personal risk factors for cardiovascular disease
- Your family history and risk of cardiovascular disease, blood clots, breast cancer and osteoporosis
- Lifestyle factors, such as your weight and whether you smoke
- Your personal preferences and risk tolerance

THE BASICS OF HORMONE THERAPY

Hormone therapy is perhaps the most controversial menopause treatment available. And it's true: There's a lot of information to navigate. Before delving into the details, here are some of the basic facts to know.

Hormone therapy is effective. There's no question that hormone therapy is the most effective treatment for moderate to severe hot flashes and night sweats. It's also the best relief for vaginal symptoms that come with menopause, such as dryness, itching, burning and discomfort with intercourse. It reduces bone loss after menopause too.

There are benefits and risks. Hormone therapy can improve your symptoms and quality of life as you go through this transition, and it may have other health benefits too. But as with any medication, there are also risks — sometimes significant — to consider. You have to look at the benefit of therapy in relation to your personal risk.

Not all hormone treatments are the same. It may be tempting to lump all hormonal therapies together and label them as good or bad. But the reality is more complex. There are different treatments available that vary in terms of the hormones used and their dosages, as well as the delivery methods. Each type carries its own benefits and risks. Regardless of the type of hormone therapy, the dosage and duration of treatment should be individualized to your preferences and treatment goals.

Hormone therapy is not recommended as a preventive measure. Hormone therapy has some proven — and some unproven — health benefits beyond treating menopausal symptoms. But it's not recommended for chronic disease prevention or treatment. The exception to this guideline is if you've experienced menopause early. See page 126 for more information on premature menopause and the use of hormone therapy.

The experts do agree. Given the available information, experts agree that the benefits of hormone therapy outweigh the risks for healthy women younger than age 60 and less than 10 years past their last period who are seeking relief for moderate to severe symptoms of menopause. After age 60, it's not recommended that you start hormone therapy. But continuing treatment may be considered based on your symptoms and risk factors.

With those basics in mind, let's get into the details.

WHAT IS HORMONE THERAPY?

Hormone therapy is the use of female hormones to treat menopausal symptoms. For a long time, it was referred to as *hormone replacement therapy* (HRT). But that term has fallen from use, as it implies that postmenopausal women need to restore their hormones to premenopausal levels.

After menopause, it's natural to have lower hormone levels. The goal of treatment isn't to get back to the levels you had at 25. The goal is to find a dose that's just enough to ease the symptoms of menopause — to give you a break from hot flashes, help you sleep, stabilize your mood and more. Now called *hormone therapy* (HT) or *menopausal hormone therapy*, the use of hormones is an effective treatment for symptoms of menopause. The main female sex hormones used in HT include estrogen and a progestogen.

Estrogen is the primary hormone that eases symptoms of menopause. One of the confusing points about HT is that many of your friends will have different types of therapies prescribed for them. Women are prescribed different types of HT based on whether they still have a uterus.

In women who have undergone a hysterectomy and no longer have a uterus, estrogen can be taken alone. This is referred to as *estrogen therapy* (ET). But women who have not had a hysterectomy need a different approach. That's because giving estrogen alone can cause the lining of the uterus to overgrow. This can lead to cell changes and ultimately to cancer of the lining of the uterus (endometrial cancer). To protect the uterine lining, a progestogen is added. This type of treatment with estrogen plus a progestogen is referred to as *combination therapy* or *estrogen-progestogen therapy* (EPT).

HORMONE THERAPY TERMINOLOGY

Here are a few terms that are helpful when learning about hormone therapy.

Estrogen is actually a class of many different compounds. The three types made in the human body are 17beta-estradiol (the most active, or strongest, and the primary estrogen produced by the ovary before menopause), estrone (the primary estrogen present in postmenopausal women), and estriol (the form of estrogen produced by the placenta during pregnancy). The terms *estradiol* and *17beta-estradiol* refer to the same chemical compound. The term *conjugated estrogens* refers to a combination of numerous estrogens initially derived from pregnant mares' urine. There are also synthetic estrogens, including synthetic conjugated estrogens and ethinyl estradiol (the form of estrogen used in most oral contraceptives).

Progesterone is a hormone produced by your ovaries. The same exact chemical compound can be synthetically derived in a laboratory. Progestins are synthetic hormones that mimic progesterone but have a different chemical structure. The term *progestogen* refers to any substance with a progesterone-like activity, encompassing both progesterone and progestins.

A HISTORY RECAP

Across several generations, millions of women have used hormone therapy to treat their menopause symptoms. The earliest hormone therapy preparation, a conjugated estrogen, was first marketed in 1942. Early studies seemed to indicate hormone therapy helped protect women against heart disease, bone loss and dementia. It became widely used as a treatment for symptoms as well as a preventive health measure. However, over the years, further studies cast doubt on some of the reported benefits.

In 1991, the Women's Health Initiative (WHI) was launched. It aimed to better understand many common health conditions women experience with age. With 161,000 postmenopausal women enrolled across the United States, the WHI was the largest controlled study to date on hormone therapy, and it looked at both estrogen therapy (ET) and estrogen-progestogen therapy (EPT).

The hormone therapy component of WHI was intended to last through 2005. However, the EPT arm was stopped in 2002 because of an increased risk of breast cancer in the group taking hormones. Researchers also observed an increased risk of stroke, heart attack and blood clots in this group. The same risks were not initially seen in the ET group. But in 2004, it became clear that women taking ET without the progestogen were experiencing an increased risk of stroke.

Both treatments indicated some benefits — a reduced risk of bone fractures with both therapies, a reduced risk of colon cancer with EPT and a slightly reduced risk of breast cancer with ET. But overall, these initial results went against the prevailing understanding that hormone therapy had protective effects. The WHI findings were understandably concerning, causing an abrupt decline in the use of hormone therapy.

WHI results in context

In the years since these initial results were published, the WHI data has had more analysis, and other studies have been done. This has led the medical community to develop a more nuanced understanding of the risks and benefits of hormone therapy. The initial fears have been allayed, or at least put into context.

For example, though the ages of women participating in the WHI

BENEFITS AND ABSOLUTE RISK OF HORMONE THERAPY

You may hear about the relative risks of certain medical treatments — that is, how much your risk of something may change as a result of treatment. But when the risk is low to begin with, even a small change can increase the risk by a significant percentage. That can make a relative risk sound scarier than it should.

Absolute risk measures how often something happens in numbers rather than percentages. The charts below compare the benefits

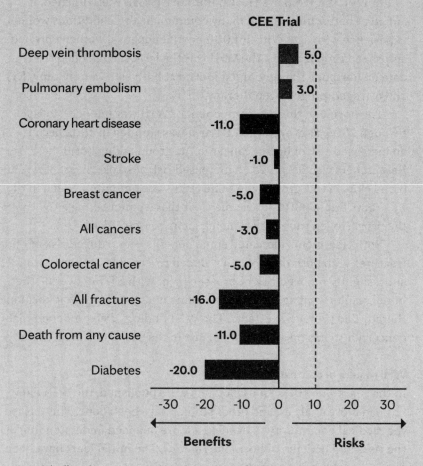

CEE Trial

Deep vein thrombosis	5.0
Pulmonary embolism	3.0
Coronary heart disease	-11.0
Stroke	-1.0
Breast cancer	-5.0
All cancers	-3.0
Colorectal cancer	-5.0
All fractures	-16.0
Death from any cause	-11.0
Diabetes	-20.0

-30 -20 -10   0   10   20   30

← Benefits   Risks →

Note: Side effects that occur in up to 10 out of 10,000 people (shown by the dashed line) are considered rare effects.

and absolute risks of two hormone therapy formulations in women ages 50 to 59, from the WHI. The gray bars show the risks that increased with conjugated estrogens (CEE) or CEE plus medroxyprogesterone acetate (MPA), a progestogen. However, the adverse events were still rare, increasing by 10 or fewer people out of 10,000.

The black bars show the benefits of therapy in each trial, including a reduction in diabetes and in death from any cause.

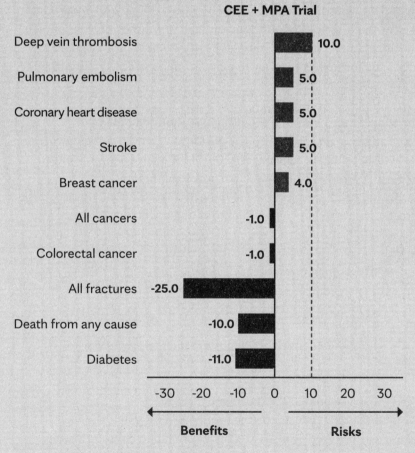

CEE + MPA Trial

Deep vein thrombosis	10.0
Pulmonary embolism	5.0
Coronary heart disease	5.0
Stroke	5.0
Breast cancer	4.0
All cancers	-1.0
Colorectal cancer	-1.0
All fractures	-25.0
Death from any cause	-10.0
Diabetes	-11.0

-30 -20 -10 0 10 20 30

← Benefits   Risks →

Source: NAMS 2022 Hormone Therapy Position Statement/Manson JE, et al.

ranged from 50 to 79, the average age was 63 years old — older than most women seeking relief from their menopausal symptoms. Some of the women in the study were smokers and had existing heart disease. In addition, because the study was designed to examine the most commonly prescribed forms of hormone therapy, it included just two regimens — a conjugated equine estrogen alone or in combination with a progestin — in only one dosage, delivered by mouth. However, we know now that different types of hormones as well as their doses and delivery methods may have different risks for women at different ages (more on that below).

The bottom line — hormone therapy isn't all good or all bad. After a period of widespread use followed by a time of fear and uncertainty, it's clear that the risks of hormone therapy vary based on your personal health history. For many younger healthy women, the risks are low, and it's the most effective way to manage menopausal symptoms and improve quality of life.

Who should use — and who should avoid — hormone therapy?

Before answering that question, let's look at what the current evidence seems to be telling us. See pages 120–121 for an overview of some of the health considerations related to hormone therapy.

Overall, study results seem to indicate that hormone therapy poses a greater risk to older women than to younger women. Evidence also indicates that, although it's required to prevent endometrial cancer, the addition of a progestogen to estrogen causes a greater risk of adverse effects than does estrogen alone — although evidence also shows that progesterone may have fewer risks than progestins. In addition, hormones delivered through the skin may have fewer risks than pills taken orally.

So who should consider taking hormone therapy, and who shouldn't?

When you may want to avoid hormone therapy

Hormone therapy may not be the best option for you if you have existing cardiovascular disease, a history of blood clots, an already increased risk of stroke, severe liver disease or abnormal vaginal bleeding that hasn't been evaluated, or if you have or have had an estrogen-dependent cancer, such as breast or endometrial cancers. Recent studies indicate that the risk of blood clot and stroke are lower with hormones delivered through the skin (transdermally) as opposed to orally. So transdermal hormone therapy might be an option for some women at risk of these conditions. Women taking hormone therapy ideally should not smoke. And if menopausal symptoms are mild and not significantly impacting quality of life, hormone therapy isn't needed to stay healthy.

When the benefits likely outweigh the risks

When menopause symptoms are frequently interrupting your sleep or impacting your quality of life, hormone therapy is often the most effective treatment. It may be a good option if you're healthy, under age 60 or less than 10 years past your last period, and you don't have specific health conditions that prevent you from using hormone therapy. Also, if you've lost bone mass, hormone therapy might be a viable option to help reduce your fracture risk. Let's take a look at the different types of hormone treatments.

TYPES OF HORMONE THERAPY

Hormone therapy is available in various delivery methods, preparations and dosages.

Delivery methods

Systemic hormone therapy refers to the delivery of hormones throughout the body to achieve relief of both hot flashes and vaginal symptoms. Systemic hormones can be delivered by mouth (oral delivery), through the skin (transdermal application) with patches, gels or sprays, or with a vaginal ring that delivers a systemic dose of estrogen.

Local therapies affect only one area of the body. In menopause, local estrogen can be used to treat vaginal dryness — part of what's known as *genitourinary syndrome of menopause*. If you're primarily seeking relief from vaginal symptoms and over-the-counter moisturizers and lubricants haven't helped or aren't enough, local vaginal estrogen therapy can be delivered by vaginal cream, tablet or ring. The lower doses of hormones used with local vaginal estrogen therapy mean that much less is absorbed into the body and a progestogen is not needed to protect the uterus. Vaginal dehydroepiandosterone (DHEA) may be another option. Low-dose vaginal hormones may even be offered to women with a history of breast cancer or cardiovascular disease, if nonhormone options haven't worked. Also, if you're taking a low-dose systemic estrogen therapy, you may still need to add local vaginal estrogen therapy or DHEA to address vaginal symptoms.

The best delivery method for you depends in part on your personal preference. You may have a hard time swallowing pills, or perhaps you find the cream messy or the adhesive on the skin patch irritating. Other considerations will have more to do with the risks of the various methods. Transdermal delivery methods have generally been shown to have fewer risks than oral. This is likely because hormones absorbed through your skin aren't metabolized by the liver. However, pills are often less expensive and may still be appropriate for some women. If you use a topical emulsion, gel or spray, you'll need to take precautions to avoid transferring the hormones to children and pets, who can be affected by the exposure. On a similar note, vaginal hormone creams shouldn't be used as a lubricant during intercourse. If you're seeking relief from only vaginal symptoms, vaginal estrogen is thought to be the most effective therapy, and you shouldn't need a systemic treatment.

Preparations

Hormone treatments for menopause symptoms will contain either estrogen alone or estrogen plus a progestogen. In perimenopausal women, hormonal contraceptives are often the recommended treatment until you reach menopause, to cover menopause symptoms and contraception. Then at the point of menopause, you would switch to a menopausal hormone therapy preparation (see "Contraceptives during the menopause transition" on page 124).

In the past, the only available hormone preparations were conjugated estrogens and a synthetic progestin. Now there are a variety of options, including the following.

Estrogens Not all estrogens are the same. The following different forms may be used in hormone therapy.

17beta-estradiol is bioidentical estrogen. It is chemically equivalent

ORAL, TRANSDERMAL AND VAGINAL ESTROGEN PRODUCTS

Common prescription estrogen therapies include:

Oral compounds	Products
Conjugated estrogen	Premarin
Synthetic conjugated estrogen	Cenestin (discontinued)
Esterified estrogen	Menest
17beta-estradiol	Estrace, generics
Estropipate	Ogen
Transdermal compounds	**Products**
17beta-estradiol matrix patch	Alora, Climara, Vivelle, Vivelle-Dot, Minivelle, generics
17beta-estradiol transdermal gel	Estrogel, Divigel
17beta-estradiol emulsion	Estrasorb (discontinued)
17beta-estradiol spray	Evamist
Vaginal therapies	**Products**
Cream, 17beta-estradiol	Estrace Vaginal Cream
Cream, conjugated estrogens	Premarin Vaginal Cream
Vaginal rings	Estring, Femring
Vaginal inserts	Vagifem, Yuvafem, Imvexxy

to the estrogen produced by your ovaries in the reproductive years.

Conjugated estrogens (CE) contain a blend of estrogens. The form used in the WHI trials, conjugated equine estrogens (CEE), is made from the urine of pregnant female horses. It contains a mixture of CE, including estrone sulfate. Synthetic CE is a blend of synthetic estrogen substances including estrone sulfate, equilin sulfate, and estradiol sulfate.

Esterified estrogens and estropipate also contain estrone sulfate, which is made into estrone and estradiol in the body.

Estetrol (E4) is a naturally occurring estrogen produced by the fetal liver. It is being studied as a treatment for menopausal hot flashes.

Ethinyl estradiol is a synthetic estrogen. It is primarily used with a progestin in hormonal contraceptives.

Progestogens These mimic the progesterone made in the body in the reproductive years to regulate the effects of estrogen and protect the uterus.

Micronized progesterone is bioidentical, structurally the same as the progesterone the body makes. It's the preferred formulation in hormone therapy.

Medroxyprogesterone acetate, levonorgestrel and norethisterone acetate (NETA), also known as norethindrone acetate, are synthetic progestins. These have a structure similar enough to progesterone that they act the same way in the body.

Selective estrogen receptor modulators (SERMs) SERMs are estrogen-like compounds that either block or allow the activity of estrogen in the tissues they act upon. (Selectively, as the name implies.) Some SERMs are used to prevent and treat osteoporosis (raloxifene) or to treat pain during intercourse (ospemifene).

Conjugated estrogens and bazedoxifene A newer type of drug combines estrogens with a SERM, called a *tissue-selective estrogen complex* (TSEC). In the drug Duavee, conjugated estrogens offer relief from hot flashes, and the SERM bazedoxifene is used in place of a progestogen. Bazedoxifene has a protective effect on the uterus, but it doesn't seem to cause the increase in breast density that's seen with some progestogens. This combination drug also reduces the risk of fractures and is approved to prevent osteoporosis. However, its long-term effect on the risk of breast and ovarian cancers is unknown.

More research is needed to fully understand the role these combined drugs might play in the treatment of menopausal symptoms. In theory, TSECs offer an alternative for those who are concerned about the irregular bleeding and health risks that come with adding a progestogen to estrogen therapy. Pairing a specific form of estrogen with a specific SERM may offer similar benefits with fewer downsides. However, the TSEC pairing still contains oral conjugated estrogens, which are associated with an increased risk of stroke and blood clots.

The truth is that these preparations all have different risks associated with them. None is inherently better or worse. And the delivery method of each preparation also affects the level of risk.

Continuous vs. cyclic regimen

The dosing schedule of hormone therapy with estrogen and progestogen depends on a variety of factors.

Typically, estrogen therapy is given continuously. In combination hormone therapy, a progestogen may be given either as a continuous regimen, which is taken daily, or a cyclic regimen, which has periods of treatment interspersed with progestogen-free intervals. There are pros and cons to both continuous and cyclic progestogen. Cyclic dosing reduces the exposure to progestogens, but it causes monthly withdrawal bleeding. That can be annoying — after all, one of the benefits of menopause is the end of the menstrual cycle. In many women, taking progestogens continuously leads to amenorrhea — the absence of any monthly bleeding. But it can often cause irregular bleeding, especially the closer to menopause you are. You might take a continuous regimen also because progestogen therapy (specifically progesterone) can help with sleep. So taking it daily at bedtime gives this benefit all the time, not just for part of the month.

Many women newly into menopause are started on a cyclic regimen because the risk of breakthrough bleeding is high and scheduled bleeding is often easier to manage than unscheduled bleeding. They can change to continuous therapy once the risk of breakthrough bleeding is lower, later in menopause. However, everyone is different, and other considerations and risk factors will affect what type of dosing regimen is best for you. If you experience any abnormal vaginal bleeding — especially after a period of amenorrhea — talk to your health care provider right away.

The hormones you might take to manage menopausal symptoms can affect your body in a variety of ways.

Cardiovascular disease Accumulating evidence suggests that the loss of estrogen plays a direct role in developing hardened arteries (atherosclerosis), one of the primary causes of cardiovascular disease. This indicates that giving estrogen to younger menopausal women does not increase — and may reduce — their risk of heart disease.

To describe this relationship, researchers have proposed a "timing hypothesis," which suggests that estrogen therapy has a beneficial effect on cardiovascular health if started soon after menopause but a detrimental effect if started later. It depends on the extent to which atherosclerosis has already developed at the time treatment is started — and older women are likely to have more-advanced atherosclerosis.

Breast cancer The relationship is complex. Numerous studies indicate that estrogen-progestogen therapy slightly increases the risk of breast cancer after about five years of use. This increase is similar to the breast cancer risk from consuming one to two glasses of wine per night, being inactive or being overweight. Some evidence indicates that estrogen alone does not increase the risk of breast cancer. However, not all studies agree.

Hormone therapy, particularly estrogen combined with a progestogen, can increase the density of your breasts, making breast cancer more difficult to detect in early stages with a mammogram.

If you have a history of breast cancer, you shouldn't use systemic HT, as it is associated with an increased risk of breast cancer recurrence. Local vaginal estrogen can be considered for vaginal symptoms.

Cholesterol Oral HTs have mixed effects on cholesterol levels. They've been shown to increase levels of high-density lipoprotein ("good") cholesterol and decrease levels of low-density lipoprotein ("bad") cholesterol. Though this is a good thing, they also increase triglyceride levels (not a good thing). Hormone therapies applied to the skin (transdermal therapies) haven't been shown to have these effects.

Stroke Evidence indicates that standard doses of oral HT can increase the risk of ischemic stroke — where a blood clot travels to the brain and blocks blood flow. For younger postmenopausal women, the absolute risk is quite low, but it's more substantial for older women.

Venous thromboembolism Venous thromboembolism (VTE) refers to a blood clot in a deep vein (deep vein thrombosis) or in a lung (pulmonary embolism). Hormone therapy has been shown to increase the risk of VTE. The risk tends to be lower in women who start the treatment early in menopause and is generally low for younger healthy women. Transdermal treatments may also carry a lower risk of VTE than do oral regimens.

Mood Recent data show strong evidence of estrogen's positive effect on menopause-related mood changes. It seems most effective for mood symptoms during perimenopause, when hormone levels are fluctuating.

Cognition The timing hypothesis may also apply here, although studies have had conflicting results. Some evidence has shown that HT has a neutral or even a protective effect on cognition and dementia when used in younger women. However, it can have a detrimental effect in older women or when used for longer periods of time.

Diabetes Hormone therapy reduces the risk of diabetes. For women who already have diabetes, the risk of cardiovascular disease should be assessed, but HT may still be an option. Choosing a transdermal form of HT, rather than systemic, is suggested to lower the risk of cardiovascular disease in these women.

Osteoporosis Estrogen has been shown to prevent and treat bone loss, reducing the risk of fractures. It's approved for the prevention of bone loss and reduction of fracture risk in postmenopausal women.

Gallbladder disease Hormone therapy may increase the risk of gallstones and gallbladder disease. The risks tend to be greater with oral therapies as opposed to transdermal therapies.

Other effects In addition, HT may have an impact on:
- **Sleep.** Hormone therapy can help with insomnia and night sweats.
- **Hair.** Hormone therapy may support hair growth.
- **Eyes.** Dry eyes in menopause may worsen or improve with HT.

Dosage and duration

Most hormone therapy preparations are available in a variety of doses. Experts recommend taking the lowest dose that eases your symptoms or reaches your treatment goals, and it may take a bit of trial and error to find this amount. Hormone therapy can have a variety of side effects, including vaginal bleeding, bloating and water retention, breast tenderness, headaches and mood swings. Using a lower dose may help alleviate these symptoms as well as reduce some of the more serious risks of hormone therapy. And though many women fear that weight gain is a side effect of hormone therapy, it hasn't been shown to have any effect on weight. And it may reduce your risk of diabetes.

Hormone therapy is generally taken for as long as required to treat symptoms. However, there's no firm cutoff time, and the duration of treatment will be an ongoing conversation between you and your health care provider based on your risks, benefits and preferences.

If you and your health care provider decide it's time to transition away from hormone therapy, you'll likely taper off of it, though the research isn't clear that tapering is any better than stopping abruptly when it comes to the recurrence of symptoms. If your symptoms are still moderate to severe after discontinuing treatment, you and your health care provider will decide whether restarting hormone therapy or trying a nonhormonal option is best for you.

Putting it all together

Women have many options when it comes to the preparation, delivery method and dose of hormone therapy to take. You may need to mix and match to find the right solution for you. Your health conditions and personal preferences can help guide your choices. And the treatment that is right for you may change over time.

ALTERNATIVES THAT AREN'T RECOMMENDED

Following the backlash against hormone therapy, other treatments gained popularity. In the vacuum of trusted menopause management options, these products promise relief with fewer risks. But in fact, their risks may be just as concerning.

Bioidentical custom-compounded hormones

When the results of the WHI study came out and caused significant concern about the effects of hormone therapy, a number of "bioidentical custom-compounded" treatments popped up that were purported to be safer than commercially available prescriptions. However, this is not necessarily the case, and these treatments should be approached with caution.

What is bioidentical? The term *bioidentical* generally means that the hormones in a product are chemically identical to those your body produces. But this definition is not used consistently. Marketers of custom-compounded treatments often call their products *bioidentical*, implying they are more natural than traditional hormone therapies. But many estradiol products approved by the U.S. Food and Drug Administration (FDA) — such as Estrace, Climara and Vivelle-Dot — are chemically and structurally identical to the compounds made by your body. These are technically bioidentical, but the FDA chooses not to use this term.

But aren't they custom made for me? Marketers of custom-compounded hormones say their products are better because they are individualized preparations, made for you based on a blood or saliva test to assess your hormone levels. However, the hormone levels in your saliva or blood can vary greatly from day to day — and even from hour to hour — and don't necessarily reflect the levels in your tissues. In addition, the treatments often try to bring every woman's hormones to the same predetermined level. Your symptoms and their severity are a better guide for determining your specific therapy needs.

For these custom treatments, you need to go through a compounding pharmacy — one that specializes in making medications in doses and preparations that are not commercially available. Custom-compounding pharmacies aren't regulated by the FDA, and their products aren't subject to the same rigorous testing and standards for safety, effectiveness, purity and consistency that traditional, commercially available hormonal preparations have to meet. One sampling of bioidentical custom-compounded products conducted by the FDA found that the ingredients varied significantly from what was stated on the label, and the FDA has provided warnings to companies about their misleading marketing claims.

Are they safe? There is no credible scientific data that indicates bioidentical custom-compounded products are safer or more effective than commercially available hormone therapies. They should be presumed to have the same health risks. And the risks may actually be

CONTRACEPTIVES DURING THE MENOPAUSE TRANSITION

Combination oral contraceptives containing both estrogen and a progestin are a good option for controlling hot flashes in peri-menopausal women who still require birth control. They lead to lighter and more-regular periods — which can be a relief if you have irregular and heavy bleeding. They also help preserve bone density, reduce the risk of ovarian and endometrial cancers, reduce painful cramps, help with acne and can help manage menstrual migraines. These contraceptives are generally safe for healthy nonsmokers who aren't overweight, and long-term use hasn't been shown to increase the risk of breast cancer. Progestin-only options can be used in women who smoke or have other health complications that prevent use of a pill containing estrogen. However, the progestin-only treatments likely won't help with hot flashes or migraines.

If birth control is your primary goal, you prefer to avoid the hassle of a daily pill and you don't need hot flash relief, longer term options such as subdermal implants that are inserted just under your skin, a copper IUD or a levonorgestrel-releasing (LNG) IUD are available. The hormonal IUD is also sometimes used to provide endometrial protection in peri- or postmenopausal women taking estrogen therapy, though it's not approved for this purpose. It can also significantly reduce menstrual bleeding.

Talk with your health care provider about your options. After menopause it's recommended that women switch to menopausal hormone therapies, which contain much lower doses of hormones, for symptom management.

greater with custom-compounded products if the levels of progesterone are not sufficient to protect women from endometrial cancer.

Though you should approach custom-compounded products cautiously, the process is useful in certain circumstances. For example, the commercially available form of micronized progesterone contains peanut oil, so your health care provider may prescribe a custom-compounded version if you have a peanut allergy.

Over-the-counter hormones

You may be curious about using nonprescription hormones and herbal supplements to treat your symptoms. These products are discussed more in Chapter 8.

REDUCING NEGATIVE EFFECTS

If hormone therapy is a good choice for you, here are some ways to reduce the risk of negative effects:

Find the best product and delivery method. Talk with your health care provider about the factors listed above to find what treatment is right for your unique situation.

Take the right dose for your needs. Work with your health care provider to find the dose that best meets your treatment goals. It may take a bit of trial and error to find the appropriate dose to manage your symptoms. If you're taking hormone therapy because you've experienced early menopause, talk with your health care provider about the dose and duration of therapy required to protect your health.

Seek regular follow-up care. See your health care provider regularly to ensure that the benefits continue to outweigh the risks and to receive preventive care such as mammograms and cervical cancer screenings (see Chapter 22). Make sure to see your health care provider if you experience any unusual vaginal bleeding, especially if you've gone for a period of time with no bleeding.

Make healthy lifestyle choices. Include physical activity and exercise in your daily routine, eat a healthy diet, maintain a healthy weight, don't smoke, limit alcohol, manage stress and manage chronic health conditions such as high cholesterol and high blood pressure.

PREMATURE MENOPAUSE AND HORMONE THERAPY

If you experience premature menopause — whether it happens naturally or is caused by medical interventions — the early loss of estrogen affects your body in a number of ways. Though premature menopause lowers the risk of breast cancer, it can increase the risk of osteoporosis, heart disease, dementia, sexual dysfunction, mood disorders and even early death.

For women who reach menopause prematurely, the protective benefits of hormone therapy almost always outweigh the risks. Hormone therapy is recommended at least until the average age of menopause (52 years). Once you reach that point, you can assess your symptoms, risks and treatment options with your health care provider.

IN PERSPECTIVE

Remember that hormone therapy isn't permanent. You can stop your treatment at any point and know that the need for it — and also the benefits — will lessen over time.

In addition, it's important to keep in mind that all medications and treatments carry a degree of risk. The risks of hormone therapy are actually similar to the risks of other common therapies for women. To put things in perspective — the increased risk of breast cancer associated with combination hormone therapy after five years is about equivalent to the increased risk you'd have from drinking between one and two glasses of wine each day. Though the possible consequences of hormone therapy shouldn't be taken lightly, the benefits usually outweigh the risks for healthy women under age 60 who start treatment within 10 years of menopause.

7

Nonhormonal prescription treatments

If you've had breast cancer or other conditions that prevent you from safely using hormone therapy — or you simply find the risks are greater than you're willing to accept — you're probably wondering what other options are out there for you. Hormone therapy may be the most effective treatment for hot flashes, but other options have also been shown to ease symptoms.

Lifestyle approaches and holistic or integrative medicine approaches may work for some women, and these are discussed in Chapter 8. In addition, a variety of nonhormonal prescription medications also are available and are discussed here.

LOW-DOSE ANTIDEPRESSANTS

Studies have shown that certain selective serotonin reuptake inhibitors (SSRIs) and serotonin and norepinephrine reuptake inhibitors

(SNRIs) — typically used as antidepressants — are some of the most effective nonhormonal treatments for hot flashes. While they're not as effective as hormone therapy, these medications may be used if hormone therapy isn't a desirable option. SSRIs and SNRIs may also be a good choice for women who need an antidepressant for a mood disorder in addition to relief from hot flashes, and they are sometimes used alongside hormone therapy for this purpose.

The SSRI paroxetine (Brisdelle) was the first nonhormonal prescription treatment approved for treating hot flashes. This treatment is a lower dose (7.5 mg) than what is used for treating mood disorders. Notably, this lower dose has not been associated with sexual dysfunction or weight gain. Higher doses (10 mg) of paroxetine (Paxil) may be used off-label for menopausal symptoms. Other SSRIs and SNRIs used for hot flashes include escitalopram (Lexapro), citalopram (Celexa), venlafaxine (Effexor XR) and desvenlafaxine (Pristiq).

SSRIs and SNRIs are known to have a range of common side effects, including upset stomach, dizziness, dry mouth, weight gain and insomnia. They can also cause sexual problems, such as reduced desire or difficulty with arousal or reaching orgasm. However, the doses needed to treat menopausal symptoms are lower than to treat depression and anxiety, and side effects are less likely. Any side effects that do occur may subside after the first couple of weeks of treatment, but some might be persistent. Talk with your practitioner to see if there are ways to minimize these impacts while still getting relief.

The effectiveness of SSRIs and SNRIs in treating hot flashes can be assessed fairly quickly — generally within 2 to 4 weeks. You may need to try a few different SSRIs or SNRIs to see if they are effective for you before deciding to switch to another type of medication. And because the only way to tell whether your symptoms have subsided naturally is to go off treatment, you'll need to stop taking these medications periodically in order to assess your symptoms.

OTHER MEDICATIONS AND TREATMENTS

Antidepressants aren't the only prescription therapies to help with menopausal symptoms. Others include:

Gabapentin (Neurontin)

This medication, used to prevent seizures, has also proved effective in treating hot flashes. It may help manage migraines or pain conditions, as well. The typical treatment requires taking pills up to three times a day, though many women can just take a bedtime dose. Gabapentin has a sedative effect in addition to helping with hot flashes, so it may be a good option to take nightly if night sweats and disturbed sleep are your primary complaints.

Pregabalin (Lyrica)

This drug is similar to gabapentin and is used to treat nerve-related pain. Though it seems to be effective in treating hot flashes, it's not been studied as extensively for use in menopausal women. It has been associated with significant weight gain, however. For these reasons, it's not a recommended therapy for menopause symptoms.

Oxybutynin

This medication treats overactive bladder and can help control incontinence issues arising in menopause. It has also been shown to make vasomotor symptoms — hot flashes and night sweats — less frequent and less severe. It's important to note that longer-term use of anticholinergic medications, like oxybutynin, is associated with an increased risk of dementia. But for some women, this medication may still be a good short-term option.

Fezolinetant

This newly developed, first-in-class medication holds great promise for relieving hot flashes. That's because it targets chain reactions in the brain that were only recently discovered to be the cause of hot flashes.

Fezolinetant targets brain cells known as KNDy (pronounced "candy") neurons, which produce kisspeptin, neurokinin B and dynorphin, in the brain's hypothalamus. The hormonal changes of the menopause transition cause the KNDy neurons to overfire, flooding the surrounding area with neurokinin B. This disrupts the body's temperature-regulating center in the hypothalamus, leading to sweaty hot flashes that seem to come out of nowhere.

Fezolinetant acts as a neurokinin-B inhibitor, controlling the flood.

> " I got my period at the tender age of 9, quickly realizing that an elementary school bathroom is not well stocked with feminine supplies. I went to the nurse, who called my mother. My mother picked me up early and gently congratulated me. My father, I remember distinctly, started crying, saying — with a degree of awe — "you're a woman now."

I was most definitely NOT a woman. I was a fourth-grade tomboy, not happy with the sudden blood and pain and the unnerving feeling that I was no longer free, not in the way men were, anyway. I knew even at 9 that I didn't want to have children (a decision that never wavered). And when it became apparent that my period would mean brutal menstrual pains each month, I instantly lamented becoming, as my father had so wistfully said, "a woman."

For the next four decades, my body — while mostly healthy and strong — was also usually either highly emotionally volatile, when experiencing PMS, or in a state of sharp and seemingly interminable pain. I described it as "like an icepick to the uterus." I took infinite amounts of ibuprofen. I laid around and groaned. I was either cranky and impatient with others or filled with tearful, moody sentiments.

Then a month after turning age 50, my body and my mind — suddenly, joyfully — transformed. For me, menopause was a bright, clear entry into a new phase of freedom: freedom from pain, from the hormonal waves of emotions, from messiness and inconvenience, and from icepicks to the uterus. An older friend had told me she called her hot flashes her "power surges," and I finally got what she meant — the heat roiling up from within, somehow psychedelic and exhilarating. I was free, finally, from my body's control over who I was and what I did. Menopause was a thrilling evolution that has finally made me welcome all it is to be a woman.

In early trials, it appears to significantly reduce vasomotor symptoms more effectively than other nonhormonal therapies. It was under review for U.S. Food and Drug Administration (FDA) approval as of early 2023.

Medications such as suvorexant (Belsomra), eszopiclone (Lunesta), zaleplon (Sonata) and zolpidem (Ambien)
These are used to treat insomnia. Suvorexant is a newer medication that some research has shown to help reduce night sweats, which may lead to fewer sleep interruptions. Eszopiclone, zaleplon and zolpidem have been shown to help improve sleep, though they don't impact hot flashes or night sweats. They may simply help you sleep through the night.

Stellate ganglion block
This procedure involves injecting an anesthetic into the stellate ganglion, a group of nerves in the front of your neck. Typically used for pain relief or to treat excessive sweating, it may also offer relief from hot flashes. The connection between hot flashes and the stellate ganglion is not quite clear. It's possible that the nerves affect blood flow to areas in your brain that regulate body temperature.

The procedure itself takes only a few minutes, and it's generally safe when performed by an experienced practitioner, particularly when done with ultrasound guidance. But it does involve some risk, and the injection can be costly. Further research is needed to better understand its effectiveness in treating hot flashes.

THE CHOICE IS YOURS

If lifestyle modifications don't help your symptoms, a prescription therapy may be the right choice for you. Keep in mind that it might take a while to find the right medication or combination of medications. Whatever option you choose, it's important to keep in touch with your health care provider. Researchers continue to learn more, and new medications may become available.

In addition, the best treatment for you may change over time. You'll need to reassess the risks and benefits of different therapies as you age, depending on your health, your symptoms and your goals for treatment.

8

Holistic and integrative therapies

Integrative medicine is an approach to health care that incorporates conventional medicine and natural healing practices. This approach emphasizes whole-person care focused on health and healing, including practices such as acupuncture, massage, yoga, dietary supplements, wellness coaching and meditation. Many integrative medicine therapies are based in traditional healing practices. As evidence of their effectiveness and safety grows, integrative treatments are increasingly being used alongside conventional practices in modern medicine.

This chapter looks at some complementary health approaches and products that may help treat common menopause symptoms. It's not an exhaustive list, as the field is very broad, but it will cover some popular products and practices you may be curious about. Some may help control menopause symptoms, and others may be helpful in treating other common health conditions that women experience in midlife.

As you explore integrative treatment options, keep in mind that the scientific evidence for their effectiveness is often weaker than that for medications. They are considered less effective than hormone therapy for treating menopausal symptoms. Still, some alternative approaches may give adequate relief in people with mild to moderate symptoms.

It's worth noting that studies investigating therapies for hot flashes generally have a 30% to 40% placebo response rate, meaning they have found that same response with a sugar pill. So some improvements seen with integrative therapies may be due to this effect.

However, not all integrative therapies are safe. Some have the potential for serious side effects or interactions with medications. In addition, using integrative therapies without seeking medical guidance could delay effective care for serious conditions. Make sure to discuss integrative treatments you're interested in with your health care provider, especially before trying new supplements.

MIND-BODY PRACTICES

Mind-body practices rely on the connection between mind and body to promote health and wellness. Although they don't necessarily target the hormonal fluctuations of menopause directly, they can ease stress, improve mood and sleep patterns, and increase quality of life and your ability to cope with this life transition.

Cognitive behavioral therapy

Also known as *CBT*, cognitive behavioral therapy is a type of mental health counseling, or psychotherapy. CBT explores the connection between thoughts, feelings and behaviors. Among holistic treatments, CBT has proven to be one of the most effective for managing hot flashes and night sweats (vasomotor symptoms) in menopause.

Through self-observation, CBT helps people identify inaccurate or unhealthy beliefs and then reframe them into more constructive thoughts. It's been shown to be effective in treating depression and anxiety and can be an effective tool for learning how to manage stressful life situations.

Studies have shown that both individual and group CBT can help with the management of hot flashes and night sweats. It's likely that the therapy reduces the perception and impact of hot flashes — perhaps by reducing anxiety and providing an increased sense of control — rather than reducing their actual frequency or severity. Regardless, research shows it can have a real benefit. CBT is generally safe and is a widely used type of therapy. In addition to individual or group therapy, many self-guided options are available, along with online programs and apps.

Hypnosis

Accumulating evidence suggests that clinical hypnosis is one of few nonpharmaceutical treatments that are truly effective for hot flash control. Hypnosis induces a state of deep relaxation that helps you concentrate and makes you more open to the power of suggestion. Some research has found that hypnosis helped reduce the frequency and severity of hot flashes.

In the past, finding a trained provider could be difficult, but some self-hypnosis options are now available through smartphone apps.

Yoga

Originating in India, this combination of physical postures, controlled breathing and meditation has become one of the most popular modern self-care practices.

Yoga is associated with a number of health benefits. It may help lessen pain, reduce your heart rate and blood pressure, ease anxiety and depression, improve sleep, reduce stress and generally improve your quality of life. It can also improve strength, balance and flexibility, though it has less effect on aerobic fitness. However, yoga probably won't cure your hot flashes. Several recent studies, including a systematic review of randomized, controlled trials, showed that yoga had limited effect on reducing vasomotor symptoms.

Tai chi

Originating as a form of martial arts in China, tai chi (TIE-CHEE) also has benefits as a health and wellness practice. It's a series of gentle, flowing movements combined with focused breathing and awareness. It's said to help facilitate the flow of qi (chee) — or vital energy — in the body. Tai chi is practiced for a variety of health benefits, including improved balance, coordination, strength and sleep. More research is needed to understand any potential benefits it may have in menopause.

Qi gong

Part of traditional Chinese medicine, the practice of qigong (CHEE-gung) incorporates meditation, physical movement and breathing exercises to restore and maintain balance. Some evidence indicates that qigong may improve sleep for women experiencing menpause-related sleep disturbances. It may also help relieve anxiety and depression.

Meditation and mindfulness techniques

Meditation is a mind-body technique that has been practiced for thousands of years. It's often used to reduce stress and create a relaxed state. Research suggests it may have many more health benefits, such as reducing blood pressure and relieving anxiety, depression and insomnia. There are many different types of meditation you can try. Most involve eliminating outside distractions, focusing your attention and adopting a nonjudgmental mindset.

Meditation alone doesn't appear to help with hot flashes, but some research has shown that other mindfulness-based practices may help reduce their impact. Mindfulness-based stress reduction, which involves meditation, yoga and body awareness, may offer some benefit for less severe and less disruptive hot flashes.

INTEGRATIVE AND LIFESTYLE APPROACHES

In addition to mind-body techniques, there are a variety of other practices that take a holistic approach to health and wellness.

Exercise

Getting regular physical activity of any kind has many benefits for your health, especially during midlife. It can help you sleep better, relieve stress, and regulate your mood. It helps build and maintain muscle mass, protects your joints and helps you avoid gaining weight.

Exercise alone doesn't appear to do much for hot flashes, however. Researchers have looked at a variety of activity types and generally, exercise doesn't seem to have a significant effect on vasomotor symptoms. Still, it remains an important tool for managing other menopause symptoms and your overall health.

Weight loss

Women who are obese are more likely to report more frequent and severe hot flashes than normal weight women. Losing weight is no simple or quick fix, but for these women, research suggests that weight loss can be an effective method to improve symptoms. Studies of weight loss from behavioral changes, as well as a pilot study of a weight-loss drug, found significant improvement in hot flashes with decreases in weight.

Acupuncture

Acupuncture is probably the most well-known energy therapy, based on the idea that natural energy fields can be balanced or adjusted to foster health. Acupuncture involves the insertion of very thin needles into your skin at specific points in the body. Though researchers are still studying how and why acupuncture might have beneficial effects, in traditional Chinese medicine the practice is said to rebalance the body's vital energy (qi).

Research indicates that acupuncture can help ease pain related to a variety of conditions, and it may prevent or reduce the frequency of headaches. Some studies suggest acupuncture may reduce hot flashes and improve sleep and mental health in menopausal women. However, study results have been mixed, and they typically have not shown an effect on hot flashes from acupuncture when compared with sham acupuncture — a kind of therapy placebo.

Acupuncture is generally low risk when practiced by a licensed practitioner. In the U.S., most states require nonphysician acupuncturists to be certified by the National Certification Commission for Acupuncture and Oriental Medicine.

Manual therapies

Manual, or hands-on, therapies such as massage involve applying physical touch to the body to improve symptoms and promote health. With a well-trained provider, massage may ease pain, foster relaxation and improve sleep — all results you may be seeking as you go through menopause. There are a variety of massage styles, ranging from gentle strokes to deep manipulation of your muscles.

Manipulative therapy — commonly practiced by chiropractors and osteopathic doctors — may be another familiar approach. It involves the application of controlled force to a muscle or joint to lessen symptoms. Other hands-on therapies include the Feldenkrais Method and the Alexander technique, which foster a heightened awareness of your posture and your body movements (although they haven't been studied specifically in menopause).

Though hands-on treatments are generally safe when practiced by an experienced and certified or licensed practitioner, women with certain health conditions may need to avoid these therapies. Talk with your health care practitioner to find out if you need to take precautions.

Ayurveda

Translated as *the science of life* in Sanskrit, ayurveda is a healing system that originated in India. It takes an integrated approach, combining practices such as yoga and massage with nutrition interventions, including herbal remedies and detoxification. The effects of ayurvedic practices on menopausal symptoms haven't been well studied. Still, some women may find the approach or its individual parts helpful.

Traditional Chinese medicine (TCM) herbal and dietary therapies

Chinese herbal and dietary therapies have been studied for relief of menopausal symptoms, and most research is inconclusive or conflicting. A small number of studies suggested TCM therapies were effective at improving mood and sleep and reducing hot flashes.However, they were less effective than standard hormone therapy and are not a recommended therapy at this time. Some of the individual herbal supplements used in this complex practice are discussed later in this chapter.

Another concept of TCM is the balance of yin and yang. Chinese dietary therapy incorporates high yin (cooling) foods such as cucumber and melon in the management of hot flashes. There's little harm in trying this method.

DIET, VITAMINS AND MINERALS

As menopause puts the focus on your health and body in midlife, you might be wondering how your diet and nutrition factor in. Recent research has suggested that how you nourish and fuel your body can have real impacts in menopause, as well as on your long term health. In particular, eating a plant-based diet and soy foods have been associated with reduced vasomotor symptoms. Similarly, eating more fruits and vegetables has been linked to fewer menopause symptoms overall.

Eat your greens
Vitamins and minerals are micronutrients essential to your body's functioning. They support a variety of internal processes, including

Vitamins	Recommended daily intake for women ages 31-70
Vitamin A	700 micrograms (mcg)
Vitamin B-1 (thiamin)	1.1 milligrams (mg)
Vitamin B-2 (riboflavin)	1.1 mg
Vitamin B-3 (niacin)	14 mg
Vitamin B-6 (pyridoxine)	1.3 mg (ages 31-50) 1.5 mg (ages 51-70)
Vitamin B-9 (folate, folic acid)	400 mcg
Vitamin B-12 (cyanocobalamin)	2.4 mg
Vitamin C	75 mg 110 mg (smokers)
Vitamin D	600 international units (I/U) (800 IU for women over 70)*
Vitamin E	15 mg or 22.5 IU
Vitamin K	90 mcg†

building strong bones and teeth, supporting healthy skin and vision, promoting immune system functioning, and much more. Ensuring you're getting enough of these compounds can help you maximize your nutrition and health.

Vitamins and minerals are found in a variety of foods, especially whole, plant-based foods. Although diets high in fruits and vegetables are associated with a reduced risk of disease, it's unclear if taking a multivitamin or supplement promotes health or prevents disease. Additionally, many vitamins and supplements have associated risks.

Minerals	Recommended daily intake for women ages 31-70
Calcium	1,000 mg (ages 31-50) 1,200 mg (ages 51-70)
Chromium	25 mcg (ages 31-50)† 20 mcg (ages 51-70)†
Copper	900 mcg
Iron	18 mg (ages 31-50) 8 mg (ages 51-70)
Magnesium	1.8 mg†
Molybdenum	45 mcg
Phosphorus	700 mg
Selenium	55 mcg
Zinc	8 mg

Source: Dietary Reference Intakes. Institute of Medicine.

*The National Osteoporosis Foundation recommends 400 to 800 IU of vitamin D a day for women under age 50 and 800-1,000 IU for women age 50 and older.

†Adequate intake — no established daily recommended intake.

It's preferable to get vitamins and minerals from dietary sources. If you're eating a healthy, varied and balanced diet, you're probably meeting your nutritional needs and don't need a multivitamin after menopause. If your diet is restricted, or if you have issues with digestion and absorption, then you may need supplements to support your intake. Your health care provider can help you decide whether vitamin or mineral supplements are a good choice for you.

With any supplement, watch out for too much of a good thing. Vitamins that are fat soluble — that is, they dissolve in fat — are stored in your body for a long time. They may have a greater potential to build up in your system. Fat-soluble vitamins include A, D, E and K.

How much do you need?

A balanced approach is required when it comes to vitamins and minerals. Too much of some may block the absorption of others or result in adverse effects. Meanwhile, certain vitamins or minerals — in the right amounts — are needed to help your body make use of others.

Thankfully, there are established guidelines known as Dietary Reference Intakes (DRIs) to help you figure out a healthy range for micronutrient needs — see pages 138–139. The standards are based on general age ranges for the average population, so talk with your health care provider to find out if your own needs might be different.

The units used for each vitamin or mineral may vary — some are measured in milligrams (mg) or micrograms (mcg) and others in international units (IU). Though this might get confusing, most supplements will tell you what percentage of the recommended daily intake is provided. If you're eating whole foods that don't come with a label, you may need to turn to reputable apps and websites to look up the nutrition information. Keep in mind that the recommended daily levels for vitamins and minerals refer to the total for everything you eat or drink.

ALTERNATIVE TREATMENTS FOR HOT FLASHES

Many women are interested to know whether over-the-counter products and supplements might be useful to help ease hot flashes. They might, but evidence is usually limited or conflicting.

Topical progesterone

Numerous creams and gels are available that claim to contain progesterone. These products are often made from soybeans or wild yam. They are promoted to have many anti-aging health benefits, including treating menopausal symptoms.

Progesterone creams are relatively safe. However, evidence does not support using them for menopause symptoms. The absorption of progesterone through the skin is highly variable. Because of this, these creams most likely do not provide enough of the hormone for uterine protection with the use of estrogen. They shouldn't be used for this purpose. Some wild yam creams are specifically marketed to contain a compound called *diosgenin*, which is advertised as a precursor to progesterone. However, your body can't actually convert this ingredient to progesterone. Topical wild yam or over-the-counter creams labeled as containing progesterone are not recommended

Supplements

If you've been searching for relief from your hot flashes, you've probably heard of supplements such as phytoestrogens and isoflavones. Phytoestrogens are a variety of plant-based compounds that have weak estrogen-like properties. Evidence does not support their use for hot flash management.

Isoflavones are one type of phytoestrogen and have been the most studied for use in treating menopausal symptoms. They're found in legumes such as soybeans, lentils, chickpeas and beans. Soy products contain the highest levels of isoflavones and thus have received the most attention.

Soy Many studies on the impact of soy isoflavones on hot flashes have been inconclusive. However, current research seems to suggest that, although not as effective as hormone therapy, soy-derived isoflavones may modestly improve hot flashes and quality of life for postmenopausal women.

Recent studies have helped researchers better understand the specific types of isoflavones that may be most beneficial for hot flashes and other health conditions. Hot flash improvement related to soy intake seems to be related to two specific isoflavones — genistein and daidzein.

When daidzein is broken down by your intestinal bacteria, it produces a compound called *equol*. Equol has estrogen-like effects on the body that may help with menopausal symptoms. Only some women have the bacteria necessary to produce equol — it's estimated that 25% to 35% of North American women are equol producers, compared with as many as 60% of women in Asian countries.

In general, studies haven't found isoflavones to be effective in preventing bone loss or conveying cognitive benefits. However, some initial evidence indicates that equol producers who consume dietary soy may see greater benefits in these realms — as well as with hot flash control — compared with nonequol producers.

With regard to cardiovascular benefits, soy isoflavones likely have a minimal impact on lowering cholesterol and blood pressure, though they might help your arteries retain flexibility. As with the use of prescription hormone therapy, there is a timing hypothesis at play, suggesting that this beneficial effect may be seen if soy is used early on after menopause. A woman's equol-producing status may also affect whether or not she experiences these cardiovascular benefits.

There's a lot more to learn about the effectiveness and long-term safety of equol and isoflavones. Currently, there's no commercially available test you can take to figure out whether you produce equol. Considering the low number of equol producers in the U.S., soy products may not give you much relief from your symptoms, and concentrated soy supplements should be approached with caution. For most women, though, there's little harm in including whole soy foods as part of a balanced diet.

Red clover Red clover also belongs to the legume plant family and is a source of isoflavones. Some studies have shown that red clover supplements are not effective in relieving menopausal symptoms. Though red clover seems safe for short-term use, there's a lack of safety evidence for long-term use and in women with a history of hormone-dependent cancers.

In addition to phytoestrogens, there are some other plant-based supplements that are sought for hot flash relief.

Black cohosh A member of the buttercup family, the black cohosh plant has been used in Europe for many years to treat menopause

ISOFLAVONES AND CANCER RISK

Because isoflavones have estrogen-like effects, studies have looked at their safety with regard to breast and endometrial cancers. So far, research suggests dietary soy doesn't increase the risk of breast or endometrial cancer. In fact, a diet high in soy has been associated with a reduced risk of breast cancer. More research is needed to understand exactly how it may lower the risk. Soy hasn't been associated with an increased risk of breast cancer recurrence, and dietary soy is likely safe for breast cancer survivors. However, women with breast cancer or at high risk for breast cancer should generally avoid soy supplements until more information is available about their long-term safety.

symptoms. However, a systematic review of studies concluded that it was no more effective at reducing or treating hot flashes than a placebo. In addition, there are various concerns about its safety, particularly the potential for it to be toxic to the liver. It is not recommended.

Evening primrose oil Native to North America, the seeds of the evening primrose plant contain gamma-linolenic acid, an essential fatty acid. Supplements are promoted for hot flash relief, but there's little scientific evidence to support their effectiveness for this or other uses. It also can have adverse side effects, including diarrhea, blood clots, reduced immune system functioning and, in women taking antipsychotic medication, seizures. It is not recommended and especially should not be used with blood thinners or antipsychotic drugs.

Sage The common garden herb you may be familiar with for culinary uses is also a traditional folk remedy. Some women use it to treat hot flashes. Small studies have shown some effectiveness, but evidence is limited and it is not recommended for this reason. Sage is generally safe, but avoid oil-based preparations, as they contain a compound called *thujone*, which affects the nervous system. It may cause vomiting, seizures, kidney damage and dizziness.

OTHER COMMON SUPPLEMENTS

In addition to hot flash relief, you may be seeking alternative approaches for other health concerns. Many of the treatments below have long been used in medicinal preparations. However, conclusive scientific data on their effectiveness and long-term safety is often lacking.

For multi-symptom "menopause relief"

Amberen, MENO, Relizen and others A growing list of supplements with various ingredients claim to provide relief for multiple menopause symptoms. These products are marketed as hormone-free and often soy-free treatments to improve hot flashes, sleep, memory, mood and more. So far, there's no strong evidence that they actually work.

Cannabis Interest in and access to the medical use of marijuana (cannabis) is increasing, including for relief of menopause symptoms. However, currently there is a lack of evidence supporting its safety or efficancy for menopause symptom management. At this time, it is not recommended as a menopause treatment.

For mood

Ginseng Some evidence suggests that the root of the Asian *Panax ginseng* plant — a mainstay of Chinese medicine — may help improve fatigue, well-being and mood, but not hot flashes. Short-term use at recommended doses seems safe, and further study is needed to assess long-term safety. Be aware that ginseng may lower blood sugar levels and increase blood pressure. It may also increase uterine bleeding, so use caution if you're taking a blood thinner.

S-adenosylmethionine (SAM-e) Though evidence is inconclusive, some research indicates SAM-e may be effective in relieving mild to moderate depression. See more information on this supplement in the joint health section on page 149.

St. John's wort The flowers of this herb have been used for centuries in medicinal preparations. Some research indicates St. John's wort is effective in treating mild to moderate depression. It's also been used to treat hot flashes, either on its own or alongside black cohosh, without evidence to support its use. St. John's wort can interact with numerous drugs, including antidepressants, as well as immunosuppressants, contraceptives, cancer treatment drugs and anticoagulants. It may reduce the effectiveness of tamoxifen. If you are taking other medications, talk with your health care provider or pharmacist before trying St. John's wort.

Valerian The valerian plant has long been used as a medicinal plant in Europe. Supplements are made from its roots and underground stems. Valerian has traditionally been promoted as a sedative and has shown some effectiveness in reducing anxiety, but it needs more study. It has few side effects with short-term use. However, its long-term safety hasn't been established.

Vitex (chasteberry) The fruit of the shrublike vitex tree has been used to treat menstrual symptoms for thousands of years. Though reliable evidence is lacking, supplements may help perimenopausal women manage PMS and irregular bleeding. Vitex is not known to cause serious side effects, though it may negatively affect sexual desire. This has earned the plant its common name — *chasteberry*. Vitex may also increase the likelihood of pregnancy. Vitex shouldn't be used alongside antipsychotic medications or those used to treat Parkinson's disease, as it may affect dopamine levels in the brain.

For sleep

Melatonin The hormone melatonin plays a role in your body's natural sleep-wake cycle. Research results on the effectiveness of melatonin supplements are mixed, and there is limited evidence to show they offer relief from menopause-related sleep issues. Melatonin supplements may be most effective when treating sleep issues related to circadian rhythm disturbances, such as shift work or jet lag. They are generally safe for short-term use, though the safest dose for long-term use isn't known. High doses are associated with a range of adverse effects and can worsen depression.

Valerian Though it needs more study, valerian may help improve sleep and is a traditional remedy for insomnia. Valerian is discussed in greater detail on page 189.

For memory

Ginkgo Ginkgo seeds and leaf extracts have been used for thousands of years in Chinese medicine to treat a variety of ailments. Supplements are primarily promoted for their cognitive benefits, but research results are generally mixed, and the evidence is unreliable. There are some reports of allergic reactions to ginkgo, and the seeds should be avoided because of toxicity concerns. It may cause bleeding, so use caution if you're taking anticoagulants. Animal studies have shown tumor development with long-term use, and more study is needed to know if ginkgo affects cancer risk in humans.

Ginseng Traditionally used to improve mental performance, Asian

SUPPLEMENT SAFETY

A vast world of products falls under the umbrella of dietary supplements. Some supplements can be part of a healthy lifestyle and are safe in recommended doses, while others have significant safety concerns. It's always good to assess supplements with a critical eye.

Keep in mind that supplements — like prescription medications — can affect your body in many ways. They may have side effects that range from mildly bothersome to potentially life threatening. And they can have harmful interactions with other supplements, prescription medications and over-the-counter drugs. Many supplements need more scientific study before their effectiveness and safety are established.

Dietary supplements are governed by different rules from those that apply to prescription drugs. Supplements don't go through the same rigorous testing and approval process to establish their safety and effectiveness. It's up to each manufacturer to ensure that product labeling is sufficient and truthful and that the product is safe and effective. Labels might not contain information about adverse effects or possible drug interactions. And though the Food and Drug Administration (FDA) can monitor products once they're on the market, it has little power to step in until after a concern is brought to light.

Some companies do make high-quality products. But it can be challenging to separate the good from the bad. Here are some tips

ginseng has been studied for use in treating Alzheimer's disease. However, research results are inconclusive. Turn to the section on mood (pages 144–145) for more information on ginseng's use for sleep and mood concerns.

For cardiovascular health
Coenzyme Q10 Coenzyme Q10 (CoQ10) is an antioxidant found in the human body and elsewhere in nature. It's necessary for proper cell

---

that will help you approach supplements safely:
- Avoid self-prescribing supplements. If you're getting information online, make sure it's from a trusted source and discuss it with your health care provider.
- Look for products labeled with the seal of a third-party testing group such as U.S. Pharmacopeia (USP), NSF International or ConsumerLab.com. This means the product has been tested to make sure it contains what's on its label.
- Don't assume something marketed as "natural" means it's safe. Many natural compounds are poisonous to humans.
- Be wary of products claiming immediate or drastic effects. If it sounds too good to be true, it probably is.
- Don't presume more is better. Even compounds your body requires, such as vitamins and minerals, can be toxic in high doses. And you might waste money on unnecessary products.
- If you're taking supplements or drugs, keep good track of the amount you take, how frequently you take it and any side effects you experience.
- Discuss your needs and questions with your health care provider or pharmacist before taking any supplements. Both can help you navigate the options available as you seek to optimize your health and wellness.

functioning, and low natural levels have been associated with a variety of diseases. CoQ10 may benefit some women with cardiovascular conditions such as congestive heart failure. More research is needed to determine its effectiveness in treating other health concerns. CoQ10 is relatively safe, though it may interfere with chemotherapy. Some side effects include insomnia, rashes, upset stomach, dizziness, heartburn and headaches.

Fish oil Fish oil has become a popular supplement because it contains omega-3 fatty acids — polyunsaturated fats that are thought to offer a wide range of health benefits. Fish oil has been found to have cardiovascular benefits — lowering triglyceride levels and blood pressure. A prescription form (Lovaza) is available to treat very high triglyceride levels. Omega-3s from fish oils may help ease pain from rheumatoid arthritis, and more research is being done on the possible benefits fish oil and omega-3s may have for cognitive health, depression and other conditions. Fish oil is generally safe, though it may cause indigestion, diarrhea and fishy-smelling breath. It can slow blood clotting, and supplements should be used with care if you're taking an anticoagulant. You can also get fish oil through your diet by eating fatty fish — such as salmon, mackerel, sardines and herring — and shellfish.

Red yeast rice A fermented rice product, red yeast rice contains a compound called *monacolin K*. This compound has the same chemical structure as lovastatin, a statin drug used to treat high cholesterol. Supplements with high amounts of monacolin K have been shown to reduce cholesterol levels. However, red yeast rice has not been proven to reduce cardiovascular events as statin drugs do. In addition, the FDA has determined that products containing more than trace amounts of monacolin K can't be sold as over-the-counter supplements in the U.S.

As with most dietary supplements, the quantity of active ingredient can vary greatly. More study is needed to determine the safety of red yeast rice. If you're concerned about your cholesterol levels, talk with your health care provider about more effective treatment options.

For joint health

Glucosamine and chondroitin Glucosamine and chondroitin are natural compounds found in your cartilage tissue. Supplements have been studied for their use in treating joint pain related to osteoarthritis; however, results are mixed as to whether they are helpful for this purpose. Glucosamine and chondroitin supplements are generally safe with few side effects, though glucosamine can enhance the effects of anticoagulants. Glucosamine supplements are made from the skeletons of shellfish, so women with a shellfish allergy should use with caution.

S-adenosylmethionine Also called *SAM-e*, S-adenosylmethionine is produced in the human body from the amino acid methionine. SAM-e plays a role in numerous body functions. It may be useful for treating depression, alleviating pain related to osteoarthritis, and preventing liver disease, but more study is needed to establish its effectiveness. SAM-e was found to be safe with few side effects during short-term use, though longer term safety information — including drug interactions — isn't yet known.

AN OPEN-MINDED, INTEGRATIVE APPROACH

Though holistic and integrative health treatments may not be as effective as other prescription therapies in alleviating common menopausal symptoms, it can be helpful to know you have options to try. That may be especially important if you have health conditions that limit other solutions. Just remember the safety tips in this chapter and be a savvy consumer as you try out what might work for you. These treatment options can be part of the ongoing conversation you have with your health care provider.

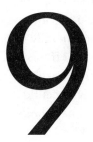

Hot flashes and night sweats

Here's the truth: Most women experience hot flashes to some degree as estrogen production decreases significantly after menopause. In fact, about three-fourths of women in perimenopause or menopause in the United States report having hot flashes. This makes hot flashes the most common symptom of the transition to menopause.

Here's what else you should know about hot flashes: They won't necessarily just go away, and they're not always simply a benign symptom of menopause.

A growing body of research shows that health care providers have long underestimated the duration of hot flash symptoms. It had been widely believed that hot flashes would diminish and stop within a couple of years of onset. But studies now indicate that women experience hot flashes for an average of seven to nine years, often starting before menstrual periods stop. And for about 1 in 3 women, hot flashes are an issue for 10 years or more.

Keep this timeline in mind as you learn more about hot flashes in this chapter and consider the strategies you may need to keep yourself cool. Then if your hot flashes don't last that long, that's great.

In addition, hot flashes aren't to be taken lightly, as they could have serious health implications. For example, research suggests that certain patterns of hot flashes, such as those starting well before periods end, may be linked with higher risk of future heart disease.

Chapter 2 discussed how the body's hormone shifts in perimenopause and menopause set off hot flashes. This chapter will dive deeper into how you can manage — or avoid — these sweaty disruptions to your daily routine, your wardrobe and your social life.

MORE THAN A FEELING

For working women, hot flashes can take a professional toll. New research shows that hot flashes account for a significant economic burden on working women and their employers. One study showed that women with untreated hot flash symptoms had a significantly higher frequency of doctor visits and absences from work and decreased productivity on the job when compared with women with no hot flash symptoms.

This isn't a revelation to any woman who has experienced hot flashes in the office, the boardroom or an important client meeting. Being red, sweaty, bad tempered and unable to concentrate throughout the workday can have a major impact on your self-esteem, your enjoyment of your work and your productivity. Even if you can shrug it off personally, it can undermine your authority if others misinterpret your symptoms as a sign of nervousness, insecurity or lack of preparation.

Hot flashes can also contribute to sexual problems and relationship strife. After all, hot, passionate, sweaty sex may have been a turn-on in your 20s, but when hot flashes are the cause of the sweatiness, it may not lead to any burning desire. And if you're struggling with night sweats, you may feel too exhausted to think about sex.

All in all, hot flashes may be very disruptive to you, your daily activities, your family, your relationship with your partner and your general quality of life. Simple sweatiness is only a small part of the problem.

RISK FACTORS FOR SEVERE HOT FLASHES

You may wonder how your particular symptoms compare with what other women are feeling. In general, doctors classify the severity of hot flashes and night sweats using these definitions:

- **Mild.** If you experience hot flashes but they don't interfere with your usual activities, they're considered mild.
- **Moderate.** Moderate hot flashes are associated with sweating and interfere somewhat with usual activities.
- **Severe.** In this case, hot flashes are so bothersome that you have to interrupt or stop what you're doing to let them pass.

Researchers don't know exactly why some women land on the severe side of this scale and others don't.

Your risk of developing severe hot flashes depends partly on the following factors. Being at higher risk in one or more of these categories doesn't necessarily mean that you will develop severe hot flashes, but it's helpful to understand your risks.

Your stage of menopause

The severity at which you experience hot flash symptoms is strongly associated with how long you've had them and where you are in the menopause process. If you begin having hot flashes while you're still having regular menstrual periods, the flashes may be mild at first. But symptoms can intensify over time, typically becoming the most extreme in the two years after your final menstrual period.

Your weight

Women who are overweight or obese typically have more frequent and severe hot flashes than women at a normal weight. There may be several reasons for this — the relationship between body weight and vasomotor symptoms is complex. But research suggests that losing weight can help relieve hot flashes.

Your habits and diet

Daily lifestyle choices and habits can impact your hot flash symptoms. For example, women who smoke are more likely than nonsmokers to report severe hot flashes. What you eat may be important too. In a recent study, women who ate a low-fat, plant-based diet including soy significantly reduced their moderate to severe hot flashes. Other research has found similar benefits for veggie-heavy diets. Simply eating more fruits and vegetables has also been linked to fewer menopause symptoms.

Your race or culture

Studies consistently show that Black women are more likely to report having hot flashes and night sweats than are Hispanic or white women. Among groups that have been studied, hot flashes are least commonly reported among women of Japanese and Chinese descent. This may be partly due to differences in biology or physiology, but the discrepancy may also be traced to the effects of structural racism as well as cultural differences in reporting symptoms. Differences in body weight, economic status, education, traditional cultural diets and other factors may play a role too.

Your mental health and trauma history

Studies show that women with a history of mood disorders may have more trouble with hot flashes.

Traumatic experiences from childhood also may lead to worse hot flashes in menopause, according to recent research.

Surgical history

Surgical removal of one or both ovaries (oophorectomy) is sometimes needed to treat ovarian tumors or cysts, ovarian cancer, or endometriosis. Or it may be done to reduce the cancer risk in women with a BRCA1 or BRCA2 mutation. If both ovaries are removed before the natural age of menopause, it results in a sudden decline in the hormones that are produced by the ovaries. This surgically induced menopause can be a much tougher transition than with a gradual loss of hormones. Severe or very frequent hot flashes may begin right after oophorectomy.

Cancer history

Women who undergo cancer treatment — including radiation, chemotherapy or bone marrow transplant — may experience an abrupt decline in estrogen. This quick shift can result in severe hot flash symptoms, similar to surgical removal of the ovaries.

In addition, many cancer medications, including tamoxifen and aromatase inhibitors, can worsen hot flash symptoms. Tamoxifen may be used before or after menopause as an additional therapy to keep cancer from returning. For women at high risk of breast cancer, tamoxifen may also be prescribed as a preventive therapy to keep cancer at bay. In contrast, aromatase inhibitors are used only after menopause. This class of medications reduces the amount of estrogen in the body after menopause to help keep cancer from returning. All these medications can be good for cancer but bad for hot flashes.

WHAT CAUSES HOT FLASHES?

Let's recap: What happens in the brain to trigger a hot flash?

The hypothalamus regulates your core body temperature, keeping you in your comfort zone. But as estrogen levels fluctuate and fall in the transition to menopause, this regulation goes awry. Recent research is finally beginning to discover why. Estrogen helps control chemical signaling from neurons in the hypothalamus that release kisspeptin, neurokinin B and dynorphin, known as KNDy (pronounced "candy") neurons. When estrogen levels in the brain drop, this signaling goes unchecked. The hypothalamus may then overreact as if you're too hot. So it trips a sudden warmth in your skin, flushing and sweating to cool you down.

Finding your triggers

Take some time to think about what may be your triggers. Review the list of common triggers in Chapter 2, including:

- Spicy foods
- Caffeinated beverages and alcohol
- Smoking
- Warm clothing or environment
- Stress

If you're not sure whether any of these affect you, consider tracking your hot flashes for a few weeks. Make sure to log any possible trig-

NEW NONHORMONAL TREATMENTS

Excitingly, recent research has identified the specific types of neurons in the brain that are involved in hot flashes. This better understanding of the underlying mechanism is helping scientists create newer, better treatments without hormones.

One new class of drugs targets neurokinin 3 receptors (NK3R) in the hypothalamus. Research has determined that the internal cascade of a hot flash is triggered by signaling between KNDy neurons and the NK3R. So new medications work by blocking the NK3R, interfering with those chemical signals. These new treatments are called NK3R antagonists or NK3R inhibitors.

Trial data for one NK3R antagonist, fezolinetant, was submitted to the U.S. Food and Drug Administration in 2022 as the first of its kind. In trials, the medication drastically reduced the number of hot flashes for women who were experiencing seven or more each day. Other recent trials showed that similar treatments also gave significant relief. More research is ongoing.

These medications may be able to offer better menopause symptom relief to breast cancer survivors, people with prior blood clots, and anyone else for whom hormone therapy isn't a good fit.

gers that might be related to your symptoms. Then you can review your log and see if you can unearth any patterns.

You may find that your love of hot sauce plays a prominent role in your symptoms. Or that the hot, stuffy meeting room in the corner of your office building is to blame. Or wool sweaters. Or too much wine. Or not enough stress-busting yoga. These insights are powerful.

Other causes of hot flashes

Keep in mind that it's possible for hot flashes or night sweats to be caused by something other than the transition to menopause. Other conditions can cause these symptoms, including thyroid disease, infections and some types of cancers. Taking certain medications, such as opioids or tricyclic antidepressants, can also cause severe sweating that may be mistaken for menopausal hot flashes. In these cases, the body processes that cause flushing or sweating are different.

HOW TO GET RELIEF

Once a hot flash is starting, there's no instant cure. The most effective way to manage frequent hot flashes is with hormone therapy or other treatment that helps avoid them in the first place. Read up on medications and complementary therapies that can help in Chapters 6, 7 and 8. Then talk with your health care practitioner about which options make the most sense for you.

If your hot flashes are mild, you may be able to manage them by revamping your environment and avoiding your triggers. If you experience moderate or severe hot flashes, controlling your diet and your weight may make a difference.

Experiment with the following strategies and tips:

Keep your core body temperature as cool as possible

This seems like simple common sense, but it's hugely important in managing hot flashes. You may need to alter your habits and your wardrobe to stay cool and help you cool down quickly when a hot flash hits.

Start by thinking about how you can remain in cooler areas as much as possible. Open windows or use air conditioning and use fans to keep cool air flowing. Lower room temperatures if you can.

If you work in an office building, for example, schedule meetings in cooler, larger conference rooms or open areas. Don't pack into a cube or tight office space to discuss an issue. In addition, avoid back-to-back meetings on opposite sides of the building that would cause you to rush from one area to the other. If you typically meet colleagues for lunch at an outdoor cafe or picnic area, look for shade or seek out a cooler indoor spot. Ask a trusted colleague to help in any way possible.

Outside the office, plan your social gatherings at breezy restaurants that aren't hot and overcrowded. Or entertain guests in your own home, where you can control the temperature. When you know you'll be outdoors — such as watching your daughter's or grandson's soccer game — pack an umbrella to shade yourself from the sun. Whatever your daily routine, plan ahead to try to keep cool.

In addition, get smart about your clothing choices. As much as possible, dress in layers so that you can remove one or two when you're hot and replace them when you're cooler. Try a jacket or cardigan over a sleeveless dress, silk shell or T-shirt. Choose light, natural, breathable fabrics and open-weave materials that allow air to circulate.

Finally, carry a cool drink with you, when you can. If you feel a hot flash coming on, take a few sips to help cool you down.

Keep cool at night

If night sweats bother you, you'll need to find strategies to stay cool while you're sleeping — or lying in bed not sleeping, as the case may be. Start by surveying your bedroom. Is the temperature too high? Can you turn down the thermostat in the bedroom? Can you open windows or plug in a bedside fan for some breeze?

Next, examine your bed. Is it made up with flannel sheets and a huge down comforter? Or do you have multiple layers of breathable bedding that can be pulled up or down as needed? Wicking sheets could help too. In addition, make sure you have comfortable, light pajamas, and consider keeping a cold glass of water on your nightstand.

If you sleep with a partner, try to find cooling solutions that don't drive a wedge in between you. Hot flashes can be tough on your relationship. Avoiding your partner's body heat, throwing covers on and off all night long, or freezing your partner into the guest room won't help build any intimacy. Instead, look for solutions that keep you cool without icing out your partner. Try keeping a frozen cold pack under your pillow on your side of the bed. Turn your pillow often so that your head is always resting on a cool surface without affecting your partner. You may also find that cooling products — such as sprays, gels or special pillows — may be helpful.

Watch what you eat and drink

Hot, spicy foods are a common trigger for hot flashes. Keep this in mind if you're about to order a fiery favorite dish. If you like bold

“ I am a retired physician assistant, with 25 years of emergency medicine experience. I am also an Army veteran. The year that my menopause symptoms started, my brain fog was so bad that I was afraid I was developing early-onset dementia.

At about 53, I started to have longer times between cycles, and I developed brain fog. I started "word finding," where I could be staring at a coffee pot but forget what it was called. Two female coworkers, both physicians a few years older, said, "That's menopause, you idiot!" (So much love in the ER.) It's funny now, but at the time, I was pretty upset. I began to question my judgment at work. Thank God the nurses I worked with knew me well, because when I would ask for "one of those thingies," they knew what I was talking about.

My wife wasn't as patient and would get aggravated at my memory lapses. My anxiety, depression and PTSD also worsened. There were some dark times. At that point, I sought care from my OB/GYN who put me on estrogen therapy, and I had a fantastic response to it. However, when I saw my primary care physician at another health care system, she took me off estrogen due to the risk of stroke and heart attack. I was pretty discouraged, but I dealt with it as I am not a fan of either heart attack or stroke. And, working in

flavors, look for dishes with fresh herbs, pungent cheeses, pickled vegetables or other ingredients that add taste and tang without adding heat and spice.

Mind your beverages too. Hot drinks, caffeinated drinks and alcoholic drinks can all be a problem when you're trying to avoid hot flashes. If you usually have your coffee at work, experiment with drinking it at home before you shower. Swap caffeinated tea for herbal tea. Or try cold sparkling water or a smoothie instead of an afternoon soda.

It may take a little trial and error to find what works best for you.

medicine, I understood that different providers have different ways of doing things.

Fast forward to about age 55, when I was having significant brain fog and hot flashes. The hot flashes and night sweats caused a lot of friction between my wife and me. The fan and AC wars were epic. I was absolutely miserable.

I decided to consolidate my health care within one system and found a new OB/GYN, a physician assistant (PA). I didn't even bother to ask for hormone therapy at first — I assumed I would be told no, and I didn't want to cause a conflict between my primary physician and PA. I waited another year and finally asked. That was when I was referred to a women's health specialist.

This physician evaluated me for hormone therapy and treatment of lichen sclerosis, a previous diagnosis. After discussing risks versus benefits and all the most recent research, she put me on an estrogen patch and progesterone pill, and vaginal estrogen and steroid ointment for the lichen sclerosis. My symptoms are now gone. I am so grateful for her care. Later, when I explained to my primary care doctor that my quality of life had been suffering, she agreed that I should remain on hormone therapy.

You may find that you can enjoy a steaming-hot latte without a hot flash as long as it's decaf. Or you may find that coffee is OK as long as it's iced instead of heated. Find the limits that keep you comfortable.

Refrain from smoking

Keep cigarettes out of your home and car. By not smoking, you may reduce hot flashes as well as your risk of many serious health conditions, such as heart disease, stroke and cancer. If you need help quitting, talk to your health care provider about the best way to go smoke-free for good.

Lose extra pounds

If you're overweight or obese, losing weight might help ease your hot flashes. A number of studies have shown that overweight or obese people who lose weight reduce the frequency of hot flashes. And it's not only about the number on the scale. People who lowered their BMI or reduced their waist size also experienced significant relief from hot flashes. In many women who are overweight, dropping 10% of body weight can reduce — or, in some, completely eliminate — hot flashes. But even losing 10 pounds may help give symptom relief.

While staying active is important, you'll likely need to focus on what you eat and drink to lose weight in midlife. But exercise can help you keep the weight off or avoid gaining it in the first place!

Reduce your stress

Finding ways to reduce your load or increase the feeling of calm and balance in your life can help with hot flashes. Try meditation, yoga, massage or whatever stress-busting activities sound good to you. Even if these approaches don't quell your hot flashes, they may offer many other benefits, including better sleep.

If you're overwhelmed by stress or anxiety, seek support. Menopause can correspond with a lot of major life changes and transitions. Some of these changes are thrilling — such as landing a big promotion at work or watching your kids go through major milestones. Other common changes during this time, such as caring for aging parents, are difficult. In all cases, big life events can cause stress. If you're struggling to manage it all, don't be afraid to lean on a good friend or family member or a therapist. Getting your stress under control is important for your health. And you'll be able to better manage all your responsibilities when you're feeling your best.

STRIKE A BALANCE

In the end, your goal isn't to stop living a full life to try to avoid or manage hot flashes. You don't necessarily have to cut out coffee entirely. But if hot flashes are affecting your daily life, it might be worth considering cutting down a bit to see if it has an effect on your symptoms. Find your individual triggers, and then use that knowledge to seize control and feel your best.

If you're unable to control your hot flashes by changing your environment and avoiding triggers, talk to your health care provider about other options, including hormone therapies that can help. Remember that your symptoms could last for a decade or longer. That's too long to rely on middle-of-the-night cold showers and a bag of frozen peas for relief.

10

Mental health and mood changes

By now, you're probably quite familiar with the connection between hormone swings and mood swings. During your reproductive years, you might have felt slightly more emotional just before your period, or maybe you could go so far as to predict the start of your period based on mood alone. These mood-related menstrual symptoms — known as *premenstrual syndrome* (PMS) — are common.

As you head into menopause, your changing hormones may, once again, be affecting your moods. However, hormones often aren't the only culprits. This chapter will explore the many causes of menopause-related mood changes and how you can manage them successfully.

MOOD CHANGES DURING MENOPAUSE

You might've hoped that any mood swings associated with your menstrual cycle would be over as soon as your period stopped. Unfortunately, this isn't always the case. Some women find that they continue to experience moodiness as they transition to menopause.

Mood changes are common especially in perimenopause, as your estrogen levels rise and fall (and then fall some more) as your body changes. These shifting hormone levels may contribute to a wide range of mood effects, including slight irritability, worry, anxiety and major depressive disorder.

However, mood changes may also be the result of other midlife changes. Navigating aging parents and growing (or adult) children and planning for your own future can be stressful and overwhelming. You may be sad over the loss of your fertility or wonder what's next for you. It's no surprise that feelings like these can lead to stress, anxiety or a depressed mood.

Other factors that may affect your mood during menopause include:

- History of depression. Most women who experience major depression during the transition to menopause have had depression before.
- Severe menopausal symptoms. Sleep problems, hot flashes and menopause-related fatigue can affect your mood.
- Nervousness or uncertainty about menopause. You may worry about your changing body and what it means for you.
- Feelings about fertility. You may be sad about not being able to have more children — even if you considered your family complete.
- Poor health habits, including smoking, eating a poor diet and not getting enough exercise.
- Relationship troubles. Relationships with your partner, children or parents may be in transition during this time. Some women may go through the death of a loved one or a divorce.
- A lack of strong social connections. After years of raising children, you may find yourself alone or with a smaller network of friends.
- Changes in employment or income. A change in employment or the prospect of retirement can weigh heavily on your moods.

Whatever the reason for your mood swings, there are actions you can take to adapt to and overcome them. For instance, getting enough sleep, eating a healthy diet and keeping up with a regular exercise program can go a long way for your mental health. And adopting a positive attitude can make a big difference too. Instead of looking at menopause for what you've lost, for instance, try to look at what you've gained. This period of life can be a great time to explore new opportunities, spend more time with your partner or friends and really define what you want your life to look like.

Sometimes the mood changes associated with menopause are more severe, resulting in depression or overwhelming stress. In these cases, coping mechanisms such as adopting a healthy lifestyle and a positive attitude aren't enough, and it's worth seeing a medical professional for help right away. We'll explore these more-serious conditions below — along with ways to manage them.

Depression during menopause
Everybody feels sad from time to time. You get in a fight with your partner, a dear friend moves away, you miss out on that promotion at work. You feel terrible — maybe for a couple of hours, maybe for a couple of days — but are able to continue on with your life.

Depression is different. Depression is a serious mood disorder that interferes with your daily life. The feelings of sadness and hopelessness that go with depression are so severe that you may not feel like eating, going to work or even getting out of bed. Depression can affect your relationships, your job and your physical health.

A combination of factors — genetic and chemical, environmental and psychological — appear to play a role in whether someone develops depression. Lifestyle changes such as illnesses, shifting work or family dynamics, or even severe menopause symptoms can lead to feelings of sadness and despair too. Some women may have trouble coming to terms with growing older and facing mounting menopausal symptoms.

Hormones, which affect the chemicals in your brain that control your mood, may also contribute to depression.

It's important to note that most women transition to menopause without experiencing depression — or any other major mental disorder. In fact, some women don't experience any mood changes whatsoever. However, you should be aware of the risks, and the signs and symptoms of depression, so you know what to look for in order to get help, if necessary.

The risk of developing a mood disorder is higher for all women in perimenopause, compared with other periods. But women who have experienced a mood disorder, such as depression, bipolar disorder or schizophrenia, are more likely to have issues at this time. Women with a history of hormone-related mood changes are at a higher risk of developing depression during menopause, as well. Other factors that can increase your risk of depression include high stress or having experienced stressful life events during childhood.

What depression looks and feels like varies from person to person and can range from mild to severe. Common signs and symptoms may include:

- Sad, hopeless or negative feelings. In depression, these interfere with daily life and don't go away.
- Feelings of anxiousness, irritability or restlessness. Or you may feel helpless or worthless.
- Loss of interest in activities that you once enjoyed, such as spending time with friends, pursuing hobbies or even having sex.
- Fatigue. You may feel this way even after a good night's sleep or even after getting more sleep than usual.
- Changes in your eating habits. Either overeating or losing your appetite can be a symptom of depression.
- Physical problems. These may include headaches, stomach pain, back pain or other physical symptoms that persist.
- Sleep problems such as having insomnia, waking during the night or sleeping more than usual.
- Cognitive problems. You may have trouble concentrating, remembering things or making decisions.
- Thoughts of harming yourself or others. This may include thoughts of suicide or lashing out at others, including loved ones.

TREATING DEPRESSION

Depression is a very real medical condition, and there are several effective ways to treat it successfully — from medications and therapy to lifestyle changes.

Depression related to menopause is treated in the same way as depression during any other time of life. The treatment that's right for you will depend on personal factors, such as the severity of depression you're experiencing. Some people with mild cases of depression benefit from therapy alone. Others, with moderate to severe depression, find antidepressants to be necessary.

Your health care provider can help you find the right treatment or combination of treatments to help you not only cope but live a healthy, active and happy life.

Antidepressants

Many menopausal women find that taking a prescription antidepressant medication is an effective way to manage and improve their symptoms. Antidepressants go to work in your brain, helping to stabilize chemicals called neurotransmitters that are involved in regulating mood.

RED FLAGS: WHEN SHOULD YOU SEEK HELP?

If you're experiencing any of the signs and symptoms of depression during menopause (or at any time), make an appointment with your health care provider.

Depression can range from feeling blue and not your usual self to having deep feelings of hopelessness and despair. Even if you just wonder if you have depression, seeking professional help is always the right choice.

Don't let embarrassment or pride convince you to manage the condition on your own. Depression can get worse if it isn't treated and can lead to other mental and physical health problems. The earlier you start treatment, the sooner you'll feel like yourself again.

If you're having suicidal thoughts, reach out to a trusted friend or family member, a leader in your faith community, or your health care provider. Or call a suicide hotline to reach a trained counselor and get help anonymously. In the United States, you can call or text 988 for the Suicide and Crisis Lifeline.

There is no good or bad antidepressant — or one that will be a cure-all. The type of medication you should take, if any, depends on your situation. The length of time you will take antidepressants differs too. When you start taking an antidepressant, it often takes 3 to 4 weeks to notice a change in your mood.

Try to be patient. It can take some time to find the right medication and dose for your situation. Sometimes you need to try two or three different medications or combinations to find a good fit. Stick with the program and work with your health care provider to find what works for you. It's worth it.

Once you start feeling better, it can be tempting to feel like you're "cured" and want to quit taking your medication. But antidepressants must be taken on a regular, consistent schedule to be effective. You should stop only under the advice of your health care provider. When it's time to discontinue your antidepressant, your practitioner may recommend that you wean off gradually to avoid withdrawal symptoms. Some people may need to continue taking antidepressants indefinitely.

Hormone therapy
For some women, hormone therapy may be enough to treat mild mood problems at menopause. This is because hormone therapy can help reduce the menopause symptoms, such as hot flashes and night sweats, that contribute to irritability and depressive moods. Research also suggests that hormone therapy may help alleviate mild depression in menopausal women by helping to stabilize fluctuating hormones.

Depending on your symptoms and their severity, your health care provider might recommend trying hormone therapy — especially if you're also experiencing significant menopause symptoms. However, hormone therapy is not a replacement for antidepressants in women who have been diagnosed with moderate to severe depression. For more information on hormone therapy, see Chapter 6.

Cognitive behavioral therapy
The thoughts you have during depression can be painful and defeating. You may feel worthless and insignificant, or even just hollow or empty inside. These can be scary feelings, especially if you keep them bottled up.

LIFESTYLE STRATEGIES FOR TREATING DEPRESSION

Medications and professional counseling are typically important parts of treating depression. But there are things you can do on your own too. Try these actions while continuing your other treatments.

- **Get enough sleep.** Practice good sleep hygiene to help you get enough, and regular, sleep. For sleep tips, see Chapter 11.
- **Exercise.** Try to get at least 30 minutes of physical activity on most days of the week.
- **Take time for yourself.** Take a break from your daily stresses by spending some quiet time, every day, by yourself. Take a bath, read a book, go for a walk, or practice the relaxation therapies suggested later in this chapter (see page 171).
- **Keep the lines of communication open.** Talk to your family and friends about your feelings, or find a support group of people who are going through the same thing you're going through. Talking about your problems and challenges can help you manage them and put them in perspective.

That's where cognitive behavioral therapy (CBT) comes in. This form of therapy can help you improve these negative thoughts and feelings and get you back on the road to good mental health. In CBT, a professional therapist helps you change your negative way of thinking — and the negative behaviors that often occur as a result.

Cognitive behavioral therapy is more than the opportunity to share what's on your mind. The process is action oriented and collaborative. Your therapist uses your sessions to help you find the relationships between your thoughts, feelings and behaviors, and then helps you set goals and learn strategies to make changes in order to meet those goals. Your therapist may even ask you to keep a journal, write down behavior patterns or do other take-home work between appointments. The objective is to work together to change your thought processes, stop damaging behavior and recover from your depression.

LET'S TALK ABOUT STRESS

Stress — that pulse-quickening, muscle-tensing, adrenaline-releasing jolt you get during times of change or challenge — often gets a bad rap. But stress isn't always bad. In fact, in some situations, it can be quite helpful.

Stress, which is your brain's response to a change or demand, can help you take action, be more alert and find energy when faced with danger. When you feel stress, your body responds by increasing (or, sometimes, decreasing) the release of certain "stress hormones" that help you manage and adapt to whatever it is that's causing your stress. It can be a great resource when you're faced with a life-or-death situation, such as dodging out of the way of an oncoming car or catching a child who is about to fall down a staircase.

But when you experience stress over the long term, it can harm both your mental and physical health. Instead of being helpful, that constant surge of stress hormones can negatively affect your body systems.

There are many reasons you may experience long-term stress during menopause. In addition to the myriad changes you're experiencing in your body, midlife can also be a time of changes in family, work and relationships. Combine hot flashes, aging parents, an empty nest or a testy teen, retirement planning, fatigue and hormone fluctuations, and you have a combination strong enough to stress out even the most centered person.

Some signs of stress are obvious — you can see or feel them. You may have headaches, stomachaches or trouble sleeping. You may tense your shoulders, clench your hands or tighten your jaw, often without even realizing it. You may jump to anger and irritability more quickly, feel down, and contract viruses — such as the flu or a cold — more frequently.

Other signs of stress are happening under the surface — with your hormones. Those hormone surges that are great for fight-or-flight situations can also cause your blood pressure, heart rate and blood sugar levels to rise. They may disrupt your menstrual cycle if you're still having your period, cause problems with your digestion, and even affect your immune system. The strain on your body from long-term stress can contribute to heart disease, high blood pressure, obesity, mental health disorders, diabetes and even skin problems, such as acne.

Signs and symptoms of stress to watch for include:

- **A change in diet.** You may eat less or more than you usually have.
- **Memory loss.** You may become forgetful or easily distracted and lack focus.
- **A "short fuse."** Your temper may flare unpredictably.
- **Sleeping problems.** You may have trouble falling asleep or trouble falling back asleep after waking at night.
- **Control issues.** You may worry that you have no control — or feel the need to exert too much control.
- **Aches and pains.** You may experience physical signs of stress, including headache, upset stomach, back pain and just general aches and pains.
- **Problems with motivation.** You may have trouble completing tasks because of a lack of energy or drive.

With all the responsibilities, obligations and concerns that you may face in menopause, it may seem impossible to get a grip on your stress. But it's not. There are many proven methods that will not only help you manage stress but help you live a calmer, happier life in the process.

MANAGING STRESS

When you manage stress well, you can prevent it from becoming a significant issue in your life. Start by recognizing your triggers. Once you do this, it's easier to avoid, or manage, situations that cause you stress.

A good first step is to write down the activities or obligations that are stressful to you. Then, write down possible solutions. For instance, if being late to appointments causes you stress, decide to leave 10 minutes earlier than usual. Or if you feel there are too many demands on your time, take a critical look at your commitments and decide what can go. Looking at your challenges and coming up with solutions in a calm, strategic way can help you feel more in control when stressors do arise.

Of course, not all stress can be avoided. And some times in your life — like the menopause years — can cause an increase in your stress levels. So if you're feeling stress creep into your life, consider these techniques to help you cope:

Practice mindfulness

There are many ways you might describe that feeling you get when your thoughts jump or wander from topic to topic and idea to idea: *Unfocused. Distracted.* And, of course, *stressed out.*

The world is full of distractions that pull your attention in multiple directions. You're in a conversation with a friend when the phone rings. You reach for your phone and notice that you just got an email from your boss. Meanwhile, a reminder pops up for that 2 p.m. meeting you scheduled yesterday. You remember you have to pick up bread before dinner, and — oh, yeah — you also need to pick up that prescription and a gift for your niece's birthday.

It's no wonder you may feel overwhelmed, anxious and stressed out. It's hard to focus on the moment when there are so many things happening at once.

That's where mindfulness exercises come in. Mindfulness is setting aside these distractions and worries and being fully present and aware in the moment. It's a way to focus on what is happening in front of you. See pages 172–173 for some suggestions on getting started.

The benefits of mindfulness are convincing. Practicing mindfulness can help reduce your stress and anxiety, manage depression, improve mood and even help you cope with illness. It can help you relax and manage the demands on your life.

Relaxation therapies

When it comes to managing stress, some specific relaxation techniques have been proven to be effective. Try the following to get through a particularly stressful moment or day — and to help keep future stress in check.

Take some deep breaths. You can practice relaxation breathing almost anywhere — at your desk, in your living room just before the dinner rush or even in bed at night before you fall asleep. The key is finding a quiet, comfortable place where you can relax and focus for a few minutes. Then, close your eyes, and with one hand resting gently on your abdomen, breathe slowly and evenly — in through your nose and out through your mouth.

As you focus on your breath, let other thoughts fall away. Focus on the air passing in and out of your body and the way your abdomen expands and falls with each breath. Feel your abdomen pushing your hand out as you fill your lungs and letting it sink back as you fully exhale.

Continue this deep breathing for several minutes. If your mind starts to drift, don't worry. This is common. Just gently redirect it back to your breathing. Practice this breathing exercise throughout the day to help you relax, focus your energy and reduce stress.

Pay attention to your muscles. Of all the physical side effects of stress, tense muscles are often the most apparent. Stress can cause you to tighten your shoulders, stiffen your neck, clench your hands, tighten your jaw muscles or grind your teeth — even when you're sleeping. In

EVERYDAY WAYS TO PRACTICE MINDFULNESS

Keep these techniques in mind when trying to work mindfulness into your daily life:

Focus on what's in front of you
Consciously practice being more aware of your daily activities. As you go about your day, take the time to really hear the sounds around you — your fingers on the keyboard, the wind blowing through the trees. Look at the familiar objects in your life — your coffee mug, your favorite pair of shoes — with fresh eyes. See if you can notice new details in them.

It would be impossible to maintain complete focus all day long. Instead, set aside time each day to pay attention to what you're doing in the moment. If you're talking to a family member or coworker, for instance, focus on what he or she is saying instead of letting your mind wander or planning what you'll say next. If you're writing a to-do list, focus on each of the items you're writing. If you find your mind wandering, gently return your focus to the present moment.

Meditate on your loved ones
Once a day, in a quiet moment, close your eyes and think of a person who is important to you. Then, remember specific details about this

fact, you may not even realize you're doing these things until you feel those knots in your shoulders or that tension headache creep up.

There are a couple of ways you can help yourself feel less tense. Flexibility exercises, such as routine stretches or yoga, can help you relax your muscles and your mind. Massage can also be a powerful tension reducer. Neck, shoulder and upper back massages target the common culprits, but hand, face and foot massages can also be relaxing.

Treat yourself. With so many demands on your time, it's easy to put yourself last. But taking the time to do things you enjoy can be a powerful and healthy way to combat stress. Each day, carve out time to

person. Picture this person's face. Hear the sound of his or her voice. Think about how you feel when you're with this person. Do this for two or three people in a row.

Practice gratitude

It's easy to take the positive aspects of your life for granted. Be more aware of your good fortune by practicing gratitude. Each morning before you get out of bed, think about three things that make you feel grateful. These may be as simple as a sunny morning or getting an unexpected phone call from a friend.

Dine deliberately

If you're like many women, when you sit down for a meal, you are often multitasking — watching TV, checking social media on your phone, maybe even working at your desk. Instead, avoid distractions while eating and focus on each bite of food. Notice how it looks. Notice its taste and how it feels in your mouth as you chew it. This simple act of being present with your food can help refresh your mind and help you be mindful about eating, as well.

focus on activities that are meaningful to you — perhaps reading a book, going for a walk, or playing or listening to music.

Practice stress-reducing exercises. Quiet and gentle exercise programs, such as yoga and tai chi, can be a great way to de-stress. You may want to consider classes that include a meditation component.

RESPECT THE BASICS

In addition to relaxation and mindfulness techniques, keep in mind the following basic practices for a healthier and less stressful life:

Prioritize your time. Take a critical look at what's most important to you. Make conscious decisions about how you're going to spend your time, then carve out space in your week for those activities.

Say no. When you try to "do it all," someone usually suffers. And that someone is often you. Make sure to leave time for your own interests and downtime. Saying no can be freeing.

Sleep. Being well rested helps promote mental health, allowing you to think more clearly and take on challenges.

Energize the right way. Caffeine or high-sugar snack foods may offer a short-term energy jolt. But when it wears off, you could wind up feeling more tired than you did before. Instead, fuel up with a healthy diet including fruits, vegetables, legumes and whole grains. Physical activity also helps increase your energy, relax your tense muscles and improve your mood.

Talk it out. Talk to family or friends about the things that cause stress in your life. Sometimes just talking about it will make you feel better. If you're still feeling overwhelmed, consider talking to a professional. A counselor or therapist can help you find ways to better manage your stress.

Avoid unhealthy coping strategies. Relaxation techniques, mindfulness practices or exercise are always better options than short-term fixes such as alcohol, drugs, tobacco or food.

“ I have named my experience "freight train menopause" because one minute I was fine, and the next I was NOT. It was a sunny Saturday morning, and I had kissed my husband goodbye as he left to play tennis. I was about to enjoy my coffee and a house all to myself when my heart started racing and I felt an overwhelming feeling of panic. Out of nowhere, I was having suicidal thoughts fueled by irrational anxiety. It was as if an alien had taken over my body. I had tears streaming down my face because I didn't know what was happening to me.

Luckily, my best friend is also my doctor, and I video called her in a panic to not be alone. My heart was still racing, and I felt so vulnerable and frightened. Through my cries of "Help me, please help me," my friend somehow was able to discern that I had just been hit by a huge wave of hormones related to menopause.

My best friend put on her doctor hat and explained that she could help me. "We have medicine that you can take to balance out your hormones, but it will take about two weeks for you to feel back to normal," she said. She put me on an estradiol patch and citalopram [an SSRI antidepressant], and after exactly two weeks I felt like a magic wand had been waved and I was back to myself. I have tried to go down on citalopram, but the panicky feeling comes back, along with thoughts that are not mine. I distinctly feel the chemical imbalance as it comes on.

In the past, I think I would've been classified as someone who had actually gone crazy and probably would've been sent away to an institution. I am SO thankful modern medicine recognizes that the hormonal imbalance of menopause causes treatable problems that are a reality for so many women.

11

When you can't sleep

What you wouldn't give to enjoy a good night's sleep again. Think back to your teens and early 20s when you may have fallen asleep the minute your head hit the pillow and would sleep so soundly that you barely moved. Those nights might seem like a faded dream. Now, sleep is often a struggle. You may have trouble falling asleep. During the night, you may toss and turn and wake up several times and find it hard to get back to sleep. In the morning, you may find yourself up with the birds, despite having a restless night. And because you aren't sleeping well, you may feel tired during the daytime.

As with other changes taking place in your life, it's easy to blame your sleep problems on menopause. But the truth is, your hormones are only partly to blame. There's no doubt that menopause can make getting a good night's sleep more difficult, but it's just one piece of a larger puzzle. Many factors affect your ability to sleep. As you age, your body and your life circumstances change. The overall effect of these changes often makes good sleep harder to come by in the second half of your life.

The good news is you don't have to live with poor sleep, dragging yourself through each day. Conditions such as insomnia, sleep apnea and restless legs syndrome can be treated. By understanding the changes happening in your life and how they may be affecting your sleep, you can take steps to help ensure that you get a good night's rest.

NORMAL SLEEP PATTERNS

As you've likely learned over the years, not all sleep is the same. When you close your eyes and drift off, your sleep follows a type of biological rhythm — a recurring sleep pattern that's known as the sleep-wake cycle.

Your sleep-wake cycle is influenced by your body's natural circadian rhythms. Circadian rhythms are changes — such as fluctuations in body temperature and hormone levels — that happen on a 24-hour cycle driven by your body's internal clock. The circadian system is heavily affected by day and night. Your natural circadian rhythms try to keep you awake during the daylight hours, and they prompt you to sleep once darkness falls.

While most people's sleep-wake cycle follows a similar pattern, our sleep needs and routines vary. Some of us need more sleep, and others need less. Some of us are morning people, while others are night owls. Some of us fall asleep the minute we get into bed, while others need to read or listen to music to coax us to sleep.

Sleep patterns also vary with age. Between the ages of 50 and 60, sleep tends to become more restless and less refreshing. This is because more of the night is spent in light sleep and less of it in deep and dreaming sleep. In other words, your sleep-wake cycle is changing.

Sleep cycles

Sleep researchers have identified several stages of sleep that make up the sleep-wake cycle. These stages are divided into two main categories:

- **NREM sleep.** *NREM* stands for nonrapid eye movement. NREM includes three stages of sleep, each deeper than the last.
- **REM sleep.** *REM* refers to rapid eye movement. In REM sleep,

your eyes actually move back and forth. This is the stage of sleep when you do the majority of your dreaming.

Your nightly sleep journey begins in the first stage of NREM sleep, called *N1*, a transition period between wake and sleep. It progresses to the next levels of NREM sleep before crossing over into REM sleep. This pattern repeats itself several times during the night.

NREM sleep	
N1 Stage: Transitional sleep	During this stage, which lasts about five minutes, you transition from being awake to falling asleep. Your eyes move slowly behind your eyelids, and your brain waves and muscle activity slow down.
N2 Stage: Light sleep	Your eye movement stops, your heart rate slows, and your body temperature decreases.
N3 Stage: Deep sleep	In this stage of sleep, your brain waves are extremely slow, your blood pressure drops, and your breathing slows. During deep sleep, you're difficult to awaken, and if you are awakened, it takes you a while to adjust.
REM sleep	
Dreaming sleep	Following NREM sleep, you enter REM sleep, where most dreaming happens. Your eyes move rapidly beneath your eyelids, your breathing is shallow and irregular, and your heart rate and blood pressure increase. During this stage, your arm and leg muscles become temporarily paralyzed.

Adults spend, on average, more than half our total daily sleep time in N2 sleep, about 20% in REM sleep and the remaining time in other stages, mainly N3 sleep. However, with age, the amount of time spent in deep sleep and dream sleep decreases, and lighter sleep increases.

So, if it seems that you just don't sleep like you used to, you're right. Beginning in your young adult and middle adult years, your sleep gradually becomes less sound. You experience more awakenings each night, and you're more aware of being awake.

Hours of sleep

Do sleep patterns change because you simply need less sleep as you get older? There's no cut and dried answer. For the most part, studies suggest that older adults require just as much sleep as younger adults do. The recommended amount is at least seven hours a night.

There is some evidence that with age, both too much and too little sleep may be harmful to your health. Sleeping less than five hours a night or over nine hours a night may be associated with increased risk of heart disease or stroke. Other studies have shown that cognitive efficiency or mental sharpness is improved in adults who sleep 7 to 8 hours a night as compared with those who sleep less or more.

WHAT HAPPENS DURING MENOPAUSE

If you're frustrated because you aren't sleeping well, you're not alone. Somewhere between 40% and 60% of women report having sleep problems during the menopausal years. This fits with studies showing that the closer women get to menopause, the more sleep troubles they experience. Common complaints include having difficulty falling asleep, waking up in the middle of the night and awakening early in the morning. It may not be surprising to you that poor sleep is often second only to hot flashes as the most common complaint of women going through the menopause transition.

The reasons behind sleep problems around this time of life are still being investigated. While some studies point to declining hormone levels as the reason you're not sleeping well, others suggest that the main culprit is the natural aging process. The most likely possibility is an intermingling of the two — your age and your hormones are both working against you.

Reduced hormones

As you've learned in earlier chapters, beginning at around age 40 — although it can happen later — your ovaries gradually begin producing decreased amounts of estrogen and progesterone. These hormones have a wide range of effects, including on specific brain chemicals (neurotransmitters) that help promote sleep. So it makes sense that as hormone production gradually declines, the simple act of falling asleep and staying asleep may become more difficult.

Related conditions

While the decline in hormone levels may impact sleep during menopause, other conditions related to these hormonal changes often play a major role.

A prime example is hot flashes. Night sweats — hot flashes that occur at night — may leave you hot and sweating one moment and cold and shivering the next, making it tough to sleep. Some women even need to get up and change their clothes after a particularly drenching episode. If you're among the many women who struggle with hot flashes, your inability to get a good night's sleep is closely tied to the hot-and-cold routine you dance to each night.

In addition, obstructive sleep apnea and restless legs syndrome are more common after menopause, and these can also interfere with sleep. At least one study found that more than half the women who complained of trouble sleeping during menopause had sleep apnea, restless legs or both.

Natural aging

Research suggests that sleep quality naturally worsens over time. In other words, loss of sleep is an effect of natural aging, completely independent of any effects from declining hormones.

Life circumstances

As you transition through midlife, there may be a lot going on. In addition to changing hormones and natural aging, you may be dealing

RED FLAGS: WARNING SIGNS OF OBSTRUCTIVE SLEEP APNEA

Some sleep problems are more than just annoying — they can be a sign of obstructive sleep apnea, a potentially harmful sleep disorder. Obstructive sleep apnea causes someone to repeatedly stop and restart breathing as muscles in the throat intermittently relax and block the airway during sleep. This disorder can have serious health consequences. People with obstructive sleep apnea are at increased risk of high blood pressure, coronary artery disease, dementia, heart attacks, heart failure and strokes.

Many people think of obstructive sleep apnea as a man's disease because symptoms like loud snoring may be more noticeable in men. But sleep apnea affects women too, and the risk increases with age. The risk goes up especially after menopause. Sleep apnea most commonly affects people who are overweight or obese. Some research suggests that you may also be at greater risk if you experience hot flashes and night sweats.

To check for other warning signs of sleep apnea, ask yourself:

- Has anyone told me I snore?
- Do I sometimes wake up gasping or choking?
- Has anyone ever told me that sometimes my breathing briefly stops during sleep?
- Do I wake in the morning with a headache, dry mouth or sore throat — or just feeling plain terrible?
- Do I often feel excessively drowsy during the daytime?

If you answered yes to one or more of these questions, there's a chance you have sleep apnea. In some cases, insomnia, anxiety and depression can also be symptoms of the disorder. If you're concerned you've developed sleep apnea, talk to your health care provider. Learn more about this condition and treatment options starting on page 193.

with all kinds of other life changes, some of them significant. Often, these changes produce stress, which in turn can mess with your ability to sleep. When you're experiencing menopause, it's easy to blame everything on your hormones — or lack of them. But is that always the true cause?

Stressful events Like many women in midlife, you may find yourself dealing with major life challenges. Job-related issues, loss of life partners through divorce or death, children moving away, and — living in the sandwich generation — caregiving for elderly parents. During the day when you're busy, you may be able to avoid dwelling on it all. But at night, when you try to rest and relax, the worry and anxiety may put on an all-night show, hampering your ability to sleep.

Changing routines You may find that as you get older, you're less physically or socially active than you once were. A lack of activity can interfere with a good night's sleep. Also, the less active you are, the more likely you may be to take a nap during the day, making it more difficult to sleep at night. Even if you're socializing more now that kids are older or gone, an extra glass of wine you're having at night could also be causing sleep difficulty.

Health issues Midlife is often when medical conditions develop that can interfere with sleep, such as back problems or arthritis. You may begin experiencing bladder problems and find yourself waking up at night to go to the bathroom. What's more, the older you get, the more likely you are to take medications, some of which can interfere with sleep. Common medications that can affect sleep are bronchodilators, steroids, thyroid hormones and certain antidepressants.

Sleep history

Has sleep always been a problem for you? Some research suggests that your ability to sleep during your younger years may predict how well you'll sleep in later years. If you had trouble sleeping in your 30s and 40s, you may be significantly more likely to experience sleep difficulties compared to someone who had an easier time sleeping when they were younger. If you also experience hot flashes during menopause, you're even more likely to have sleep issues.

THE NEXT STEP

The key message here is that often it's not just one thing that's making sleep harder as you enter menopause but several issues all mixed together. The bigger question, of course, is, What can you do about it?

The first step is to try and peel back the layers to find the source of the unrest. Is it stress? Hormones? Aging? Is it a combination of several things? If your sleep troubles are moderate to severe, you may need the guidance of your health care provider to help decipher the possible causes and determine potential treatments.

A number of options exist to treat menopause-related insomnia. For milder symptoms, a few changes to your daily and nightly routines may do the trick. Alternative therapies to improve sleep are also coming to the forefront. For more-severe symptoms, cognitive behavioral therapy or medications may be helpful. If your difficult nights are a result of obstructive sleep apnea or restless legs syndrome, those conditions can be successfully treated too.

OVERCOMING INSOMNIA

If you have a hard time falling asleep, staying asleep or both, you have insomnia. With insomnia, you may wake up feeling groggy and unrefreshed, which can take a toll on you during the day. Insomnia can not only drain your energy level and your mood but can also affect your health, work performance, relationships and quality of life.

For insomnia that happens during menopause, your health care provider may ask some questions, and you may even be asked to take part in a sleep study to figure out if there's a specific cause for the problem. For example, what you think is insomnia may actually be obstructive sleep apnea. Once a diagnosis of insomnia is made, you and your health care professional can decide on the best form of treatment.

Cognitive behavioral therapy for insomnia

As with so many other aspects of your life, your habits are important. Good sleep habits help promote sound sleep. Cognitive behavioral therapy for insomnia (CBT-I) is a structured program that teaches you good sleep behaviors and specific strategies to improve your sleep. The cognitive part of CBT-I teaches you to find and change thoughts that cause or worsen your sleep problems. This type of therapy can help you control or cut out negative thoughts and worries that keep you awake. The behavioral part of CBT-I helps you replace behaviors that keep you from sleeping well with good sleep habits.

Numerous studies have shown the effectiveness of CBT-I in relieving insomnia. That's why medical associations such as such as the American College of Physicians and American Academy of Sleep Medicine recommend the therapy as the first choice of treatment for chronic insomnia.

Many people with insomnia can benefit from CBT-I, including women experiencing sleep problems during and after the menopause transition. In one recent study, postmenopausal women who received CBT-I were less exhausted and sleepy during the day, felt more energized, and functioned better at work. The women also reported improved well-being and a greater ability to bounce back from physical and emotional problems.

CBT-I may be a good choice if you have long-term sleep problems, if you're worried about becoming dependent on sleep medications, or if medications aren't effective or cause unpleasant side effects. Unlike medications, CBT-I addresses the underlying causes of insomnia rather than just relieving symptoms, making it more effective than medications in many cases.

The following techniques may be part of a CBT-I program, whether using an app at home or working with a sleep therapist:

Stimulus control This strategy helps change habits that cause your mind to resist sleep. For example, you might be coached to set a consistent bedtime and wake time, avoid naps, use the bed only for sleep and sex and leave the bedroom if you can't go to sleep within 20 minutes, returning only when you're sleepy.

Sleep restriction Lying in bed when you're awake can become a habit that leads to poor sleep. This treatment reduces the time you spend in bed, causing partial sleep deprivation, which makes you more tired the next night. Once your sleep has improved, your time in bed is gradually increased.

Sleep hygiene This method of therapy involves changing basic lifestyle habits that influence sleep, such as smoking, drinking too much caffeine late in the day, drinking too much alcohol or not getting regular exercise. It also includes tips that help you sleep better, such as ways to wind down an hour or two before bedtime.

Sleep environment improvement To get some z's, it helps to create a comfortable sleep environment, such as keeping your bedroom quiet, dark and cool, not having a TV in the bedroom and hiding the clock from view.

Relaxation training This method helps you calm your mind and body. Approaches include breathing exercises, meditation, imagery, muscle relaxation and others.

Remaining passively awake Also called *paradoxical intention*, this involves avoiding any effort to fall asleep. Paradoxically, worrying that you can't sleep can actually keep you awake. Letting go of this worry can help you relax and make it easier to fall asleep.

Biofeedback This technique allows you to observe biological signs such as your heart rate and muscle tension and shows you how to adjust them. Your sleep specialist may have you take a biofeedback device home to record your daily patterns. The information can help find patterns that affect sleep.

Prescription medications

Sometimes a change in sleeping habits may not be enough. Or it may take a while for you to master various CBT-I techniques. The next

---

GOING DIGITAL

In recent years, a number of effective CBT-I apps have cropped up. These digital offerings may be available as part of an in-person program or used as an entirely self-paced, at-home experience. Like traditional CBT-I programs, the apps teach techniques to help you reset your thought patterns and sleep habits to relieve insomnia. Many of these digital programs are accessible, convenient and effective. The trick is sticking with it.

option is usually medication. In general, long-term use of prescription medications to promote sleep isn't recommended because the medications can produce side effects and some may be habit-forming. But your provider may suggest medications on a short-term basis to help you through an especially rocky period. A number of different options exist.

10 STEPS TO BETTER SLEEP

You might not be able to control all the factors that interfere with your sleep, but you can adopt habits that help.

1. **Nix the naps.** Naps can make it more difficult to fall asleep at night. If you can't get by without a nap, limit it to no more than 30 minutes, and don't nap after 3 p.m.
2. **Check your medications.** Talk to your health care provider or pharmacist to see if any medications you're taking may be contributing to your insomnia. Also check the labels of nonprescription products to see if they contain caffeine or other stimulants, such as pseudoephedrine.
3. **Get physical.** Activity helps promote a good night's sleep. Get at least 30 minutes of vigorous exercise each day, but make sure you do so at least 5 to 6 hours before bedtime. Exercising too close to bedtime will keep you awake.
4. **Lay off the caffeine and alcohol.** Caffeine and alcohol can make it more difficult to achieve sound sleep. Make it a point not to have any caffeine after lunchtime. Besides coffee, caffeine is found in tea, energy drinks, some sodas and chocolate. Also limit or avoid alcohol in the evening. Initially, alcohol may make you sleepy, but it also causes you to awaken during the night.
5. **Avoid heavy dinners or eating late, and keep your bedtime snack small.** Eating too much late in the evening can cause stomach upset and digestion problems that keep you awake. Also don't drink too much fluid before bed if you don't want your bladder to give you middle-of-the-night wakeup calls.

Hormone therapy Hormone therapy is the most effective treatment for relieving menopausal symptoms. If your sleep difficulties are severe and accompanied by other menopausal symptoms, such as hot flashes, your health care provider may recommend hormone therapy to provide symptom relief. Whether you're a good candidate will

6. **Relax before bed.** Try to put your worries and concerns aside when you get into bed. Even better, plan a time during the early part of the day to address your worries so they don't weigh on you when it's time to sleep. Create a relaxing bedtime ritual. A warm bath before bedtime can help prepare you for sleep. Other options include reading a book or participating in breathing exercises, yoga or prayer. Don't bring laptops, your cellphone or other screens into your bedroom. The light can interfere with your sleep-wake cycle, and the stimulation can prevent you from falling asleep. Remember, your bedroom is only for sleep and sex!

7. **Make your bedroom comfortable.** Close your bedroom door or create a subtle background noise, such as a running fan, to help drown out other noises. Keep your bedroom temperature comfortable — make sure it's not too warm, especially if you're experiencing hot flashes.

8. **Stick to a schedule.** Keep your bedtime and wake time consistent from day to day, including on weekends.

9. **Hide the clocks.** Set your alarm so that you know when to get up, but then hide all clocks in your bedroom, including your cellphone, so you don't worry about what time it is if you wake up.

10. **Don't "try" to sleep.** The harder you try, the more awake you'll become. If you can't fall asleep, get out of bed and read (but not on a screen) or listen to soothing music in another room until you become drowsy, then go back to bed.

depend on your personal and family medical history. Hormone therapy can offer relief for disruptive symptoms, including disturbed sleep, especially in the first few years after menopause. For more on hormone therapy, see Chapter 6.

Prescription sleeping pills These medications may be prescribed for a short time, such as a couple of weeks, to help break a cycle of insomnia.

- **Short-acting nonbenzodiazepines.** These medications include eszopiclone (Lunesta), zolpidem (Ambien, Edluar, ZolpiMist) and zaleplon (Sonata). They act on brain receptors to slow down your nervous system and help you fall asleep and stay asleep. Zolpidem is the first medication for which the FDA recommends different doses based on sex, as women metabolize it more slowly than men do.
- **Benzodiazepines.** They include the older medications clonazepam (Klonopin), diazepam (Valium) and lorazepam (Ativan, Loreev XR). Benzodiazepines can help you both fall asleep and stay asleep, but they may have significant side effects, such as next-day drowsiness, and they can lead to dependence.
- **Melatonin agonist.** Not to be confused with the supplement melatonin, the prescription medication ramelteon (Rozerem) works like the natural hormone melatonin produced by your body, helping to regulate your sleep-wake cycle (circadian rhythm). Some small trials have found ramelteon beneficial in helping people fall asleep more quickly and slightly increasing their total sleep time.

Antidepressants The drug doxepin (Silenor) has been approved for the treatment of chronic insomnia. Other antidepressants generally aren't recommended as a treatment for insomnia in people who don't have depression.

Nonprescription medications

Common over-the-counter sleep aids, such as diphenhydramine (Tylenol PM, Advil PM, Aleve PM, others) and doxylamine succinate (Unisom SleepTabs), contain antihistamines that cause drowsiness. They aren't intended for regular use because you can develop a tolerance to their sedating effect quickly. That means the longer you take these sleep aids, the less likely they are to make you sleepy. What's more, some over-the-counter sleep aids can leave you feeling groggy and unwell the next day. This is the so-called hangover effect, and it can be worse in older adults.

Medication interactions are possible too, and much remains unknown about the safety and effectiveness of over-the-counter sleep medications. Before taking a sleep aid, ask your provider what dosage to take and if it might interact with other medications or underlying conditions.

Supplements and botanicals

As an alternative to prescription or over-the-counter sleeping pills, some people turn to supplements, teas and extracts. While most of these products are considered safe, evidence of their effectiveness is limited. Some studies show modest benefits, while others indicate that these sleeping aids perform no better than placebos.

Supplements and other botanical products generally haven't gotten the same scientific scrutiny as medications and aren't as strictly regulated. Yet these products — including those labeled as "natural" — can have strong effects in the body and may interact with medications. Before taking a new supplement, it's a good idea to discuss it with your primary care provider.

- **Melatonin.** If you're recovering from jet lag or trying to fall asleep earlier at night, melatonin may be just the ticket. Melatonin is a hormone that's secreted by the brain's pineal gland to help control your natural sleep-wake cycle. The hormone is sold as a supplement and marketed as a treatment for insomnia. Research suggests melatonin may improve jet lag symptoms, help shift the time of day or night you fall asleep and slightly reduce the time it takes to fall asleep. But its effects on sleep quality, total sleep time and insomnia aren't clear.

- **Valerian.** This botanical supplement is sold as a sleep aid because it has a mildly sedating effect that may help when racing thoughts or worry keep you awake. Valerian is one of the most well-studied supplements for sleep, but the evidence is conflicting. While some studies suggest that valerian may improve how well you sleep, others indicate that the supplement has little to no effect on sleep quality or insomnia. Discuss valerian with your health care provider before trying it. High doses and long-term use may increase the risk of liver damage.

- **Hops.** Surprise! This plant supplement might do more than flavor beer. On its own, hops may not make much difference when it comes to sleep. But a few small studies suggest that when combined with valerian, hops may help you fall asleep faster and stay asleep longer. In one study, menopausal women who took a supplement that included hops, valerian and other herbal extracts reported significantly improved sleep.
- **Lemon balm.** Most often sold as a tea or extract, this herbal product may quiet a busy mind by helping you relax. As with most other supplements, the jury is still out on whether lemon balm helps improve insomnia.
- **Skullcap.** The extract of this flowering North American plant is often sold as an anxiety reliever and sleep aid, but scientific evidence of its benefits is scarce.
- **Kava.** While research supports the anti-anxiety effects of this plant-based product, kava has been linked to a risk of severe liver injury, even with short-term use. Use extra caution and consult with your health care provider if you're considering taking it.
- **L-tryptophan and 5-hydroxytryptophan (5-HTP).** These two supplements are sometimes marketed as sleep aids. L-tryptophan and 5-HTP are thought to work by boosting levels of serotonin, a natural chemical in the brain that may affect mood and sleep. It's unclear, though, whether the supplements help improve insomnia.
- **Chamomile.** Humans have been using this botanical for thousands of years. Drunk as a tea, chamomile may help encourage a better night's sleep, but more research is needed.

Other treatments

You may prefer help for your sleep troubles that doesn't involve the use of medication or supplements. If you have chronic insomnia, CBT-I might be your best bet. But these alternative therapies might also be worth a try.

Acupuncture During an acupuncture session, a practitioner places many thin needles in your skin at specific points on your body. There's some evidence that this practice may be beneficial for people with insomnia, but more research is needed. If you choose to try acupuncture, ask your health care provider how to find a qualified practitioner.

Yoga Some studies suggest that performing yoga regularly can improve your sleep. There are many beneficial styles, including hatha, restorative, Tibetan yoga and yoga nidra. You might want to try a few types to find what works best for you. Be sure to start slow, listen to your body and work with an instructor who helps adapt poses to your needs.

Tai chi Tai chi is an ancient Chinese tradition that today is practiced as a graceful form of exercise. It involves a series of movements done in a slow, focused way and accompanied by deep breathing. Some evidence suggests that practicing tai chi may improve how well you sleep, especially as you age.

Meditation There's evidence that meditation also may improve sleep in some individuals by promoting relaxation and reducing anxiety. Like yoga, it may be worth experimenting with this technique to see if it might alleviate your restless nights. Again, seek out a qualified instructor. Other positive health effects from regular meditation include reduced stress and reduced blood pressure.

Relaxation techniques Do you often lie awake at night rehashing your day or dwelling on tomorrow's to-do list? Relaxation techniques such as breathing exercises, progressive muscle relaxation and guided imagery can help slow down your mind and your body at bedtime. (See the sidebar for some useful tips!)

Bedtime stories They're not just for children anymore! Recorded stories designed to lull grown-ups to sleep are available on meditation or sleep apps and bedtime podcasts.

Mindfulness-based stress reduction (MBSR) Mindfulness involves being present to what you're sensing and feeling in the moment, without interpretation or judgment. MBSR is a structured program that trains you in mindfulness, using techniques such as yoga and meditation. In multiple studies this therapy significantly improved sleep quality in people with insomnia. And, bonus! MBSR can reduce stress, anxiety and depression, improving your overall mental health.

Aromatherapy Try making your bedroom a peaceful sanctuary with essential oils such as lavender, rosemary, orange peel, tea tree or peppermint. Using plant-based scents to improve well-being is called *aromatherapy*, and it just might help you sleep better. Essential oils may be inhaled directly or indirectly or rubbed on the skin through massage or lotions. Just be aware that some people who use aromatherapy on

RELAXATION TIPS

Try these tips at bedtime to prime you for a good night's sleep. Be patient. The more you do them, the more natural they'll become.

Relaxed breathing
Sit or lie in a comfortable position. Rest one hand comfortably on your abdomen and the other hand on your chest. Inhale slowly through your nose for a count of four while pushing your abdomen out. Hold your breath for a count of four. Then slowly exhale through your mouth for a count of four while pushing your abdomen in. Concentrate on breathing this way for a few minutes and become aware of the hand on your abdomen rising and falling with each breath.

Progressive muscle relaxation
Sit or lie in a comfortable position and close your eyes. Allow your jaw to drop and your eyelids to be relaxed but not tightly closed. Tighten the muscles in one area of your body and hold them for a count of five. Release the tightness completely and move on to the next part of your body. Start by tensing and relaxing the muscles in your toes and progressively working your way up to your neck and head. Alternatively, you can start with your head and neck and work down to your toes. Smartphone apps are available to guide you if you'd prefer to just follow along.

Guided imagery
Sitting or lying comfortably, start breathing slowly, regularly and deeply. Once you're more relaxed, imagine a calming place — somewhere you feel safe, happy and comfortable. Use all your senses to notice every detail about this great place. What do you see, hear and smell? What do you feel with your hands and under your bare feet? After five or 10 minutes, rouse yourself gradually.

their skin experience allergic reactions, skin irritation or sun sensitivity. If you're considering aromatherapy, consult your health care provider or a trained aromatherapist about the possible risks and benefits.

The bottom line

You may find that you need to experiment with a couple of different approaches to find a combination that works for you. The most important first step is to talk to your health care provider and discuss what strategies might work best. Try to be patient. It often takes a few weeks for some treatments to become effective.

TREATING OBSTRUCTIVE SLEEP APNEA

If you're dealing with insomnia, breathing problems could be behind your interrupted sleep.

Obstructive sleep apnea is a potentially serious sleep disorder in which your breathing repeatedly stops for brief periods of time. The most common form of sleep apnea, obstructive sleep apnea, happens when the tissues and muscles in the back of your throat relax. Your airway narrows or closes, and you can't take in enough air. Your brain senses this inability to breathe and briefly rouses you from sleep so you can reopen your airway. The awakening is usually so brief that you don't remember it. The trouble is, this generally happens multiple times per hour, so the reality is that you aren't getting uninterrupted, good-quality sleep because your brain has fire alarms going off all night. The result is that you wake up feeling like you haven't slept, even if you've been in bed for eight hours.

Among women, sleep apnea is most common in midlife and beyond. After menopause, women develop sleep apnea at a rate similar to men. Most often, the reason is related to weight gain or hormonal changes.

In both men and women, the strongest risk factor for obstructive sleep apnea is obesity. As you may already know, during and after menopause, women tend to gain weight. This includes weight gain in your neck, which can place pressure on your airway. Additionally, the hormonal changes associated with menopause increase your risk of developing sleep apnea.

For milder cases, your health care provider may suggest lifestyle changes, such as losing weight, to improve your sleep. If your symptoms are moderate to severe, other treatments are available.

Devices and procedures

There are a number of different products out there to treat sleep apnea. You can get the following devices from your health care provider.

Continuous positive airway pressure (CPAP) With this treatment, a machine delivers air pressure by way of soft prongs that go into the nostrils or a mask that's placed over your nose while you sleep. The air pressure is just enough to keep your upper airway passages open, preventing apnea. CPAP is the most common and most effective method of treating sleep apnea. Some people, however, find the device cumbersome or uncomfortable, and it takes a while to adjust to wearing it. You may need to try more than one type of mask to find one that's comfortable. A humidifier attached to the CPAP system can help prevent a dry throat or stuffy nose.

Other PAP machines If you can't tolerate CPAP, talk with your doctor about changing to a positive airway pressure machine that delivers a lower pressure when you breathe out (exhale) than when you breathe in (inhale), which may be more comfortable. This is known as a bilevel positive airway pressure (BPAP) machine.

Oral appliances Another option is to use an oral device that positions your lower jaw slightly forward, resulting in a more open airway. Some people find oral appliances to be easier and more comfortable than CPAP. However, the oral appliances may not be effective in everyone, and some patients develop changes in their bites with long-term use. A sleep specialist or qualified dentist can help decide if an oral appliance is right for you.

Upper airway stimulation This new device is approved for use in people with moderate to severe obstructive sleep apnea who can't tolerate CPAP or BPAP. A small, thin impulse generator (hypoglossal nerve stimulator) is implanted under the skin in the upper chest. The device detects your breathing patterns and, when necessary, stimulates the nerve that controls movement of the tongue. Studies have found that upper airway stimulation leads to significant improvement in obstructive sleep apnea symptoms and quality of life.

STRATEGIES FOR OVERCOMING SLEEP APNEA

If your sleep apnea is very mild, you may be able to treat it on your own with some changes to your diet and daily routine. These strategies can improve your sleep:

- Lose excess weight. This step is key. Even a slight loss in weight may help improve sleep apnea. In some cases, returning to a healthy weight can resolve the problem entirely. If you need to lose weight, talk to your doctor about the best type of program for you and how to get started.
- Exercise. Each day, try to get at least 30 minutes of moderate activity, such as a brisk walk. Exercise may help ease obstructive sleep apnea symptoms by helping you lose weight.
- Avoid alcohol and certain medications. Alcohol and medications such as benzodiazepines and sleeping pills relax the muscles in the back of your throat, interfering with breathing.
- Don't sleep on your back. Sleeping on your back can cause your tongue and soft palate to rest against the back of your throat and block your airway. To prevent sleeping on your back, try sewing a tennis ball in the back of your pajama top to keep you from rolling onto your back. Using a body pillow can also help keep you on your side when you sleep.
- Keep your nasal passages open. Use a saline nasal spray or nasal rinse before bed to help open your nasal passages, improving breathing. Don't use nasal decongestants or antihistamines without talking to your doctor. They're generally recommended only for short-term use.

Surgery

Sleep apnea surgery is generally performed only in individuals with severe disease who cannot tolerate CPAP. Surgery may also be recommended for those with certain jaw structure problems. The goal of surgery is to enlarge the airway by removing or tightening tissues and muscles that may block your upper air passages. These procedures may be combined with removal of enlarged tonsils or adenoids.

DEALING WITH RESTLESS LEGS

Restless legs syndrome is a disorder that becomes more common with age. Although the condition hasn't been linked to menopause, it may occur more frequently in women experiencing hot flashes. For some women, part of the reason they have difficulty falling asleep at night is because their legs feel restless and uncomfortable.

People with restless legs syndrome have an uncontrollable urge to move their legs during rest, often with unpleasant sensations in their legs or feet. Symptoms typically develop in the evening or at night while sitting or lying down. Often, getting up and walking will temporarily ease the unpleasant feelings, which are often described as crawling, creeping, antsy, pulling, throbbing, aching or itching.

Medications
Several prescription medications are available that may help reduce the restlessness in your legs. If your symptoms are severe, see your health care provider. You may also be tested for iron deficiency, which can be associated with restless legs symptoms. Some common medications for this condition include:

Anti-convulsants Anti-seizure medications (anti-convulsants) were originally designed to treat people with epilepsy. But the nerve-calming qualities of some of these medications, including gabapentin (Neurontin, Gralise), gabapentin enacarbil (Horizant) and pregabalin (Lyrica), work for some people with restless legs syndrome.

Dopamine-boosters Certain medications increase levels of the chemical messenger dopamine in the brain. Rotigotine (Neupro) and pramipexole (Mirapex) are approved by the FDA for the treatment of moderate to severe restless legs syndrome.

Simple lifestyle changes
The following strategies may help alleviate your symptoms.

Soak in a warm bath. Soaking in a bath and massaging your legs

PERSONAL STORY: CARLISE | AGE 53

" I started menopause at the age of 25 after having a complete hysterectomy. In 1994, I had no clue what life would be like without having ovaries or a uterus. Did not know the meaning of hot flashes or that having low hormone levels would mean my body would be out of its senses. So, as I experienced different types of hormone therapies, I noticed changes in my body, but again I was young and did not really know what the different medications had to do with those changes.

Life went on, and as I reached my late 40s and early 50s, I had started having conversations with my doctor about discontinuing hormone therapy because of the talk of it causing breast cancer. The cancer risk did frighten me a bit, but we decided that we would revisit the conversation later. So, for over 25 years I had been taking [esterified estrogens and methyltestosterone], and I felt fine. Sometimes during the night I would experience some hot flashes.

Fast forward to age 53. At my yearly visit we talked again about me stopping estrogen. I agreed to it. A few weeks later I thought, *what is going on with me*? I was getting up all during the night to pee rivers. I would wake up at 2 a.m. and be up until the next night. My body temperature would hit 100+ degrees without sweating. I was miserable and could not function at all. It was hard for me to concentrate, I was forgetful, and I was moving at a slow pace and very fatigued! It was bad. I sent my doctor an email to inform her I was putting myself back on estrogen, and it was the best decision I ever made. I told her I will die taking this medication because I feel great, and I'm back to feeling 100%.

in the evening can help relax your muscles and ease the restless symptoms.

Apply warm or cool packs. Use of heat or cold, or alternating use of the two, may help lessen the uncomfortable sensations in your legs and feet.

Establish good sleep hygiene. Fatigue also tends to worsen symptoms. If you're overly tired, your symptoms are likely to be worse. Practice good sleep habits (see pages 186–187).

Exercise. Get at least 30 minutes of moderate exercise most days of the week. Exercise helps prevent symptoms.

Avoid caffeine and alcohol. Sometimes cutting back on caffeine improves symptoms. Avoid products with caffeine, including chocolate, coffee, tea and soft drinks, for a few weeks to see if this helps. Also see what happens if you cut out alcohol. Alcohol worsens symptoms in some individuals.

STAY POSITIVE

When you're worn out and grumpy because you're not sleeping well, it's easy to feel down. You might think you'll never sleep well again. Keep in mind that this is a phase in life you're going through. Also keep in mind that the journey doesn't have to be miserable. If a few changes to your evening and nighttime habits aren't helpful, talk to your health care practitioner. Prescription therapies or medication might help get your sleep back in sync so that you can get out and enjoy your life.

12

Changes in sexual health

Menopause is no reason to stop having sex. Women can and do enjoy satisfying sex and intimacy well into old age.

That said, it's common to face some challenges along the way. The transition to menopause may bring about changes in your sex drive, your vagina or your feelings about your own sex appeal. Other aspects of aging can complicate your sex life too. And factors such as depression, the presence of your partner and how important sex was for you before menopause may play an even bigger role than any physical changes.

Sex may be the last thing on your mind right now. If you've been with your partner for a long time, you may actually be grateful that the frequent, feverish trysts of your younger years have transformed into a cooler, easier companionship. Just remember that there's no time limit on feeling sexy or being sexual. Every long-lasting relationship can benefit from butterflies, longing, spontaneity, fun and physical closeness. Sex isn't the only thing that holds two people together, but it can help strengthen your connection.

Of course, women without partners aren't excused from this conversation either. Even if you're not having sex with a partner now, you might continue to be sexual on your own, and you may decide to engage in a sexual relationship at a later time. All women deserve to enjoy sex long after their last menstrual period if they want to.

THE MYTH OF MIDLIFE CHASTITY

Most often, the couples kissing, shedding their clothes, or having sex on TV or in the movies are younger adults. Films featuring older couples are less common. Off-screen, real-life examples of a red-hot older sex life can be hard to come by too. Many people grow up believing that their parents and grandparents aren't having sex. And few parents and grandparents go out of their way to dispute this belief.

Given this dearth of role models, you might think sex naturally ends at a certain point. Nonsense. The truth is that your parents and grandparents probably were (or are!) having sex. People can (and do) have sex right up until they die. In fact, older women may be having sex a lot more than you think. In a study of more than 2,000 women, nearly 60% of those age 60 and older who were married or living with a partner were sexually active. Even among those age 80 and older who had a romantic partner, 37% were sexually active.

Give yourself permission to be sexual well into your golden years. If you need help, talk to your health care provider, a counselor or a sex therapist.

COMMON SEXUAL CHANGES DURING MENOPAUSE

While the belief that all older adults are celibate isn't true, there are some genuine changes that happen during menopause that can alter your sex life. For some women, sex is more enjoyable. Not having to worry about getting pregnant can be liberating and sexy. Some couples also become empty nesters around the time of menopause, and this can add to the sense of feeling uninhibited. When grown children move out, privacy and sexual spontaneity may return. Spur-of-the-moment sex on the couch becomes a real possibility again, even in the afternoon!

However, many women find that they think about sex less often or don't enjoy it as much after menopause. Menopausal changes can contribute to these feelings: For example, decreasing estrogen levels can cause drier vaginal tissues and thinning of the vaginal wall, resulting in painful or uncomfortable sex.

In addition, night sweats can disturb your sleep and make you feel too exhausted or sweaty for sex. Emotional changes can make you feel too stressed for sex. And weight gain can make you feel too uncomfortable with your body image for sex.

How do you know if you have a problem? There's no magical number of times you should have sex each week. The real key is whether sexual changes are troubling to you or your partner. If sexual changes associated with the menopause transition bother you or cause strife in your relationship, that's a problem, and it's time to focus on solutions.

Here's a summary of some of the most common sexual issues that occur at this time.

Low sex drive (low libido)

Fluctuations in your sex drive are a normal part of every relationship and every stage of life. It's common to feel revved up at the beginning of a new relationship or while on a romantic trip. On the flip side, your sex drive may drop after you have a baby or get bored with a relationship.

You should know that there are two types of sexual desire. One is spontaneous desire — this is the biological drive or craving for sex. With this type of desire, you may have sexual thoughts after watching a steamy movie and want to initiate sex with your partner. The other type of desire is called *receptive desire*. In this type of desire, sex isn't on your mind, but the ingredients are in place for you to be willing when your partner initiates or when the right circumstances arise.

Spontaneous desire relies heavily on hormones, and it can plummet for some women as hormone levels shift during menopause. Men also experience a decrease in spontaneous desire with age, but it happens at a much slower rate — more like a slow leak.

If your spontaneous desire for sex declines, it can be difficult to recover. But you can make up for any loss in spontaneous desire by maximizing your receptive desire. How? Optimize all the ingredients that contribute to your willingness to have sex. These ingredients differ among women and are different over time, but they usually fall into four general categories — biological issues, psychological issues, relationship issues and life issues.

Review the list on page 203 and check every issue that's impacting your willingness to be sexual. Add in extra factors of your own. Ask yourself: Which issues on this list jump out? What are the big things that are getting in the way of being sexual? Could I enjoy sexual activity if any of these barriers were removed? For example, could you let everything else go if you felt close to your partner again or if you didn't have pain during intercourse?

Create a plan to address your turnoffs and take full advantage of your receptive desire. When your spontaneous desire was kicking, this conscientious approach to sex probably wasn't necessary. But now, it's essential to recalculate your desire equation. As part of your plan, meet with your health care provider to identify any health conditions or medications that may curb your desire.

Also, be sure to discuss your feelings with your partner. Low sex drive can be very difficult on your relationship. Low desire can make your partner feel rejected, which leads to conflicts or avoidance of the situation. And this type of relationship turmoil can further reduce your desire for sex. Help your partner understand what you're feeling and identify how he or she can help.

Even if you're able to increase your receptive desire, your partner may need to initiate sex for you to be receptive. If this isn't your usual pattern, you may need to change things.

Problems with arousal
Like desire, arousal can also change with menopause. *Arousal* refers to your readiness for sex. During arousal, your breathing and heart rate speed up, your nipples become tingly and erect and the blood flow to your genitals increases. This causes your labia, clitoris and upper vagina to swell in anticipation of sex.

For many women, all of these processes are thwarted during

Biological issues

☐ Vaginal dryness
☐ Sexual pain
☐ Other chronic pain or arthritis
☐ Other health concerns or illnesses
☐ Incontinence
☐ Sleep problems
☐ Low energy or fatigue
☐ Hot flashes
☐ Cardiovascular disease
☐ Medication side effects
☐ Other: _____

Psychological issues

☐ Anxiety
☐ Depression
☐ Stress
☐ History of unwanted sexual experiences
☐ Low self-esteem
☐ Poor body image
☐ Substance abuse
☐ Other: _____

Relationship issues

☐ Unresolved relationship conflicts
☐ Inadequate sexual stimulation
☐ Partner's loss of interest in sex or sexual dysfunction
☐ Partner's renewed interest in sex
☐ Lack of emotional closeness or connectedness
☐ Poor communication
☐ Lack of privacy
☐ Opposing schedules
☐ Other: _____

Life and socioeconomic issues

☐ Stress from caregiving
☐ Work deadlines
☐ Busy schedules
☐ Limited sex education
☐ Conflict with personal, family or religious values
☐ Other: _____

menopause. The decline in estrogen can cause vaginal dryness and reduced blood flow to the vulva, clitoris and vagina, causing arousal to take longer or be harder to achieve.

The sensations and pleasure that you typically experience during sex may change significantly. You may need more time for foreplay and more emphasis on strong clitoral stimulation before jumping into intercourse.

Changes in orgasm

In addition to arousal struggles, there can be changes in orgasm. In particular, the clitoris — a key pleasure zone for most women — can become less sensitive. If you do reach orgasm, it may not be as long or intense as it used to be.

It can be frustrating if your usual lovemaking routine suddenly doesn't do it for you anymore. Take comfort in knowing that there's nothing wrong with you or your partner. This is a normal part of the menopause transition. You can also consider it a license to experiment with new tricks and positions. In addition, you may benefit from vaginal lubricants and moisturizers as well as vibrators to give extra stimulation.

Sexual pain

The medical term for painful intercourse is *dyspareunia* (dis-puh-ROO-nee-uh), which is defined as persistent or recurrent genital pain that occurs just before, during or after intercourse. Many women experience painful intercourse at some point in their lives. Treatments — discussed later in this chapter — focus on the underlying cause of the pain. They can help eliminate or reduce this common problem.

No matter how much you love your partner and want to be intimate, sex should never be painful. If you can't get relief on your own, seek help from your health care practitioner.

Vaginal dryness As you read in Chapter 2, insufficient lubrication is a very common, early sign of menopause. For some women, this early symptom grows to be a severe, distressing problem. And dryness can cause significant discomfort and pain during initial penetration.

Vaginal dryness is commonly part of a larger condition known as genitourinary syndrome of menopause (GSM). As discussed on pages 58–59, in this condition, the vulvar skin becomes thin and dry. Ongoing burning, itching, irritation and even spotting or bleeding can also occur. All these signs and symptoms can dampen your desire or arousal and make sex painful.

Vaginal moisturizers and lubricants are often used as an initial treatment for these conditions. Vaginal estrogen or vaginal treatment with the medication prasterone (Intrarosa), a synthetic version of the hormone dehydroepiandrosterone (DHEA), may be prescribed for moderate to severe cases of GSM. For women taking systemic hormone therapy to manage hot flashes or other symptoms, sometimes a local hormonal treatment is still needed to manage GSM symptoms. The oral medication ospemifene (Osphena) may be another treatment option.

In addition, regular sexual activity or use of a vibrator may be recommended, if you can engage in these activities without pain. Regular, painless sexual activity — including massage and oral stimulation — can help increase arousal and promote blood flow to the genital area, which can help rejuvenate it.

Vulvodynia Chronic pain in the area around the opening of your vagina (vulva) with no observable, physical reason is called *vulvodynia*. The pain, burning, stinging or irritation associated with vulvodynia may be constant or occasional and can last for months to years. You may feel the pain in your entire vulvar area (generalized), or it may be localized to a certain area, such as the opening of your vagina (vestibule). The latter is called *vestibulodynia*. Symptoms can make you so uncomfortable that sitting for long periods is difficult and sex is unthinkable.

Treatment depends on the severity of symptoms but often starts with self-care measures. Try to avoid any vaginal irritants, including soaps, detergents, dryer sheets, moistened wipes, perfumes, douches, spermicides, scented toilet paper, bubble baths and flavored or warming vaginal lubricants. Tightfitting pantyhose and nylon underwear can be problematic too, restricting airflow to your genital area and leading to increased moisture and irritation. Switch to cotton underwear, and consider sleeping with no underwear to promote ventilation and dryness. Clean the affected area with plain water and apply a preservative-free emollient, such as plain petroleum jelly, to create a protective barrier. Cold compresses or warm water baths also may help.

You may need vaginal lubricants and moisturizers to make sex more comfortable. Topical lidocaine may be another option. Your doctor may recommend applying this numbing medication before sexual activity or as needed for comfort. For moderate or severe cases that don't respond to these treatments, it may be necessary to consider topical or oral medications for chronic pain, pelvic floor physical therapy, or even surgery. Pain control takes time, up to 6 weeks or more. You may need to work with a gynecologist or women's health specialist to find the right mix of therapies for you.

Other conditions and surgeries Many conditions and surgical side effects can cause sexual pain. Pain with initial penetration can be caused by scarring from a cut made during childbirth to enlarge the birth canal (episiotomy) or an infection in your genital area or urinary tract. Deep pain can be caused by scarring from pelvic surgery, including hysterectomy, or by cancer treatments. In addition, many gynecological conditions can be to blame, including pelvic floor dysfunction. Work with your health care provider to identify and treat the cause of your pain.

LESBIAN RELATIONSHIPS

Navigating menopausal sex may be significantly harder for lesbian couples than heterosexual couples. Unless there's a big age difference, both women can hit menopause at about the same time. There are many experiences in life that are fun to share with your partner, but menopause may not be one of them.

If you and your partner simultaneously experience menopausal symptoms — including trouble sleeping, irritability, weight gain and vaginal dryness — it can put a lot of stress on your relationship. Plus, you may both lose your spontaneous desire for sex at the same time as estrogen levels drop. So no one is initiating anything.

If you're in this situation, it's important for you and your partner to figure out how to maximize willingness for both of you. A high level of mutual willingness can help offset a loss of spontaneous desire. Review all the issues that can undo your desire for sex, and work diligently to remove these barriers. Working with a counselor or sex therapist can help.

STRATEGIES FOR MORE-SATISFYING SEX

No matter what sexual setbacks you face during menopause, there are many treatments out there. Your health care provider can guide you to the best solution for your situation, but there's little harm in trying a few measures on your own. Think of menopause as an opportunity to revive your sex life and your relationship.

Self-care measures

If you have minor sexual symptoms, this is a good place to start. You can also use self-care measures to protect your sexual health before symptoms begin.

Avoid products that irritate your vagina. This is particularly important for vaginal dryness or irritation, but it's good advice all-around. As mentioned earlier, skip douches, bubble baths, dryer sheets, moistened wipes, perfumes and other irritants. Remember that nylon underwear can be irritating too. Find something sexy in 100% cotton.

Practice pelvic floor (Kegel) exercises. These exercises can increase blood flow to your vagina and strengthen the muscles involved in orgasm. If you need help finding your pelvic floor muscles, stop urination in midstream. But don't do Kegel exercises while you're urinating — only use this technique to isolate the correct muscles. Then, lie on your back and practice contracting the muscles for five seconds and then relaxing them for five seconds. Work up to keeping the muscles contracted for 10 seconds at a time, with 10 seconds in between. Repeat three times a day. Once you've got the technique down, you can do Kegel exercises discreetly just about anywhere.

Exercise. Physical activity can increase your energy, lift your mood and help you feel good about your body.

Avoid smoking and alcohol. Cigarette smoking can reduce blood flow to the vagina and contribute to vaginal dryness. Alcohol can slow down your biological sexual response. You may think that alcohol helps put you in the mood, but the result can be the opposite.

Adjust your attitude. Remember that your brain is your most powerful sexual organ. Focus on your attitude and mindset about sex.

Intimacy boosters

Studies show that postmenopausal women often have better, more frequent sex and fewer sexual symptoms when they have a new lover. This underlines the fact that novelty, excitement and emotional closeness can increase sexual intimacy. If you've been in a relationship for a while, focus on rekindling some magic with your partner:

Make your partner a priority. Take time to enjoy each other and nurture your relationship. Go for a long walk or bike ride together. Make a date night at your favorite restaurant. Solve the Saturday crossword puzzle together. Any of these activities that you enjoy are good foreplay. Even a morning kiss, a funny midday text exchange, an evening walk or a shared dinner can help you feel more connected to your partner, which can lead to better sexual intimacy.

Make sex a priority. Try to have sex more often. Plan an overnight trip so you have time to rediscover one another without the distractions of home and work. Or set aside time at home when both of you like to have sex. That might mean changing your schedule so that you can have sex in the morning when you're both well rested.

In general, your vagina will lose elasticity if you don't use it. Regular sexual activity can increase blood flow to your vagina and help keep tissues healthy. Just remember that you shouldn't tolerate painful sex. If you have pain during intercourse, prioritize other ways to be sexual while you treat the source of your pain.

Communicate your needs. Take time to understand the physical and emotional changes that you and your partner are facing and how they impact your sexual needs. You should be able to talk about sex just like you talk about finances or housework. However, both men and women often have difficulty expressing their sexual preferences out loud. If you're struggling to talk about your desires and needs, start by talking about what you don't want. Which positions no longer feel good? What time of day would you prefer not to have sex? This is often an easier way to start talking about sex, and the conversation can broaden from there.

Good sexual communication is the process of realizing that you can share your desires with your partner without judgment. Talking with your partner can strengthen your sexual relationship and your overall connection. Good communication is also associated with higher sexual satisfaction. If you need help, consider scheduling an appointment with a counselor or sex therapist.

Take it slow. If your partner wants to have sex as soon as he gets an erection, you are likely being deprived of the extended foreplay that you need to feel aroused and satisfied. Try slowing things way down.

If you're not sure how, try sensate focus exercises. These exercises involve a series of progressive touching activities designed to help build intimacy. Sensate focus exercises generally follow several phases. In the first phases, you and your partner focus on touching and caressing each other and exploring the sensations and emotions you feel. In a later phase, you may add in nonpenetrative sexual activities, followed by penetrative sexual activities in the final phase. Sensate focus exercises are a good way for you and your partner to schedule quality, intimate time together. They purposely take away the pressure of penetrative sex and orgasm and help you become comfortable with physical intimacy. See pages 210–211 for instructions.

Venture beyond your usual. Try having sex in new positions or different rooms in your house — or outside your house (perhaps a hotel, your backyard or the back of your car). Buy some new lingerie. Plan an erotic surprise, such as a candlelit bath for two or a racy movie. Rekindle your sense of daring and excitement.

Broaden your definition of sex. Many heterosexual couples define sex as penile-vaginal penetration. That's a very narrow definition. There are many other ways to be sexual and sensual. If you have vaginal pain and your partner has erectile problems, you're going to have to rethink what "sex" means for your relationship. If you're not having problems with penetration, you may still find it enjoyable to broaden your horizons as you age.

Need some ideas? The shortlist might include giving or getting a hickey, tickling, massage, dry humping, masturbating in front of your partner, mutual masturbation, oral sex, manual sex (with hands or fingers) or allowing your partner to ejaculate on your stomach. Biting, spanking, blindfolds, toys and objects that restrict movement can also be part of a satisfying nonpenetrative sexual encounter. Not "going all the way" doesn't have to be G-rated. In fact, taking penetration off the table can force you to be more adventurous and creative, which can also enhance arousal.

Share the work of having good sex. If you're struggling with menopausal symptoms, you may be exhausted at the "chore" of figuring out how to rehab your sex life. Shoulder the load with your partner. Split the duties of buying lubricants or a vibrator or scheduling an appointment with a sex therapist. It takes two to tango.

Lubricants, moisturizers and vibrators

Many couples find that lubricants are a must for midlife sex. If you haven't needed a lubricant before, don't be timid about trying it now.

SENSATE FOCUS EXERCISES

Sensate focus exercises may be one tool to help couples feel connected and revive or expand sensuality. The goal is not to experience erotic feelings or even feelings of pleasure. Rather, it's meant to help you learn about your own bodily responses and feelings. It can also help you stay tuned into your body when your mind is active or distracted.

In addition, sensate focus can help you accept both giving and receiving. It shows that touching can be just as intimate as intercourse — sometimes even more so. Eventually, a couple may experience erotic feelings arising from touch without pressure. But in the first phases of sensate focus, outlined below, try not to let it turn into a sexual experience.

Instructions for sensate focus:
1. Arrange for one hour of complete privacy when you are not exhausted.
2. Set the mood for relaxation by sitting on the couch together, perhaps sharing a meal. Mood music and low lighting are OK.
3. The temperature should be arranged for comfort.
4. Alcohol or recreational drug use is not suggested.
5. Clothing should be off as much as possible; electronics should be off and pets elsewhere.
6. Relax together first, then have one person touch the other for 5 to 15 minutes, then switch. Using hands and fingers only, focus your attention on the sensations of temperature, texture and pressure as you touch your partner for your interest, not for his or her pleasure.
7. Do this without words, kissing or full-body contact.

Pay particular attention to:

Temperature. Where is your partner warmer or cooler? Does that change?

Texture. Of hair, of skin. Where are they smoother and rougher? What are the textures?

Pressure. How does it feel to you when you use a firmer or lighter touch?

Tips for the *giver*:
1. Position your body to comfortably touch your partner.
2. Initiate by saying "I'd like to touch now." The receiver can decline, but he or she is then to set another time.
3. Be concerned with your own feelings and sensations rather than those of your partner. Trust that your partner will protect you from doing anything uncomfortable by communicating that to you — nonverbally if possible.
4. Bring any wandering thoughts back to temperature, texture and pressure.
5. Touch long enough to get over any initial feelings of discomfort but not so long as to get tired or bored (at least 3 to 5 minutes).

Tips for the *receiver*:
1. Get as relaxed as possible. Begin in any position that's comfortable, and move as you wish.
2. Focus on your feelings coming in, and don't be concerned with what your partner is experiencing. Bring yourself back from distractions and protect your partner by acknowledging — nonverbally if possible — if something is psychologically or physically uncomfortable.

After the exchange of touch, spend time as a couple talking about the experience. Sensate focus exercises should be made a priority one or two times a week.

Relying on a bottle for adequate lubrication is not a failure on your part — or your partner's.

Vaginal lubricants reduce the friction associated with thin, dry genital tissue. They're an effective way to provide temporary relief from vaginal dryness and pain before and during sex.

Steer clear of oil-based lubricants (such as petroleum jelly or baby oil); they can cause vaginal irritation and are not compatible with latex condoms. Instead, choose a water- or silicone-based lubricant. The silicone version lasts longer and is generally slicker, which may be good if you have significant vaginal dryness. Silicone lubricants may also be better for water play and for anal sex. However, if you use a sex toy made of silicone, the silicone lubricant may degrade the silicone toy. In addition, the long-lasting extra-slipperiness of a silicone-based lubricant may be enjoyable for you but could negatively affect your partner's erection, especially if he has trouble with erectile dysfunction. In these cases, water-based lubricants may be better.

Many women are hesitant to use lubricants because they believe pausing to worry about gel can kill the moment. However, there are many ways to make adequate lubrication part of your sexual activity, rather than a disruption to the main event. For best results, you'll want lubricant in your vagina, on your vulva and on your partner's penis right before sex. Experiment with applying lubricant on one another as part of your foreplay. Your partner may also enjoy watching you apply lubricant.

If you have vaginal dryness, GSM, arousal difficulties or pain during sex, you may also need a vaginal moisturizer. You apply this product several times a week to moisturize vaginal tissues over time. This can offer longer term relief from vaginal dryness. However, you'll still need a vaginal lubricant right before sex.

Vibrators are another thing to stash in your nightstand drawer, next to the lubricant. As your vagina and clitoris become less sensitive over time, you may need more stimulation to achieve arousal and orgasm. This is where a vibrator comes in handy.

Look for a silicone, battery-powered version that can be used for internal and external stimulation. Try it out on your own before you bring it into bed with your partner. There is no wrong way to use a vibrator. You can use it all over your vulva, thighs, clitoris and other erogenous zones. Experiment with different intensities and areas of your body to see what feels good to you. If you have a waterproof vibrator, the bathtub can be a relaxing, private space to practice. Once you're comfortable, introduce the vibrator into your relationship and show your partner what you like. The more you practice on your own and teach your partner, the easier it will be for you to reach orgasm. Your vibrator can also be used to stimulate your partner.

If vibrators seem risqué to you or you're concerned that they don't align with your values, give it some thought. What are your sexual values? Do you value monogamy? Do you value mutual sexual pleasure? What else? List your values and think about whether a vibrator fits in or not. Many women decide that using a vibrator with a committed partner in a consensual, enjoyable way is actually in line with their sexual values.

MEDICATIONS

If you can't get sufficient relief from other measures, you may benefit from a prescription medication. Many medications for sexual symptoms are also remedies for other symptoms of menopause and are discussed in greater detail in Chapters 6 and 7. But here's a brief overview.

Estrogen

Since declining estrogen is at the heart of vaginal dryness related to menopause, it's no surprise that estrogen can help restore vaginal moisture and reduce pain with sex. It's unclear if estrogen can help boost libido and sex drive.

Estrogen can be delivered throughout your whole body (systemically) by pill, patch, spray or gel. However, there are some risks associated with systemic estrogen. As a result, it's typically reserved for women who need it to treat other menopause symptoms, such as hot flashes and night sweats.

If vaginal dryness is your only symptom, a better option is a smaller dose of estrogen concentrated right where you need it — in the form of a vaginal cream or a slow-releasing suppository or ring that you place in your vagina. These forms can restore blood flow to the vagina and improve the suppleness and stretchiness of vaginal tissues in postmenopausal women. Low-dose vaginal estrogen can also reverse thinning and dryness and give longer term relief than do vaginal lubricants or moisturizers. All these benefits come without the risks associated with systemic estrogen. You'll need a prescription for any form of vaginal estrogen.

A vaginal cream is applied in the vagina in small amounts, daily for the first two weeks and then 2 to 3 times a week. It's best to avoid using it within a couple of hours before sex with your partner. You may still need to use a vaginal lubricant right before sex.

A softgel capsule or a tablet is placed into your vagina using your finger or an applicator. Initially, a new capsule or tablet is inserted once a day for two weeks, then twice a week. The capsule or tablet dissolves inside your vagina.

A low-dose vaginal ring is inserted into your vagina and worn for three months before being removed and replaced. (*Note:* There is also a ring that delivers a systemic dose of estrogen. Don't confuse a low-dose vaginal ring with a systemic estrogen ring.)

Another option is the drug ospemifene (Osphena). This medication is approved to treat moderate to severe pain during sex caused by vaginal dryness. Ospemifene is a selective estrogen receptor modulator (SERM) that acts like estrogen on the vaginal lining in some ways. But the risks are not quite the same, and hot flashes may be a side effect.

Dehydroepiandrosterone (DHEA)

DHEA is a natural substance produced by your adrenal gland and ovaries that your body then turns into estrogen and testosterone. Vaginal preparations of DHEA have been shown to be effective for treating vaginal dryness. A vaginal insert DHEA, prasterone (Intrarosa), is approved by the FDA. It is inserted nightly.

However, there is little solid evidence for oral DHEA supplements or products available without a prescription, which have been promoted for anti-aging properties and for boosting sexual desire.

It's worth noting, though, that if you're trying to bolster your sexual arousal along with relieving dryness, you'll need to find and treat any other potential causes — such as stress or anxiety — as well.

Testosterone

Traditionally, testosterone has been referred to as a male sex hormone. But testosterone is also present in women, in smaller amounts. Testosterone has been shown to improve sexual interest, desire and orgasm in some postmenopausal women.

Prescription testosterone skin patches and gels developed for men contain doses that are inappropriately high for women. However, topical testosterone may be recommended for women in one specific circumstance: if they have been diagnosed with low sexual desire with no underlying cause. In this use, it has been shown to be effective.

There are still concerns about the long-term safety and effectiveness of testosterone in women. For this reason, it isn't recommended for most women in menopause.

WHEN YOUR PARTNER HAS ERECTILE DYSFUNCTION

Erectile dysfunction (impotence) is the inability to get and keep an erection firm enough for sex. It's common in older men.

If you're fortunate enough not to have sexual problems of your own, your partner's erectile dysfunction can still be a problem, leaving you both frustrated and dissatisfied.

Sexual dysfunction in either partner also can contribute to the other's problems with arousal or orgasm. It can be a cycle. Treating your partner's erectile problems can be a critical step in improving your sexual satisfaction.

Ironically, the cure can bring about a new set of issues. If you haven't had intercourse for a while because of erectile dysfunction, the vagina may have lost some of its elasticity and lubrication. You may not be ready for sex as quickly as your partner is. You and your partner may need to ease back into the saddle and learn how to be sexually active again in a way that is pleasurable for both of you.

SAFE SEX

The hot sex of a new relationship doesn't depend on age — you can get swept up in the moment at 55 just like at 25. But if you're having sex of any kind with new sexual partners or with a partner who has other partners, protection is a priority.

In fact, if you've been through menopause and you're not using some form of estrogen, your vaginal tissue may be more vulnerable to a sexually transmitted infection (STI) than it was before menopause. That's because the vaginal walls can be thinner and more delicate after menopause, leaving them prone to small tears and cuts that can act as pathways for infection.

Make sure you're taking steps to have safer sex:

Test for STIs and communicate openly. Ideally, you should both get tested for STIs before having sex. If that's not going to happen, then it's critical to discuss sexual history with your partner.

Insist that male partners always use a new latex condom for each sex act. Do this until you're sure that your partner is disease-free and your relationship has developed into a long-term, mutually monogamous thing. Condoms aren't foolproof, but they're highly effective for reducing transmission of some STIs when used correctly.

Use dental dams. A dental dam is a thin square of latex rubber that you place over your vagina to enjoy oral sex without exchange of bodily fluids. It should be used for oral sex with both female and male partners.

Have an annual physical exam, and get screened for STIs. Sexual infections often have no signs or symptoms until serious complications develop, so regular testing is the best way to detect a problem. Also talk to your doctor about other ways to protect yourself from STIs. You may need a Pap test and HPV testing or a hepatitis B vaccine, if yours isn't up to date.

Limit your cocktails. When you're under the influence of alcohol, you're more likely to take sexual risks.

Flibanserin

The medication flibanserin (Addyi) was approved by the FDA in 2015 to treat a small, select group of premenopausal women who have been diagnosed with low sexual desire. In these women, the switch is just turned off for no clear reason. This drug is not recommended for women who take certain medications that are metabolized by the liver or have liver impairment. And it shouldn't be taken within two hours after drinking alcohol.

Vyleesi

Bremelanotide injection (Vyleesi) is another prescription medication to boost women's libido, approved by the FDA in 2019. It can treat low sex drive in some women who don't have other problems contributing to low sexual desire. However, this drug is only approved for use in premenopausal women.

BE PATIENT WITH YOURSELF

The female sexual response is complicated. Sexual desire for women depends not just on blood flow and biological issues but also on psychological issues, relationship issues and life issues. In addition, the female sexual response is far more subjective and less measurable than the quality of a penile erection. So as potential new treatments are tested, achieving a meaningful sexual effect might mean different things for different women.

Try to be patient. If the entire pharmaceutical industry hasn't found a cure-all for women's sexual dysfunction, you can't possibly be expected to remedy your own problems overnight.

Take time to identify your symptoms and try out various self-care measures and other treatments. You can have satisfying sex long after menopause, especially if you're willing to adjust your ideas about sex and try new things. It may not be exactly as it was in your younger years, but it can still be mind-blowing.

13

Pelvic issues

The hormone estrogen has wide-ranging effects. During perimeno-pause and menopause, when estrogen production begins to decline, a number of changes can take place in a woman's body. In addition to the conditions discussed in previous chapters, menopause may lead to changes in your urinary system, resulting in bladder control problems and greater susceptibility to urinary tract infections. If you haven't been bothered by bladder problems before, this can be frustrating. Fortunately, there are many options for treating and managing urinary conditions. Bladder-related troubles shouldn't in any way slow you down or interfere with your daily life.

Meanwhile, other conditions that plague some women during their reproductive years, such as uterine fibroids and heavy menstrual bleeding, typically improve during perimenopause and menopause. If you continue to experience vaginal bleeding or pelvic pressure or pain during menopause, it's important to see your health care provider to find the cause of your symptoms.

AN ANATOMY LESSON

To better understand urinary incontinence and other pelvic conditions, it helps to have some basic knowledge of key organs and structures.

Urinary tract

Your urinary system has two main parts — upper and lower. The upper urinary tract consists of two kidneys, each attached to a long, muscular tube called a *ureter*. The kidneys are your body's primary filtration system, removing excess fluid and waste from your bloodstream to make urine. The ureters carry the urine to the bladder, delivering it in small, steady amounts.

Your lower urinary tract consists of the bladder, a slender drainage tube at the bladder's base called the *urethra* and two ringlike bands of

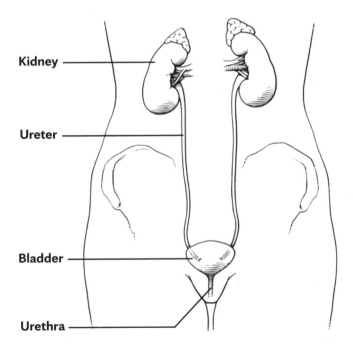

Kidney

Ureter

Bladder

Urethra

The upper urinary tract consists of two kidneys, each attached to a long, muscular tube called a *ureter*. Your lower urinary tract consists of the bladder and two ringlike bands of muscles known as the urethral sphincters.

muscles at the junction of the bladder and the urethra known as the internal and external urethral sphincters. Nerves carry signals from your bladder to your brain to let you know when your bladder is full. Your brain responds back to your bladder when it's time to urinate.

When you urinate, your bladder muscle contracts, pushing urine out of the bladder and through the urethra. The urethral sphincters help control the release of urine. The internal sphincter, composed of muscles that you can't control, keeps your urethra closed while your bladder is filling. The external sphincter, operated by muscles that you can control, helps you keep your urethra closed until you can get to a bathroom. At that time, both sphincters relax, allowing urine to flow out of the bladder and into the urethra.

Pelvic floor muscles

The pelvic floor muscles play a supporting role in the storage and release of urine. This hammock-like network of muscles extends from

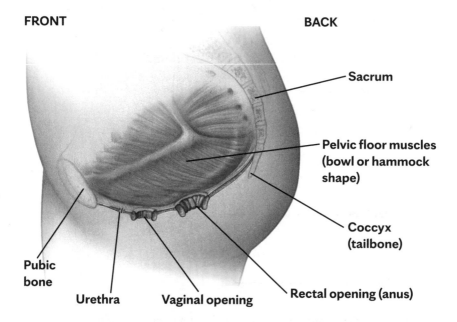

FRONT   **BACK**

Sacrum

Pelvic floor muscles (bowl or hammock shape)

Coccyx (tailbone)

Pubic bone

Urethra   Vaginal opening   Rectal opening (anus)

The pelvic floor muscles are a hammock-like network of muscles that extends from your pubic bone in the front of your pelvis to your tailbone at the base of your spine.

your pubic bone in the front of your pelvis to your tailbone at the base of your spine. The muscles also extend sideways and attach to the inside of your pelvic bones.

Strong pelvic floor muscles are very important for normal bladder function. When you urinate, the pelvic floor muscles relax, allowing urine to pass out of your body easily. When you're not urinating, the pelvic floor muscles lightly contract, holding urine in. These muscles have several other functions. They help support your abdominal organs and your back, they contract and relax in order to maintain normal bowel function, and they help make sexual intercourse satisfying and pleasurable. Because these muscles are under voluntary control, they can be strengthened with exercise.

Female reproductive system
The female reproductive system is composed of those organs associated with childbearing. It's largely located behind the bladder and just

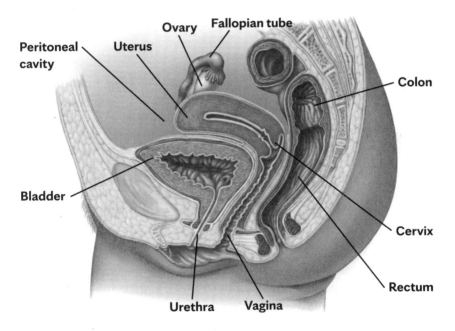

The female reproductive system consists of two ovaries, two fallopian tubes, the uterus and the external genitals.

above the pelvic floor. This system consists of two ovaries, two fallopian tubes, the uterus and the external genitals.

The ovaries produce the hormones estrogen, progesterone and testosterone and house the female eggs (ova). Each month during ovulation, one of the ovaries releases an egg into the adjacent fallopian tube. The egg travels down the tube and into the uterus.

The uterus is a pear-shaped organ with thick walls, primarily composed of powerful muscles. When a fertilized egg reaches the uterus, it implants itself within the uterine wall and begins to develop into a baby. If the egg isn't fertilized, it degenerates and the lining of the uterus is shed during menstruation. The narrow neck of the uterus, which opens (dilates) to allow the passage of a baby, is called the *cervix*.

The external genitals — the mons pubis, labia majora and labia minora, clitoris and vaginal opening (vestibule) — are called the *vulva*. These structures are composed mainly of fatty tissue. They also contain glands that secrete substances to lubricate the vaginal opening.

URINARY TRACT INFECTIONS

Urinary tract infections (UTIs) are a well-known problem for millions of women. You may have first experienced a UTI when you became sexually active. Perhaps you didn't experience a UTI for several years after learning a few basic steps to help prevent such infections. Now, as you enter menopause, you're experiencing UTIs again. Why?

During menopause and in the years that follow, some women experience an increase in the frequency of UTIs. Menopausal changes in hormone levels can cause urethral tissues to become more vulnerable to infection, which can then spread up to the bladder. You're also more likely to experience UTIs after menopause if you battled recurrent UTIs in your younger years or if you have a health condition that increases your susceptibility to infection, such as diabetes.

Infection limited to your urethra and bladder can be painful and annoying. However, serious consequences can occur if the infection spreads to your kidneys. So, if you experience signs and symptoms of a UTI — a strong and frequent urge to urinate, a burning sensation when you urinate, urine that appears cloudy or has a strong odor — don't ignore them.

Getting treatment

Antibiotics are typically used to treat UTIs. The type of drug prescribed and how long you need to take it will depend on the type of bacteria found in your urine and your overall health. Usually, symptoms clear within a couple of days. Drink plenty of fluids, and make sure to take the entire course of antibiotics prescribed by your health care provider to ensure that the infection is completely gone.

If UTIs become a frequent problem, your health care provider may recommend a longer course of antibiotic treatment. If your infections are related to sexual activity, he or she may recommend that after sexual intercourse you take a single dose of an antibiotic.

Another option to help minimize UTIs is vaginal estrogen therapy. Vaginal estrogen helps restore the health of urinary tract tissues, making them less vulnerable to infection. It's also thought to encourage the production of infection-fighting substances in the bladder. Vaginal estrogen is available in the form of a cream, a gel capsule or small tablet inserted into the vagina, or a ring.

CRANBERRY JUICE AND SUPPLEMENTS

There's some indication that cranberry juice may have infection-fighting properties, and drinking it daily may help prevent UTIs. In healthy women who have had a UTI in the past, drinking one 8-ounce serving may be enough to have a benefit. Limited research also suggests that 500 milligrams (mg) of a cranberry dietary supplement could help reduce the chance of future UTIs. If you like 100% cranberry juice and you feel it helps prevent UTIs, there's little harm in continuing to drink it, but watch the calories. For most people, drinking cranberry juice is safe, but some people report an upset stomach or diarrhea.

With vaginal therapy, a minimal amount of estrogen is absorbed into the bloodstream, but much less than with oral (systemic) estrogen therapy. The absorption generally happens in the first few weeks of treatment when the tissues are very thin and dry. After vaginal tissue becomes more plump and full, absorption of estrogen in the bloodstream is thought to be minimal. As a result, there's a much lower risk of potential side effects.

UNDERSTANDING INCONTINENCE

Another problem that becomes more common around the time of menopause is urinary incontinence, the leakage of urine as a result of decreased bladder control. It can be frustrating and embarrassing, but it's a common issue. And it's treatable, so discuss your situation with your health care provider.

About half of women who are middle-aged and older experience some degree of urinary incontinence at some point. In addition, women may experience fecal incontinence, the leakage of stool.

There are several reasons incontinence is so common in women. First off, a woman's urethra is much shorter than a man's. That means urine has a shorter distance to travel to cause leakage.

For many women, incontinence may develop because of a combination of the following factors.

Pregnancy and childbirth They can weaken or damage the pelvic floor muscles, which support the uterus, bladder and bowel. Pregnancy and childbirth can also weaken the urethral sphincters and the anal sphincter. In addition, childbirth can damage nerves in the pelvis, affecting the overall function of the pelvic floor muscles. Oftentimes, the nerve damage doesn't become noticeable until later in life when women begin to lose muscle mass. The change in muscle mass tips the scale enough to cause leakage.

Family history Your genetics may play a role in bladder control. Women whose mothers or older sisters are incontinent are more likely to develop urinary incontinence.

Menopause Some studies suggest a direct link between decreased production of estrogen and the development of incontinence. The

TYPES OF URINARY INCONTINENCE

Not all incontinence is the same. Bladder leakage can happen for different reasons. The most common types of incontinence include:

- **Stress incontinence.** Urine leaks when you exert pressure on the bladder by coughing, laughing, exercising or lifting something heavy.
- **Urge incontinence.** You have a sudden, intense urge to urinate followed by an involuntary loss of urine. You may need to urinate often, including throughout the night. These symptoms are often referred to as an *overactive bladder*.
- **Overflow incontinence.** You experience frequent or constant dribbling of urine due to a bladder that doesn't empty completely.
- **Mixed incontinence.** You have more than one type of incontinence.

decline in estrogen associated with menopause is thought to affect the organs and tissues of the lower urinary tract. The linings of the bladder and urethra become less elastic, and the urethral sphincters (internal and external) are less able to stay closed. But not all studies agree with this theory. Instead, they point to natural aging as the main reason women become incontinent. And other recent research suggests that oral hormone therapy may increase the risk of urinary incontinence.

Aging Urinary incontinence isn't a normal part of aging — that is, it doesn't naturally occur in all individuals — but it is more common with age. As you get older, the muscles in your bladder and urethra can lose some of their strength. Because of this, your bladder may not be able to hold as much urine as it once did, meaning you have to urinate more often or risk leakage. In addition, with age, your pelvic floor muscles may weaken, making it more difficult to hold in urine. Some research also suggests that your bladder muscle can become overactive as you age. An overactive bladder muscle creates the urge to urinate, even when your bladder isn't full.

Weight gain In general, the more you weigh, the more likely you are to experience urinary incontinence. Being significantly overweight puts increased pressure on your bladder and surrounding muscles, structures and nerves, weakening them and allowing urine to leak, especially when you cough or sneeze. This type of incontinence is known as *stress incontinence.*

Weight gain is a common problem among women going through perimenopause and menopause. If your weight has increased and you're finding yourself dealing with more problems related to bladder control, there may be a link between the two.

FINDING RELIEF FROM INCONTINENCE

Whether your incontinence is more of an annoyance or severe enough that you're afraid to leave the house without a change of clothing, there are steps you can take to manage or treat the problem. Bladder leakage is not something you need to live with, and it shouldn't keep you from leading an active life.

There are a variety of treatments for incontinence. The one that's best for you depends on the type of incontinence you have and how much it affects your daily life. Most health care providers begin with conservative treatments that are noninvasive or minimally invasive and that have few side effects. If this approach doesn't work, you and your provider may want to consider other treatment options.

Lifestyle changes
It's possible that changes in your daily routine may be the only treatment needed to manage your incontinence. Many times, some fairly easy changes can improve symptoms.

The types and amount of fluid you drink each day, as well as the types of food you eat, can influence your bladder habits. Too much or too little fluid can lead to or worsen incontinence. Certain foods can also irritate the bladder and increase urinary frequency, urgency and leakage.

Pay attention to fluids. Drinking too much fluid can make you urinate more often. Excess fluid can also overwhelm your bladder and create a strong sense of urgency — that feeling of needing to go, now! In general, aim for 40 to 60 ounces of fluid daily (about 5 to 7 8-ounce glasses) spread throughout the day. If you get up several times at night to urinate, try drinking most of your fluids in the morning and afternoon.

Surprisingly, drinking too little fluid can cause problems too. Too little fluid can cause your urine to become overly concentrated with your body's waste products. Concentrated urine can irritate your bladder, increasing the urge and frequency with which you need to urinate. It may also put you at risk of a urinary tract infection.

Avoid irritating foods and beverages. Certain foods and beverages can irritate your bladder. Caffeine and alcohol both act as diuretics, which means they increase urine production. This can lead to problems with needing to go to the bathroom often and quickly.

Consuming too many acidic fruits and juices — orange, grapefruit, lemon, lime — may also irritate your bladder. So may spicy foods, tomato-based products, sparkling water and other carbonated drinks.

If any of these items are a regular part of your diet, try eliminating them for a week or two and see if your symptoms improve. Cut out only one food or beverage at a time so that you can tell which one might be causing the problem.

It may also help to pay attention to any foods that cause constipation. Constipation can make urinary incontinence worse.

Check your medications. Some medications, including high blood pressure drugs and heart medications, contribute to incontinence in a variety of ways. They may relax the bladder muscle or the urethral sphincters, cause overproduction of urine, or trigger a chronic cough that can worsen stress incontinence. If you're taking a medication that you think may be contributing to your bladder problems, discuss this with your health care provider.

Lose weight. As mentioned earlier, being overweight can increase the pressure on your abdomen and the structures in your pelvis, including your bladder. Losing weight has been shown to improve symptoms of incontinence, especially in women with stress incontinence. In one study in which overweight women with stress incontinence took part in a weight-loss program, the women experienced more than a 70% reduction in episodes of urine leakage as their weight decreased.

Behavioral modification

In addition to conservative measures, there are a few other strategies that can help bladder control problems. Your health care provider may suggest the following techniques.

Bladder training Bladder training is intended to improve symptoms related to needing to go to the bathroom frequently. Its purpose is to delay urination when you get the urge to go. You may start by trying to hold off for 10 minutes every time you feel an urge to urinate. The goal is to lengthen the time between trips to the toilet until you're urinating only every 2 to 4 hours.

Double voiding Double voiding is used among women who feel they aren't able to empty their bladders completely when urinating. The

MAKE SURE IT'S THE RIGHT PAD

Protective pads can help you stay dry and remain active while you take steps to manage and improve your bladder control problems. Most absorbent pads are no bulkier than normal underwear, and you can wear them easily under everyday clothing.

Make certain you purchase products specifically for urine leakage. Don't use menstrual pads because they don't absorb the urine and keep it away from your skin as well as pads designed for bladder control problems. Also avoid pads that contain dyes or perfumes, which can be irritating to your skin.

Absorbent products for urinary incontinence include liners, pads, disposable underwear and reusable underwear. In addition to pulling the moisture away from your skin, these products help control odor. Look for products with a natural odor-absorbing compound, such as baking soda.

process involves urinating, then waiting a few minutes and trying again.

Scheduled toilet trips This technique can help with all forms of incontinence. Instead of waiting for the feeling that you need to go to the bathroom, make it a habit to urinate every 2 to 4 hours.

Pelvic floor muscle exercises

A big part of relieving incontinence, especially stress incontinence that becomes more common with menopause, is to develop strong and well-coordinated pelvic floor muscles. The pelvic floor muscles help control the release of urine, and like other muscles, they can weaken over time as a result of childbirth, surgery and aging. By strengthening the muscles, you can improve bladder control and reduce urine leakage. When done properly, pelvic floor muscle exercises, also known as Kegels, can be as effective as medications in improving symptoms, if not more so.

How to do them The first step is to know which muscles to tighten. To find them, imagine that you're urinating and you need to stop the urine flow. Squeeze and lift your vaginal area without tightening your buttocks or belly. You should sense a pulling up and in or closing in of your genital area when you squeeze. These are the muscles you want to tighten. One way to figure out if you're using the right muscles is to place a finger inside your vagina and then squeeze so that you feel the muscles tightening around your finger.

There are different types of strengthening exercises for your pelvic floor muscles. Some promote muscle endurance, while others are designed for a rapid response.

- **Holding (endurance) exercises.** Once you know which muscles are involved, practice tightening (contracting) them every day. Slowly, tighten, lift and draw in your pelvic floor muscles and hold them for a count of 10. Relax, then repeat. At first, you may not be able to hold the contractions for a full 10 seconds. Start by holding them for one or two seconds, and gradually increase the contraction time over a period of several weeks. Your goal is to be able to do 10 contractions in a row, holding each contraction for 10 seconds at a time and resting for up to 10 seconds between contractions. Do this exercise three times a day, every day if possible, but no less than four days a week.

- **Quick flick (coordination) exercises.** With this variation, you contract and release your pelvic floor muscles without holding the contraction. Quickly tighten them, lift them up and let them go. Do this 10 times in a row. You want to do quick flicks after doing endurance exercises. Try to do them three times a day.
- **Urge control ("freeze and squeeze") exercises.** This technique can be used when you feel a sudden, strong urge to urinate. First, stop and stand very still. Sit down if you can. Contract your pelvic floor muscles and hold for 10 seconds. Take a deep breath and let the air out. Try to think of something other than going to the bathroom. Contract your muscles again if you need to. When you feel the urge has lessened, walk normally to the bathroom. If the urge happens again on the way, stop and repeat the exercise.

When to do them You can do pelvic floor muscle exercises any time and place: while you're standing by the sink washing dishes, while you're in the car traveling to and from work, when you're watching TV or talking on the phone, or when you're in the shower. A simple way to get started is to do your first round of exercises while getting ready in the morning, with another round after lunch and the last set of repetitions in the evening while relaxing. If you find yourself forgetting to do the exercises and need reminders during the day, there are apps for that!

If you're having trouble If you're finding it difficult to identify and contract the right muscles, your health care practitioner may suggest that you work with a pelvic physical therapist. When you meet with a therapist, he or she will examine your pelvic floor muscles and experiment with various techniques to help you learn how to contract these muscles. The two of you will set up a plan of care individualized to your specific needs. Treatment options may include education, behavioral modification, muscle exercises and instruction in breathing and relaxation techniques.

Benefits Studies show that if done correctly, pelvic floor muscle exercises can be effective in reducing or preventing urine leakage when you cough, sneeze or laugh. When you feel a sneeze or cough coming on or you know you're going to laugh, contract your pelvic floor muscles to hold in urine. The exercises can also help hold in urine when you have a sudden urge to go to the bathroom.

WHEN THE MUSCLES ARE TOO TIGHT

Some women experience a condition in which the opposite happens. Instead of relaxing and losing their strength, the pelvic floor muscles become too tight. Called *nonrelaxing pelvic floor dysfunction*, this condition often develops gradually. It may result from an injury to the pelvic floor due to trauma or surgery. Some cases are thought to result from chronic holding — think of nurses on a long work shift. Conditions that cause intercourse to be painful (dyspareunia) may lead to involuntary tightening of the muscles.

Symptoms of nonrelaxing pelvic floor dysfunction generally include pain and problems when passing stool or urine, pain during or after intercourse and low back pain. Some women experience symptoms early in life, others not until later on. During menopause, changes in the pelvic floor are common.

If you're experiencing these symptoms, your health care provider may recommend that you see a pelvic physical therapist. A therapist can help you learn how to relax and gently stretch your pelvic floor muscles. Devices and processes sometimes used to help stretch the muscles include dilators and the deep heating of tissues (diathermy).

Most women begin to notice an improvement after a few weeks of practicing pelvic floor muscle exercises regularly. It's the same as going to the gym — it takes time to build muscle! If you have severe leakage, the exercises may be less helpful, and you may need other forms of treatment to improve your symptoms.

Medications

Sometimes medications are prescribed to help treat incontinence. In general, medications are more effective for reducing symptoms of urge incontinence than stress incontinence. A class of medications known as anti-cholinergics may be recommended to help calm an overactive bladder. Examples include the drugs oxybutynin (Ditropan XL), tolterodine (Detrol) and solifenacin (Vesicare).

The drug mirabegron (Myrbetriq) may also be used to treat urge incontinence. It relaxes the bladder muscle and can increase the amount of urine your bladder can hold. It may also increase the amount you're able to urinate at one time, helping to empty your bladder more completely.

A low-dose, topical estrogen in the form of a vaginal cream, ring, gel capsule or tablet may be used to help restore the health of tissues in the urethra and vaginal areas. Topical estrogen is generally more effective in reducing symptoms of urge incontinence than of stress incontinence. Estrogen taken orally in pill form (systemic therapy) isn't effective for treating incontinence and may actually make it worse.

Devices and injections
Other treatments for incontinence include devices intended to block urine flow and procedures to bulk up urinary tissues and structures.

Urethral insert Before an activity that can trigger incontinence, such as a game of tennis, you insert a small, tampon-like disposable device into your urethra. The insert acts as a plug to prevent leakage. You remove it when the activity is finished.

Pessary This is a silicone ring that you insert into your vagina and wear all day. The device helps hold up your bladder, which lies in front of the vagina, to prevent urine leakage. You may benefit from a pessary if you have incontinence due to a prolapsed bladder or uterus, a condition in which the structures drop out of their normal positions and protrude into the vagina.

Bulking agents A synthetic material is injected into tissue surrounding the urethra. The bulking material helps keep the urethra closed and reduces urine leakage. This procedure can be less effective than more-invasive treatments such as surgery, and it may need to be repeated. A bulking agent also may be used around the anal sphincter to help with fecal incontinence.

OnabotulinumtoxinA (Botox) Injections of Botox into the bladder muscle may benefit people who have an overactive bladder. Botox causes the bladder to relax, increasing its storage capacity and reducing episodes of incontinence. It's generally prescribed only if other first line medications haven't been successful.

Surgery

If other treatments aren't working, surgery may be able to treat the underlying cause of your incontinence. There are several surgical procedures that may be considered, depending on your circumstances and the severity of your symptoms. Surgery offers high cure rates for stress incontinence. It may also bring relief to some women with urge incontinence or fecal incontinence.

UTERINE FIBROIDS

Uterine fibroids are noncancerous growths of the uterus, a common condition that often appears during childbearing years. If you've dealt with uterine fibroids, you should begin to notice relief from your symptoms as you enter menopause. During menopause, when menstrual bleeding stops and steroid hormone levels decrease, symptoms of uterine fibroids typically improve.

If your symptoms persist once you've experienced menopause, see your health care provider. Also be aware that use of systemic hormone therapy during menopause can cause some women to continue to experience problems associated with uterine fibroids, but the symptoms are generally mild.

Uterine fibroids develop from the smooth, muscular tissue of the uterus (myometrium). A single cell divides repeatedly, eventually creating a firm, rubbery mass that's distinct from nearby tissue. Also called *leiomyomas* or *myomas*, uterine fibroids aren't associated with an increased risk of uterine cancer. But they can be unpleasant.

Fibroids range in size from seedlings, undetectable by the human eye, to bulky masses that can distort and enlarge the uterus. As many as 3 out of 4 women have uterine fibroids sometime during their lives. Most are unaware of the growths because they often don't cause any symptoms. In women who do experience symptoms, the most common are heavy menstrual bleeding, prolonged menstrual periods, pelvic pressure or pain, frequent urination and trouble with bladder emptying.

Studies of women with a history of uterine fibroids who take hormone therapy to lessen other symptoms of menopause, such as hot flashes, indicate that the therapy generally causes only small fibroid growth and mild symptoms, if any at all. If you experience vaginal bleeding — whether you're on hormone therapy or not — don't simply chalk it up to fibroids. Make sure to see your health care provider to have it evaluated.

VAGINAL BLEEDING

Once you've completed menopause — that is, you've gone without a period for more than a year — you shouldn't have any menstrual bleeding. After menopause, even a little spotting isn't considered normal. With any type of postmenopausal bleeding, it's important to make an appointment to see your health care provider.

Causes

Various conditions may cause vaginal bleeding after menopause. Most of them aren't serious, but some are. That's why it's important to know what's behind the blood loss.

Tissue changes The most common reason for postmenopausal bleeding is the thinning and drying of tissues that make up the uterus, vagina and vulva. Because the surfaces of the tissues contain little moisture after menopause, they may bleed easily. Bleeding may result from intercourse, irritation of the tissues or an infection. In one study, thinning of the tissues of the vagina and uterine lining (endometrium) was responsible for almost 60% of postmenopausal bleeding.

Tissue thinning and drying may begin to bother you during the years leading up to menopause, or it may not become a problem until several years into menopause. Some women are never bothered by it.

Polyps and fibroids Benign growths such as uterine polyps and uterine fibroids are another cause of vaginal bleeding. Uterine polyps are growths on the inner wall of the uterus that extend into the uterine cavity. Overgrowth of cells in the lining of the uterus (endometrium) leads to the formation of uterine polyps, also known as *endometrial polyps*. These polyps most commonly occur in women who are going through or have completed menopause, although younger women can get them too. Their exact cause is unknown, but hormonal factors appear to play a role.

As mentioned earlier, uterine fibroids are benign growths that often occur during childbearing years and tend to disappear during menopause. Sometimes, however, the condition may continue into menopause, causing postmenopausal bleeding. The main difference between uterine polyps and uterine fibroids is that fibroids are composed of muscle tissue and polyps are made of endometrial tissue.

Hormone therapy Some women who take estrogen to ease symptoms of menopause, such as hot flashes and sleep difficulties, experience some vaginal bleeding while taking hormones. In fact, vaginal bleeding is the most common side effect related to hormone therapy. It often occurs right after starting therapy. The frequency of bleeding depends on the regimen used. If the bleeding is unscheduled — occurring at times in your cycle when you're not expecting it — or it's heavy, talk to your health care provider. Also make an appointment to see your care provider if you experience other bothersome symptoms, such as bloating or pain. You want to make certain the bleeding isn't related to another cause.

Cancer In about 5% to 10% of women who experience postmenopausal bleeding, the bleeding is a result of uterine (endometrial) cancer. If cancer is detected early, surgery to remove the uterus often cures the cancer. If the cancer is more advanced, other treatments may be necessary. Other types of cancer, such as cervical and vaginal cancer, can also cause vaginal bleeding, though they're a less common cause than endometrial cancer.

Endometrial hyperplasia Endometrial hyperplasia refers to the abnormal growth (thickening) of the uterine lining. If not treated, the condition can lead to cancer of the uterus. Endometrial hyperplasia usually occurs in early postmenopause, when ovulation stops and production of progesterone declines. It can also occur during perimenopause, when ovulation may not occur regularly. Obesity or use of medications that act like estrogen may also lead to the condition.

Abnormal bleeding is the most common sign of endometrial hyperplasia. If you experience abnormal bleeding resulting from the condition, your health care provider will likely suggest treatment to prevent the condition from becoming cancerous. Options include a progestin medication, which may be given in the form of a pill, shot or intrauterine device (IUD). Another option is surgery to remove the uterus (hysterectomy).

Infection An infection of the uterus, such as endometritis or cervicitis, occasionally can cause bleeding.

Evaluation

Two tests used to help find the cause of abnormal uterine bleeding are an endometrial biopsy and a transvaginal ultrasound. In an endometrial biopsy, a sample of the lining of the uterus (endometrium) is removed and examined under a microscope for abnormal cells. This procedure may be done to find the cause of abnormal bleeding, check for overgrowth of the lining (endometrial hyperplasia) or check for cancer.

With a transvaginal ultrasound, an ultrasound probe is placed inside the vagina to look at your reproductive organs and pelvic area. This test may be done to look for abnormalities causing abnormal bleeding, such as polyps and fibroids, or in cases when an endometrial biopsy isn't preferable or possible.

Treatment

If tests reveal cancer or an increased risk of cancer, surgery may be performed to remove the cancer or the abnormality that's putting you at increased risk, such as with endometrial hyperplasia.

If the condition isn't serious and you aren't experiencing significant symptoms, you may not need any other treatment. For thinning and drying of vaginal tissues, your health care provider may recommend a vaginal estrogen cream, gel capsule, tablet or ring. These use a much lower dose of estrogen than do systemic hormone therapies and thus limit your overall exposure to estrogen and its associated risks. Vaginal estrogen therapies help to reverse vulvar and vaginal tissue changes by restoring the vagina's normal pH balance, thickening surface tissue and increasing lubrication. Use of moisturizers to help maintain tissue moisture and lubricants during sexual intercourse may also help (see Chapter 12).

If the bleeding worsens or changes, make sure to see your health care practitioner as soon as possible.

GOING FORWARD

During menopause, a variety of changes may take place. If these changes are difficult or disruptive to your life, don't simply accept them. Often, conditions associated with menopause can be managed or possibly even eliminated with a few lifestyle changes or interventional therapies. Don't be afraid to speak up and ask questions. You may find the topic a bit embarrassing, but it's likely a conversation your health care provider has had with many other women in the same situation. There's no reason to be ashamed or embarrassed. Once you've taken this important first step, you'll be well on your way to a more relaxed and enjoyable daily routine.

3

Owning it and looking ahead

14

Finding balance, setting boundaries and embracing your power

Today, the average woman has more than one-third of her life ahead of her after menopause. That makes menopause a good time to take stock of your life and your priorities and consider: What do you want to do when you grow up? Who do you want to be?

This new phase of life can be as relaxing and free or busy and fulfilling as you would like to make it. This is your chance to reset, reconnect, rearrange, reschedule and retune.

Of course, you can change your life's course at any time. But for most people, meaningful change often happens on the heels of a clear defining moment — college graduation, marriage, parenthood, divorce, the death of a loved one, illness, a major job promotion, a cross-country move or retirement. Menopause can be in this category, and it often coincides with other major life changes as well — such as sending children off to college.

You get only a handful of these major milestones throughout your life, so it's wise to make them count. Take the time to pause and honor this transition in life. Then summon your inner strength and go for the life you really want. It's time.

EMBRACE YOUR THIRD ACT

By the time you reach your late 40s and 50s, you've got decades of real living behind you. You've seen your fair share of places and presidencies and new technologies. You've had your heart broken. You've made mistakes and learned from them. You've fallen down and gotten back up and dusted yourself off. You've taken a leap. You might've raised your babies — or helped raise someone else's. You've earned accolades, compliments and scars. You've forgiven and forgotten. You've learned what makes you tick and what brings you joy.

That all sets you up for your postmenopausal years to be your best yet. As you write your own life story, use your time and energy wisely and embrace your years ahead. It's time to focus on your inner self, your values and your priorities for the future.

It all starts with your attitude and your perceptions about this new phase of life. These are powerful tools for building the life you want — and they are within your control.

What if you're dreading growing older? With some work, you can reshape your attitude. Here are some specific techniques to cultivate productive thinking and embrace the years ahead:

Challenge your negative thoughts
Argue with them. Challenge their accuracy. Every time you challenge negative self-talk with facts, your negative thoughts lose their power. By changing your thoughts, you will eventually change the way you feel. You'll see that feelings of hopelessness, fear and anxiety can give way to feelings of power, courage, compassion and hope.

You can start by identifying any faulty thought patterns that get in your way and undermine your happiness. For example, maybe you tend to magnify the negative in a situation and filter out the positive. Say you're well prepared for and articulate in a work presentation and receive many compliments for a job well done. But you stumble on the answer to one minor question from a challenging younger coworker.

That evening, you focus only on the misstep and forget about the accomplishment. Another common negative thought pattern is automatically jumping to conclusions and anticipating the worst in any situation. For example, you begin having hot flashes and immediately assume they're going to ruin your life.

In both these situations, you can counter exaggerated negative self-talk (*My body is falling apart*) with realistic thoughts (*I'm starting to have hot flashes; I should figure out self-care techniques or treatments that can help*). Find areas of your life that you're often negative about and think of ways to see them in a more positive, factual light.

Focus on what you can control

Don't dwell on the menopausal changes that you can't control. Instead, control your reaction to them. Reframe the situation as a challenge — not a catastrophe. Then summon your inner strength to face it.

Take sleep problems, for example. You could keep yourself up all night worrying about sleep. Instead, control your reaction to the situation.

Problem-solve as much as possible. Buy cooler sheets and pajamas, if it's within your budget, and get out your fan. If you still have a bad night's sleep, reflect on what worked (the new pajamas were more comfortable) and what didn't (the fan was old and loud). Learn from your experiences (time to buy a new fan) and try again. Don't be discouraged if things don't always go your way. Shift your attention to planning mode. Commit to carrying out your plan before giving up or trying something else.

Practice optimism

That doesn't mean pretending menopause and all its annoying symptoms are fine when they're not. You don't have to ignore the hard truths about this stage of life. Optimism is about looking for solutions and silver linings in times of hardship and stress.

Optimists experience disappointments just like everyone else, but they're able to view them as temporary events or roadblocks to get around. When optimists have a setback, they confine it to a specific event and don't allow it to contaminate every aspect of their lives. When optimists encounter a negative event, they don't take it as a personal insult or blame themselves for life's misfortune. Try out this worldview and see if you can make it stick. It will help you live through your postmenopausal years with balance and joy.

EXAMINE YOUR VALUES

Menopause is a time of change in many areas. You experience physical change as your body stops producing estrogen, setting off a ripple effect of bothersome symptoms. But menopause can also be a time of tumultuous life changes, when women are sandwiched between the needs of aging parents, growing children and midlife partners. Career success and responsibilities can be at an all-time high too, leaving women stretched in all directions and feeling guilty that they're not doing everything right. As all of these demands converge, it can be tough to make yourself and your values a priority in your own life.

It's critical to use menopause as your opportunity to reflect and reassess your values and priorities. You get only 24 hours each day. How you spend that time is up to you. However, if you don't plan your time with clear intention, it's likely that others will fill up your time for you.

Sketch out your "time pie"

Try the following exercise to record how your time is currently spent and what you would like to change. This exercise requires a sheet of paper, a pencil and 15 to 60 minutes. Pour yourself a cup of tea or a glass of wine, and plan to take your time with this.

Draw a circle on a sheet of paper. Then divide it up into segments that represent the number of hours you spend on various activities on a typical day, adding up to 24 hours. Fill in the number of hours you spend for:

- Sleep
- Work
- Chores
- Eating
- Hygiene
- Commute
- Caregiving
- Errands

- Family time
- Significant other relationship
- Technology and device use
- Exercise
- Fun

Label each slice of the pie with the activity and the number of typical hours you spend doing it each day. Be as accurate as possible.

Now, take a good look at the pie you've sketched. Do the results surprise you? Is there a slice that's much bigger or smaller than you would like?

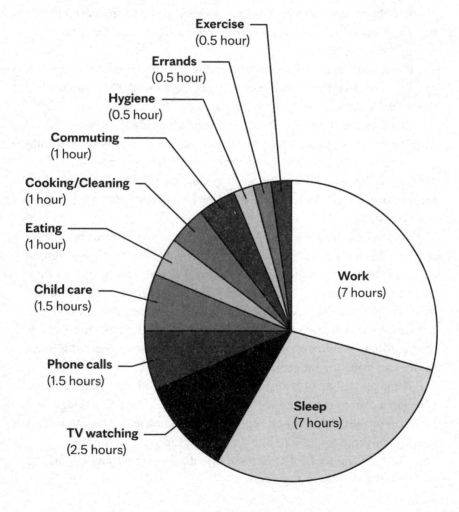

Give some thought to the following questions to help you identify what experiences and values are most important to you:

- What are your most important relationships?
- Where have you found comfort?
- What do you most value in your life?
- Which people give you a sense of community?
- What inspires you and gives you hope?
- What brings you joy?
- What are your three most memorable experiences?
- What are your proudest achievements?

How does your pie compare to your answers to the questions above? Are the things that bring you joy part of your pie? What about the things you value most?

If your typical day and your values don't match up, create one more pie that represents your ideal day. In your ideal world, how would you devote your time and energy? How would you like to spend your day?

Chances are, your typical day and your ideal day are not the same. That's a natural consequence of being an adult and having responsibilities and commitments. However, there should be some overlap and synergy. When you don't have time to spend on the things that really matter to you, it can be a source of stress that keeps you from being your best self.

Think about lifestyle changes you can make so that your typical pie and your ideal pie are a little closer. You probably can't quit your job to spend more time with the people you love. But you may be able to find more time for your family by slimming down the work slice of your pie by cutting back on nighttime work emails. Or perhaps you could outsource some errands or limit social media time to make more room for the things that bring you joy. Aligning your daily choices with your values can bring meaning and purpose to your days.

Think about one or two specific changes you would like to make. Develop a plan to make these changes, and take action. Consider saving your pie drawings and repeating this exercise in a month or two to see your progress. It will take time and effort to shift the sizes of your slices. Be patient with yourself. Monitor how your plan is working, and make adjustments as you go.

Know your "big rocks"

Of course, there are many ways to rethink your priorities. If the time pie exercise doesn't resonate with you, try reflecting on the following story, which has been told for years in many different versions. It provides another way to visualize your values:

> One day, a college professor put a mason jar on the table in front of his students. Then he produced a bucket of big rocks and began placing them into the jar. When the jar was filled to the top and no more rocks would fit inside, he asked the students, "Is the jar full?" The students said yes.
>
> But the professor proved them wrong by unveiling a bucket of pebbles and adding them to the jar. The professor was able to fit a lot of pebbles around all the big rocks. "Is the jar full now?" he asked. By this time, the students were a bit wiser, and they shook their heads no.
>
> This was the correct response, as the professor then produced a bucket of sand and poured sand around all the big rocks and small pebbles. "Now is it full?" he asked.
>
> "Probably not," the class said. And they were correct. The professor took out a pitcher of water and filled the jar to the brim.
>
> "Now the jar is really full," the professor declared. His intention was to show how important it is to start with the big rocks. "If you put the water, sand and pebbles in the jar before the big rocks," he told the students, "you would never accommodate the big rocks."

Menopause is an opportunity to identify your big rocks and build your life around them. It's important to choose your big rocks carefully and anchor them firmly.

Ask yourself: What are your big rocks? Your family? Your faith? Your job? A hobby you're passionate about, such as biking or playing the piano? A cause that's near and dear to your heart?

You have a lot of responsibilities, but only some are big rocks. The rest are pebbles and sand. Know the difference. There is not enough time to get everything done every day. But you can mitigate a lot of stress in your life if you focus on the big rocks and do the things that really matter to you.

LEARN TO SAY NO

As noted earlier in this chapter, the years surrounding menopause are often very busy in women's lives, full of competing priorities. Some of your frenzy may be the result of very good things that happen at this stage of life, such as celebrating a child's graduation, taking on a leadership role at work or accepting a position on the board of a favorite charity. Other responsibilities may not be so uplifting, such as caring for aging parents, helping a friend through a divorce, or planning how to finance your retirement or children's college educations. All of these stressors — good and bad — can take a toll. You will find balance and happiness only when you protect your time and set limits, according to the values and "big rocks" you have identified.

When to say no

At this time in life, you may receive a lot of requests for your hard-earned wisdom and expertise. This can be flattering. Sometimes it's tough to decide which activities deserve your time and attention. Use these strategies to evaluate obligations — and opportunities — that come your way.

Focus on what matters most. Remember your big rocks. When an opportunity or commitment comes your way, think about whether it is a big rock that's worthy of your time and attention. Is the new commitment important to you? Or would it be just another item on your to-do list?

Assess the time commitment. Is the new activity you're considering a short- or long-term commitment? Even if a volunteer commitment passes the "big rock" test, it's important to remember that signing up for a single Saturday event will take far less time than heading up the whole fundraising committee. Be realistic about what you can handle. Don't overcommit yourself at home, work, church or in your community.

Let go of guilt. Don't agree to a request out of guilt or obligation if you'd rather decline. Saying no is not a sign of rudeness. There are times when you have to say no, even to people you love. If your parents or in-laws want to get together for an impromptu dinner when you've already scheduled a quiet evening at home with your partner, it's OK to decline their offer. Set realistic goals for what you can — and want — to accomplish.

Sleep on it. Stop saying yes to requests on the spot. When someone asks you to do something, get in the habit of saying that you're flattered and you'll respond with a firm answer in the next day or so. Or ask them to send you an email with this request. If they do send you an email (often they won't!), this buys you time to mull over a new opportunity and decide if it really fits into your current commitments and priorities. You may find that your excitement for a new opportunity waxes or wanes overnight. This is a good indicator of whether you should sign on.

How to say no

Sometimes you have to say no in order to say yes to things that matter most. Still, it can be difficult to disappoint people who want your help and time. Sometimes the people who request your assistance are in a vulnerable spot; handle your response tenderly.

Be clear about saying no. Be careful not to use phrases such as "I'm not sure" or "I don't think I can." These can be interpreted to mean that you might say yes later.

Practice full disclosure. Don't make up reasons to get out of an obligation. The truth is usually the best way to turn someone down.

Let them down gently. It can be tough to turn down good causes that land at your door. Compliment the person or group's effort while saying that you're unable to commit at this time. A respectful approach shows that you're just turning down a commitment, not snubbing the group's mission or accomplishments.

Cushion your response to a loved one. Try using the "sandwiched no": yes-no-yes. Begin with initial honest enthusiasm ("I would love to"); follow with a polite no that includes a proper explanation ("I have too much going on"); and finish with a second-best option that partially compensates for your no ("How about next Monday?"). Your no then becomes a half yes, which is easier to swallow. Another option is to soften your no with a follow-up gesture that shows you care.

With practice, saying no will get easier over time. Remind yourself that learning to say no is an important way to shine in your postmenopausal years.

CARE FOR YOURSELF

Why is it so critical to reclaim your time and your priorities as you navigate the transition to menopause? The physical symptoms of menopause and aging are exacerbated when you don't take care of yourself. In addition, if you don't take steps to preserve or improve your health, you're at higher risk of illness and health problems that often appear in midlife or later.

Where do you fall on your own priority list? In your 30s and 40s, you may have relegated yourself to a mere sliver of your time pie, as you focused your attention on building a nest, a family and a career. While common, this tactic won't serve you well as you age. A healthy balance between work, caring for others and taking care of yourself is important to your well-being. It's time to find your voice and be an advocate for your own wants and needs.

Other chapters in Part 3 cover many lifestyle changes that can protect or improve your health at this time of life. As you may guess, the shortlist includes moving more, eating well, quitting smoking, limiting alcohol, establishing a healthy sleep routine and keeping up on regular preventive health care. Beyond these important habits, the following steps are key in caring for your body and spirit during this stage of life:

Take a break from caregiving

If you are a caregiver for aging parents, give yourself some time off. Many women who are actively caring for older adults don't identify as a "caregiver." Recognizing this role and the emotional and physical demands involved with it can help you seek out support.

Let those in your care be as independent as possible. It's tempting to go with Mom and Dad to every doctor's appointment and to be at their beck and call for household chores. But it's important to differentiate between the things your parents can handle on their own and the tasks they need you for. This distinction is good for both of you.

In addition, accept help from others. If siblings, neighbors or family friends offer to assist, say yes. Be prepared with a list of specific ways that others can help, such as taking your parents to the grocery store or mowing their lawn. Don't be too proud to accept help for yourself as well. Allowing others to help you actually helps your parents.

In addition, be sure to take advantage of resources and tools in your community that can help you help your loved one. Many communities have classes and services, such as transportation and meal delivery, that could ease your load. Your health care provider, your parent's provider or a support group for caregivers can help you find resources and solve common caregiving problems.

Many women who are caring for aging parents are also caring for teenagers or young adults and are divided in their responsibilities. If you're in this situation, try to let go of guilt and be realistic about what you can manage. Find balance in caregiving over a period of time. Don't compromise your sleep, your time for exercise or your healthy-eating habits trying to do it all. Remember, if you don't take care of yourself, you won't be able to care of those who need you.

Take time to do the things you want to do

Too often, women don't take time to do the things they really want to do until they've finished all their responsibilities and commitments to others. Doing things in this order leaves too little — sometimes zero — time for the things you really want to do.

Instead of saving your passions and hobbies for that rare free moment, schedule them into your day. Book a block of time for gardening. Schedule a meeting with your favorite book and your favorite sunny spot. Get up early and make a trail run or yoga class the first thing you do, rather than the last. Time spent doing the things you love allows you to recharge and attend to your responsibilities with new energy.

Pamper yourself

Treat yourself to a massage, manicure or bubble bath. Escape to a local concert or theater performance. Meet your best friend for coffee. Buy a new novel or a pair of earrings you've been coveting. Enjoy an alfresco glass of champagne with your partner. Shower yourself with something special — it doesn't have to be expensive or fancy.

Take care of your spirit

This is different for everyone. For some, it takes the form of religious observance, prayer, meditation or a belief in a higher power. For others, it is found in nature, music, art or a secular community. Staying connected to your inner spirit and the lives of those around you can enhance your quality of life, both mentally and physically. Your personal concept of spirituality may change with your age and life experiences, but it always forms the basis of your well-being, helps you cope with stressors and affirms your purpose in life.

Stay curious

Stretch yourself by trying new things as you age. Take a class at your local art or pottery studio or look into adult or continuing education classes in your area. If you've always wanted to try the banjo or a gourmet pasta-making class, maybe now's the time. Traveling is another way to expand your horizons and gain new perspective. If you can't book a trip to a far-flung destination right now, at least consider a reservation at the new Thai restaurant in town.

Laugh

Loud. And often. It really is the best medicine. Be silly with your kids, grandkids, nieces or nephews. Spend time with friends who keep you giggling. Or watch a movie that you know will get you laughing.

Try to let go of any guilt that you feel when you take time for yourself. It's not selfish or lazy to prioritize a bubble bath or an afternoon of painting. Think of these activities as part of your doctor's orders to take care of yourself. If you find that you can't let go of the guilt, practice mindfulness. Notice the guilt, be curious about it and then redirect your attention back to the present moment — the paint on your canvas or the warmth of the bubble bath.

NOURISH YOUR RELATIONSHIP WITH YOUR PARTNER

At this stage in life, another way to take care of yourself is to take care of your relationship with your partner. Your relationship can take a hit at this time if you don't pay special attention to it. As you learned in Chapter 12, sexual problems and relationship issues are common during midlife. If you want to grow old with your partner, you may need to work to add spice and cultivate a relationship of support — especially through midlife changes.

It's worth noting that choosing to divorce after age 50 is increasingly common. In recent decades, the divorce rate for this age group has grown to about twice what it was in 1990. If ending a marriage is what best suits your personal goals for your postmenopausal years, you're certainly not alone.

Find novelty

Novelty is your appreciation of uniqueness. Something novel is new, interesting, original, contrasting or beyond expectations. By finding novelty with your partner, you can keep your relationship fresh.

How can you develop a fresh relationship each day — especially if you've been together for decades? Try this: Imagine being apart for a 10-day trip. When you come home, are you more likely to meet your partner with a loving presence, at least for the first 15 minutes?

When you see your loved ones every day, they become familiar,

RED FLAGS: INTIMATE PARTNER VIOLENCE

Intimate partner violence (IPV) occurs between people who are or have been in a close relationship. It may be emotional, verbal, sexual or physical abuse, stalking or threats. It can happen in heterosexual or same-sex relationships. And it's common. About 1 in 4 U.S. women will experience IPV in their lifetimes. The risk of IPV is increased for people who are transgender or part of other marginalized communities.

Women with a history of IPV have an increased risk of more severe menopause symptoms, as well as other serious physical and mental health consequences. If you're in an unsafe relationship, help is available. The National Domestic Violence Hotline (800-799-7233) provides crisis intervention and referrals to resources. A trusted friend or relative or a doctor or nurse also can help you get the support you need. Intimate partner violence is never your fault. No one deserves to be abused.

HOW TO HELP YOUR PARTNER HELP YOU

If menopause caught you off guard, you're not alone. The range of changes that can occur as estrogen gradually declines can be surprising.

Now, think about your partner. If you were caught off guard by the changes that are happening in your body, your partner may be too. It can be confusing or disorienting when the person you love changes dramatically — even if the changes are a normal part of the aging process. If you're more moody, overheated, exhausted, anxious, dejected or private than you've ever been before, your partner may not know what to do.

One recent survey found that men were generally aware of their partner's menopause symptoms. Talking openly with your partner may help them know how to give you the support you need and be an active partner in helping you manage your symptoms. You may need to have an estrogen 101 talk. Briefly explain the changes you're feeling (refer back to Chapters 1 and 2 if you need to). Be honest. Let your partner know that you may need a little extra support, patience and kindness as you work your way through the challenges of menopause.

Talk to your partner about specific changes in your home and relationship that might help your symptoms. For example, let your partner know if you need to cool down your bedroom for a good night's sleep. Discuss how more lubrication or a vibrator may help during sex. Be honest if weight gain is bothering you and you want to shift your schedule around a new class at the gym.

Depending on cultural and family norms, these conversations about your health may look different for everyone. But if open, honest talks aren't a hallmark of your relationship, consider working with a counselor to facilitate better communication. Research shows that a supportive, loving partner can help reduce menopausal stress and ease symptoms.

even bordering on boring (to your brain, at least). When you haven't seen them for 10 days, the novelty draws the mind's attention.

Could you greet your partner each day as if you're seeing him or her for the first time after 10 days? Can you give your partner the same undistracted attention that you'd give a friend? Can you make a point to celebrate a little when you meet your loved ones at the end of the day? Show your excitement at being together. Take a break from folding laundry, cooking or scanning through email during the first 15 minutes of reconnecting. Do your best to give your partner your full attention.

Take 15 minutes to talk about your day, flirt and catch up. You may be amazed at the difference that these 15 minutes can make.

Practice positivity

In addition, keep a close eye on your positivity-negativity (P-N) ratio, a concept used by psychology professor and marriage researcher John Gottman. *Positivity* refers to encouraging positive feedback you give to others, while *negativity* represents negative feedback. The higher your P-N ratio, the more you thrive in a relationship. Gottman's research suggests that you need five instances of positive feedback to neutralize one instance of negative feedback. He found that most teams with excellent dynamics, including successful marriages, have a high P-N ratio (typically greater than 5), while marriages at risk of divorce have a low ratio (often less than 1).

Think back to yesterday. Did you compliment your partner's new shirt? Did you kiss your partner before you left for work or went to sleep? The little things that you do make a profound difference. Showing understanding, meeting expectations, making good on promises and sincerely apologizing all enhance the P-N ratio.

Share this idea with your partner, and work together to keep the positivity flowing at your home and boost your ratio. Yes, there are times where honest criticism is appropriate. But you really can't have too much positivity. Intentionally upping your positive instances and noting your negative instances will allow you to strengthen your connections and energy.

Also, remember that not everyone is good with words. Some people are kind with words, while others are kind with deeds. Only a rare few are kind with both. If your partner isn't good with words, take note of his or her deeds — such as making you a cup of coffee, snuggling up next to you on the couch or filling up the gas in your car. Recognize these deeds as acts of praise and love for you. These are just as powerful as a verbal compliment or profession of love.

Invest your time

Finally, invest in quality time with your partner. If you've been in your relationship for a long time, you may feel as if you've grown distant, even if you're regularly in the same room. This is common. Your time together may be stuffed with chores and obligations, and it feels like that's all you have time for.

How can you change that? Could you schedule a date night once a week? Could you buy season tickets to a concert or theater series so that you have several evenings out planned ahead of time? Could you take a spin class or a wine-tasting class together? Could you commit to setting aside just 10 or 20 minutes every day to talk or go for a walk or do something enjoyable together?

You get only so much time with the people you love. When you spend it wisely, you'll make deeper connections and foster intimacy, and your life will be better for it.

MOVING FORWARD WITH THE NEW YOU

Today is your day. Tomorrow is your day too. And the next day after that.

Yes, it's a time of change — physical changes, emotional ups and downs, and social adjustments. But it's also a time to take the reins and make changes of your own. The choices you make now can help you transform your health, your relationships and your life for decades to come. Your expectations are powerful — set them high. Use them to carve out the life you really want.

It's never too late to turn out some of your best work. For consideration: At the age of 88, actress Betty White became the oldest person to guest-host *Saturday Night Live*. She earned glowing reviews and an Emmy Award for her appearance.

What triumphs might you achieve in your third act of life?

What dreams can you dream for yourself?

15

Embracing midlife changes and body image

If you find yourself wondering why you can't have the hard-earned wisdom of midlife and rock-hard abs all at the same time — well, you're not alone. Today's society has collectively duped people, adopting a standard of beauty for women over 50 that bears no resemblance to how most women age naturally.

Menopause is a time of unbelievable change, and it takes a while to get comfortable in your new (older) skin. Plus, there are few true depictions of this stage of life in the media to help guide or reassure you. People in magazines or movies are often much younger or hiding behind a pair of SPANX and a team of makeup and photo-editing artists (or both).

It's normal to feel self-conscious or embarrassed about some of the changes that happen in menopause. It's not shallow or silly if you struggle to accept some of the things that are happening to your body. This chapter gives you practical ideas for finding a realistic, positive perspective and being kind to yourself — at least most of the time.

AGING VS. MENOPAUSE

Aging and menopause go hand in hand, so it can be difficult to tease them apart and figure out which physical and mental changes stem from the natural aging process and which are directly linked to a decline in estrogen. For the most part, it doesn't really matter. But it can be helpful to understand what natural aging really looks like. Improvements in health care and changes in the environment have significantly slowed the aging process over time, but a 60-year-old woman still isn't going to look like a 20-year-old model. The truth is that the natural aging process simply isn't all that glamorous, despite all the airbrushed images of older women that you've seen over the years.

Aging is different for everyone. There's no single, chronological timetable that all women follow. Genetics, lifestyle and disease affect the rate at which you age.

However, there are some typical changes that occur with healthy aging — even in the absence of any serious condition or disease. It's normal to gain some weight with age, especially around the waist. It's normal to lose some hearing with age, even if you have no evidence of hearing disorders or noise-induced hearing loss. You may also notice that you have trouble falling asleep or staying asleep, learning new things or remembering familiar words or names. The normal aging process also affects your eyes, your teeth and gums, and your skin.

The human mind has an innate instinct to focus on imperfection, so if one thing isn't right, it can pull your attention like a magnet. During the aging process, it's natural for women to see physical imperfections to focus on. But this certainly isn't productive.

Remind yourself that every age is a package deal — you get something and you lose something. You don't gain wisdom without a few wrinkles. You can't be discerning and perceptive without a few scars or spots. In the end, these trade-offs are worth it.

AGING WITH GRATITUDE

Gratitude represents your thankfulness for every experience, because each step of life can help you grow — sometimes materially, but almost always emotionally and spiritually. According to research, a daily practice of gratitude can boost your energy, improve your mood, generate optimism, enhance your well-being and self-esteem, and much more. During menopause and beyond, gratitude can help you gracefully accept the things that you cannot change. And this is one of the keys to successful aging.

An occasional grateful thought is helpful. But your goal is to make it a habit. Here are some ideas for sprinkling gratitude throughout your day:

- **Start your day with gratitude.** Before you even get out of bed, let your first thought be one of gratitude. Start with a few deep breaths and then think about five people in your life you're grateful for. While breathing in slowly and deeply, choose one of these people and bring that person's face in front of your closed eyes. Try to "see" this person as clearly as you can. Then send him or her silent gratitude while breathing out, again slowly and deeply. Repeat this exercise with all five. This practice will help you focus on what's most important in your life and give context to your day.

- **Start a gratitude journal.** As you close your day, write at least one thing you're thankful for — your morning yoga class, lunch with a girlfriend, your daughter's smile, the fact that your computer didn't crash during an important meeting. Gratitude can be used for your body image as well — if you think about it, there's much about your body to be grateful for. Be as specific as possible. On a rough day, refer back to this journal for some respite from negative feelings.

- **Collect gratitude sayings.** You'll find poignant quotes about gratitude in many novels, great speeches and spiritual texts. When you stumble across a saying that you like, write it down. You can place quotes in antique frames and display them at your house or office. Or you can simply jot quotes on Post-it Notes and hang them on your refrigerator, corkboard or car visor. When you have a bad day, call on these grateful thoughts to redirect your mind.

- **Be grateful to those you help.** Say thanks to people who seek your help. At this stage in life, your wisdom and unconditional love are a gift to others — be grateful that you can share them.

- **Look for the positives in the negatives.** Focusing on the positive doesn't mean you overlook a problem — it means you take a compassionate stance. Take hot flashes, for example. They're no fun. But without them, you wouldn't be enjoying so many delicious lemon ice pops. You may not have discovered your favorite new air-conditioned bookstore. And you wouldn't have laughed so hard over hot flash stories and wine with your best friends.

Which gratitude ideas might work for you? Feel free to adapt these strategies to fit into your life and your routine. For instance, if you already start your day with an early-morning run and a cup of coffee, try practicing gratitude in the shower. Let the hot water overhead be your cue to send gratitude to five people or five things. Experiment with all these ideas until gratitude becomes second nature.

Your 40s, 50s and 60s are a very wise, productive time of life, when women typically feel very settled and confident at work and in their relationships. So you have a choice: You can be a harsh judge of the person in the mirror and make yourself miserable by squeezing your body into a pair of jeans that's a size too small. Or you can focus on taking advantage of the opportunities and wisdom that you have earned.

PREVENTABLE VS. INEVITABLE CHANGES

Let's just be clear: Your goal is to gracefully accept the changes that come with normal aging, not to throw in the towel.

Remember, normal aging and disease are distinct. Your body will naturally change with age. But adding candles to your birthday cake doesn't inevitably lead to disease. There are several keys to reducing your risk of the diseases and disabilities that can occur with age. They include the following:

Maintain a healthy weight

Health problems linked with being overweight or obese include type 2 diabetes, high blood pressure, heart disease, stroke, some types of cancer, sleep apnea and osteoarthritis.

Since most people tend to gain some weight with age, it's important to keep an eye on your waistline and your body mass index (BMI). A couple of extra pounds may be OK. But a couple of extra pounds every year will be significant over the long haul. Focus on maintaining a healthy weight, not necessarily your premenopausal weight, and commit to making it happen. Being overweight is a serious health risk.

Get regular physical activity

Research suggests that people who exercise regularly actually live longer and live better. Staying active can also help you continue to do the things that you enjoy and stay independent as you age. Choose a well-rounded physical activity program that includes balance exercises, flexibility or stretching exercises, and strength training in addition to cardio time.

Eat a healthy diet

What you eat can either support healthy aging or cause health problems. Of course, eating a healthy diet will help you maintain a healthy weight. But your food choices are important in other ways as you age too. Eating unhealthy foods may increase your risk of some diseases. In contrast, eating well can help protect you from age-related problems caused by deficiencies of certain micronutrients and vitamins.

Be tobacco-free

It's never too late to enjoy the benefits of quitting smoking. There are clear benefits to quitting no matter what your age or how long you've smoked.

Limit alcohol

If you drink alcohol, keep it to one drink a day or less. Drinking this amount may have some heart-health benefits. But even light alcohol use increases your risk of several types of cancer, particularly breast cancer.

Don't be a stranger to health care

Checking in with your health care practitioner on a regular basis will ensure that you're getting the screening tests and preventive therapies you need. In addition, taking an active role in your health can help you feel more competent and in control of your own body.

These habits are the same ones that stave off health problems in your younger years. You may just have less wiggle room on them in the years after menopause.

MAKING PEACE WITH YOUR CHANGING BODY

Body image refers to your mental image or perception of your own physical appearance. It's formed by many factors and experiences, including your physical appearance, your weight, your values, your ethnic background, what you see in the media and what feedback you hear from others.

Menopause may also play a big role in your body image, just as puberty, pregnancy and other major life milestones altered how you felt in your own skin. Some women find the menopause transition to be liberating. Other women mourn the loss of their ability to have children and may feel less desirable. Often, women experience complex, conflicting feelings of relief and sadness all at once.

During menopause, weight gain can also be a major concern and a major obstacle to a positive body image. For many women, menopause and aging affect metabolism, causing an uptick in weight without any real change in activity or diet. This feeling of a loss of control of your own weight can be frustrating, disheartening and inhibiting. You may find that you no longer feel comfortable in your favorite clothes — or without your clothes. In fact, many women say that weight gain gets in the way of feeling sexy and sexual.

Unfortunately, weight gain is unlikely to go away without significant effort. Even if you're able to maintain your premenopausal weight, you may carry it differently and feel thicker around your middle. So it's important to show yourself some compassion. In fact, studies show that having a positive body image and practicing self-compassion during menopause can actually result in fewer symptoms, including fewer hot flashes or night sweats that interfere with daily activities.

If you're struggling to be kind to yourself, try focusing on nonjudgmental presence and mindfulness. Look at your body and take note of the nooks, crannies and wrinkles. Look at them and describe exactly what you see without opinion or judgment. For example, instead of "I see flabby arms," say, "I see a larger patch of skin below my right arm. It feels soft, and when I touch it, it moves from side to side." If judgment or the internal critic creeps in your mind, let these negative thoughts go by, rather than letting them consume you or undermine your self-worth. These are just thoughts. You are not your thoughts.

Let them float by like clouds in the sky and go back to the present moment. This is mindfulness. Keep practicing.

Although it's wise to focus on other things besides your looks as you age, a positive body image is still important. Having a positive view of your own body is essential for your confidence, sex life and self-esteem. Learning to take care of and love your body is crucial to your happiness.

PRACTICAL STRATEGIES FOR A BETTER BODY IMAGE

If you don't like what you see in the mirror, it's time to make a change. Try new physical activities, and look at your body with a new perspective. These strategies can help:

Get moving!
Exercise tends to make women feel better about their bodies, whether they lose weight or not. The type of exercise doesn't matter. Find something you like to do, and find a time to do it.

If you need extra motivation and accountability, sign up for an exercise class, work with a trainer or make plans to meet a friend at the gym or park.

Focus on physical accomplishments
Go rock climbing or paddle boarding. Take a cycling class or ballroom dancing class. Try pickleball or snorkeling with your kids or grandkids. Master a headstand or handstand. Jump off the diving board or the lakefront dock. Focus on all the things that your body can do, not just how it looks.

If you're up for a challenge, sign up for a physical test that you've never tried before — such as a 5K walk or run, a dance class or even a sprint triathlon. Just make sure it's within your grasp, based on your abilities and physical health.

Don't apologize for your body
Didn't your mother ever tell you that if you can't say anything nice, you shouldn't say anything at all? If you're not ready to be positive, try thinking of ways you have gratitude for your body. Maybe you can

appreciate your fingers' muscle memory for a hobby, or the nose you inherited from a favorite grandparent.

Pay attention to your body language too. The way you move your body can seem like an apology even if you never say it out loud. You are allowed to take up space. Even after menopause. Even when you're in a swimsuit. No exceptions.

Don't critique another woman's crow's-feet

When you make snarky comments about how other women are aging poorly, you contribute to the culture of unrealistic expectations about how women age. In addition, gossiping about other women affects your own body image. Pay attention to how you talk about the appearance of other women — girlfriends, neighbors, coworkers, actresses and celebrities, aging female politicians and other public figures. Your inner self can hear you.

Wear things that make you feel good about yourself

Cultivate your own style — one that makes you happy. If you feel good in jeans, make them your signature style. If you love dresses, don't bother saving them for fancy occasions. Accessories, perfume, cowboy boots and other small luxuries all count. Play to your strengths. You know what they are.

Don't draw your body image from what you see in the media

Remember, these images are carefully produced by a huge team of experts who are trained to sell products or show celebrities in a positive light. The final result often bears little resemblance to reality. Don't be tempted to use these images as a yardstick to measure your own body.

Accept and value your genes

You probably inherited a lot of physical traits from your family. You might have your grandmother's hands or your favorite aunt's dimples. You probably have the same thick thighs and spider veins that these women had too. Try to view these inherited traits as part of your pedigree and lineage. Embrace them just as you would embrace these beloved family members.

Take a good look at your own body

Sometimes, the only way to move past a negative body image is to desensitize your feelings about your body. You can do this by really looking at your body in the mirror. Start by taking a hand mirror and looking at the different parts of your body. Begin with an area you're comfortable with — such as your hands. Look at your hands with curiosity. State the facts ("I see lines that extend from my wrist to knuckles that are raised and slightly darker than the rest of my hand"), not opinion ("I see veiny hands"). Really notice them. Then continue on to different parts of your body. Over time, you might be able to look in a larger mirror. This exercise may feel uncomfortable or awkward at first. That's OK. Keep practicing until you can experience your body factually and without judgment.

Think about your partner's body

Has your partner's body changed as you've aged together? Have these changes made your partner less lovable? What would you tell your partner if he or she were struggling to accept some of the changes that have occurred with age? Try listening to your own advice.

These strategies aren't meant to minimize the difficult task of loving your body as it ages. It's OK to grieve the loss of your younger features. Just remember that the stages of grief end with acceptance. So, if you find yourself stuck in the stage of anger or depression for a long time, it's a good idea to talk to your health care provider.

In fact, if you've struggled with your body image throughout your life, you may find that menopause triggers a recurrence of old feelings. You may benefit from counseling or other treatments to help with this transition. Support groups can also supply valuable information and help you connect with other women who share your experiences.

YOU ARE MORE THAN YOUR BODY

The best way to fully embrace your postmenopausal self is a dichotomy. It's essential to foster a positive body image, even as your body changes in ways that you don't expect. Your goal is to accept your own figure, to stand tall in the mirror and be comfortable having sex with the lights on. But it's equally important to recognize that you are much more than your body.

In fact, your best inner qualities may stay with you forever and actually improve with age. Studies suggest that qualities such as kindness, willpower and enjoyment of humor tend to increase as we get older. So if your greatest personality asset is your sharp wit, your knack for telling a great story or throwing a great party, your kindness to strangers, your stubborn streak, your passion for your work or your unwavering loyalty to friends, that's unlikely to change.

As you work to embrace the woman in the mirror, remember to take a step back and think about all the things you can't see in your reflection. Focus on your whole self. Some days this may be more difficult than others. When that's the case, consider these final tips to help you gain a new perspective.

Keep a list of positive qualities that have nothing to do with your appearance. It's easy to be critical and focus on your flaws. Instead, focus on what makes you shine brightest. Write down a compliment or two for yourself and refer to it when you find yourself obsessing about your least favorite features. If you're not sure what to write, take note the next time a friend, neighbor or coworker pays you a compliment. Or ask your partner to help you name your greatest strengths.

Surround yourself with people who make you feel good about yourself. As a teenager, you probably had a few mean girls in your life — those spiteful, superficial girls who would smile nicely while making fun of your jeans. There may have been some benefit to making nice with the mean girls because they had so much influence in your social world.

At this stage in your life, there's no advantage to spending time with anyone who doesn't make you feel good about yourself. If you still have friends or family members in your life who constantly critique your choices or rain on your parade, it may be time for a breakup. At the very least, consider limiting your exposure to anyone who brings you down. Menopause is your license to close in your inner circle and to bask in the relationships that buoy you up.

Engage in hobbies or activities that you enjoy. If you had a free afternoon with absolutely no obligations or limitations, how would you choose to spend it? On your bike? In your garden? At the theater? On a stool at the local wine bar with a friend? With your nose in a new book? Baking bread? Playing the piano? There is no wrong answer here.

People who are involved in hobbies and leisure activities may be at a lower risk of some health problems. In addition, social activities and relaxing hobbies can help get rid of the stress and anxiety that contribute to some women being critical of their bodies. Make time for the passions and pursuits you enjoy. Consider scheduling time for your hobbies on your calendar just as you would an important meeting so they don't fall to the bottom of your priority list.

Also, consider sharing your hobbies or passions with your community in the form of volunteer work. If you love to cook or garden, you might volunteer at your local farmers market or soup kitchen. If you're a reader, you might relish a regular stint at the library. Older adults who participate in meaningful activities report feeling healthier and happier.

Talk to older women you admire. It's tough to feel bad about your aging body when you spend time with older women you hold in high regard. Consider scheduling a semiregular coffee or lunch with one or two older women whom you think highly of. It might be a favorite aunt, a longtime neighbor, a work mentor or someone you've met through your hobbies or religious affiliation. You don't necessarily have to talk about the trials and tribulations of getting older, although you certainly could. Often, just spending time with older women role models will assure you that you're on the right path. If you don't have any women to fill this role in your life, consider reading biographies of accomplished women that you admire.

You may not be your own best cheerleader every day of the week. As your body changes, you're bound to have days when you don't feel very poised or confident. That's perfectly normal. Dust yourself off, be kind to yourself and keep going. With practice, you can develop a newfound confidence and richly deserved sense of empowerment as you embark on this next stage of your life.

PERSONAL STORY: PENNY | AGE 65

" I was a late bloomer when it came to menopause. In my late 40s and early 50s, I watched my friends go through perimenopause and, eventually, menopause — and there I was, still having periods. When I had my annual physical, my doctor would ask, "Are you still menstruating?" Grudgingly, I'd say yes, and he'd say, "Well, you know, the average age for menopause is 51, so somebody has to be on the high side to make that average!"

We had that same exchange, every appointment, for years.

When I finally did start perimenopause, at age 53, I really only had two symptoms: hot flashes and, oddly enough, regular periods — which, for me, were irregular. Ever since puberty, I'd had erratic menstrual cycles. I could go six, eight, even 10 weeks between periods. Then, at 53, I started having periods every month, like clockwork.

For years, I had hot flashes and those strangely regular periods. Then, as I neared my late 50s, my periods changed again. I could go several months without one — and then only have a period for a couple of days.

I also started noticing other symptoms. Extra hairs began to crop up on my face. Extra weight settled in my belly. I had to cross my legs when I sneezed to keep from leaking urine (that was fun). And my hot flashes became more persistent. There were times when I'd stick my head out the door in the middle of winter just to cool off!

I finally went through menopause at age 58. When I got what ended up being my last period, I remember thinking, "This is so wrong that I'm 58 and still doing this!"

The years since have been anticlimactic. Sometimes I still feel kind of unbalanced. But for the most part, it's nice not to worry about having a period. It may be one of the great perks of growing older!

16

Weight management

Your overall health is a complex picture of countless factors. Among those factors, a healthy weight — one in which you have an appropriate amount of body fat compared to your overall body mass — can go a long way. Statistically, a healthy weight reduces your risk of cardiovascular and other diseases, and it can help you have enough energy day to day. It may also help improve your menopause symptoms, like hot flashes and poor sleep. In addition, weight management is a key strategy to combat belly fat and muscle loss in midlife.

Think of weight management as a solid foundation for any other menopause symptom treatment options you might try. For example, if you want to consider hormone therapy, you need to be generally healthy and free of certain conditions such as cardiovascular disease.

Even if you're already at a healthy weight, you may find the changes that come with menopause and age make it harder to maintain rather than gain. Now is a good time to focus on your well-being and form healthy habits that will last you the rest of your life.

YOUR HEALTHY WEIGHT

How do you know if you're at a healthy weight? To answer that question, you need to consider more factors than just the number on the scale.

Body mass index

You're probably familiar with the body mass index (BMI). It's a measure of your body weight in relation to your height. Look at the table on pages 270–271 to find your BMI. You can also find many BMI calculators online. This index has become the routine way to identify excess weight.

THE IMPACTS OF EXCESS BODY WEIGHT

Excess body weight has serious health implications that can affect your quality of life and longevity. For women entering menopause, being overweight or obese is associated with more-frequent hot flashes. And although obesity is generally associated with a lower risk of osteoporosis, this hasn't been found to reduce the risk of fractures. Obesity is also a risk factor for cardiovascular disease — the leading cause of death in women, and a disease that becomes more prevalent after menopause. Obesity can increase your risk of insulin resistance, type 2 diabetes, high blood pressure, elevated cholesterol levels, stroke, gallbladder disease, liver disease, sleep apnea, osteoarthritis, certain types of cancer and your overall risk of dying. It may also increase the risk of Alzheimer's disease. Your risk of developing these weight-related health problems increases with age. But beyond these disease risks, being obese can have a significant impact on your overall well-being and self-esteem.

The good news is that you don't need to achieve a bodybuilder's physique in order to improve your health. A weight loss of even 3% to 5% of your body weight can yield health benefits — and it may reduce the number of hot flashes you experience.

A BMI of 25 or greater is classified as overweight, and 30 or greater is classified as obese. However, your BMI doesn't differentiate between weight due to fat mass versus muscle mass. Also, BMI doesn't offer any information about the distribution of excess body fat — whether it's around the belly or in the lower body, or both. BMI and distribution of excess body fat are both important factors that have significant implications for your health.

Despite these limitations, your BMI still provides useful information in understanding whether you're at a healthy weight.

Fat distribution

You may have heard about the increased health risks that come with having an "apple-shaped" body type, where fat is carried around the waist, compared to a "pear-shaped" body type — where fat is stored in the hips and thighs. Belly fat, or visceral fat, is stored deeper in your abdomen, surrounding your organs, and affects your body in more adverse ways than does subcutaneous fat, which is stored under your skin. Excess visceral fat is associated with a greater risk of diseases such as type 2 diabetes, hypertension and high cholesterol and with higher rates of death — even in individuals with a normal BMI. Storing fat in your legs or hips is generally associated with lower cardiovascular risks, even in individuals classified as obese by the BMI scale.

Genetics play a role in your fat distribution, and you also tend to store more fat around your middle as you age. And as you learned in Chapter 2, the loss of estrogen at menopause is also associated with greater fat accumulation around your middle. Measuring your waist circumference is an easy way to figure out whether you're carrying too much belly fat. Using a flexible measuring tape, stand and measure around your stomach area just above your hipbone. Pull the tape measure until it's snug but doesn't press into your skin, and make sure it's level all the way around. For women, a waist measurement of 35 inches (89 centimeters) or more indicates an unhealthy concentration of belly fat. However, there is nothing magic about that particular number. In general, the greater the waist measurement, the greater the health risks. And though the health impacts of visceral fat are serious, the good news is that when you lose weight, abdominal fat tends to be lost first, and at a higher rate than fat elsewhere in your

WHAT'S YOUR BMI?

To determine your body mass index (BMI), find your height in the left column. Follow that row across until you reach the column with the weight nearest yours. Look at the top of the column for your approximate BMI.

	NORMAL		OVERWEIGHT		
BMI	19	24	25	26	27
Height	Weight in pounds				
4'10"	91	115	119	124	129
4'11"	94	119	124	128	133
5'0"	97	123	128	133	138
5'1"	100	127	132	137	143
5'2"	104	131	136	142	147
5'3"	107	135	141	146	152
5'4"	110	140	145	151	157
5'5"	114	144	150	156	162
5'6"	118	148	155	161	167
5'7"	121	153	159	166	172
5'8"	125	158	164	171	177
5'9"	128	162	169	176	182
5'10"	132	167	174	181	188
5'11"	136	172	179	186	193
6'0"	140	177	184	191	199
6'1"	144	182	189	197	204
6'2"	148	186	194	202	210
6'3"	152	192	200	208	216

Source: National Institutes of Health, 1998

People of Asian descent with a BMI of 23 or higher may have an increased risk of health problems.

OVERWEIGHT			OBESE			
28	29	30	35	40	45	50
Weight in pounds						
134	138	143	167	191	215	239
138	143	148	173	198	222	247
143	148	153	179	204	230	255
148	153	158	185	211	238	264
153	158	164	191	218	246	273
158	163	169	197	225	254	282
163	169	174	204	232	262	291
168	174	180	210	240	270	300
173	179	186	216	247	278	309
178	185	191	223	255	287	319
184	190	197	230	262	295	328
189	196	203	236	270	304	338
195	202	209	243	278	313	348
200	208	215	250	286	322	358
206	213	221	258	294	331	368
212	219	227	265	302	340	378
218	225	233	272	311	350	389
224	232	240	279	319	359	399

body. Exercise also plays an important role in targeting visceral fat — more on that later.

Body composition

When determining obesity, the BMI scale isn't able to take into account your body composition, which refers to the relative percentages of fat and lean muscle mass in your body. Especially in the middle ranges of the index, it may misdiagnose some people as obese when they actually have a high amount of lean muscle mass and low body fat.

The BMI scale may also classify some people as being at a normal weight when in reality they have too much body fat and a low muscle mass. This is called *normal weight obesity*. And in fact, it poses the same or greater health risks as obesity according to the BMI scale. Often, normal weight obesity is combined with excess abdominal fat. This toxic combination leads to greater cardiovascular risks. People with normal weight obesity are specifically at a greater risk of soft plaques in the arteries, which can lead to heart attacks. In particular, women who have normal BMI but a high body fat percentage may be at risk of early death due to cardiovascular disease.

If you have a BMI within the normal range but are carrying excess body fat, you will have low muscle mass. And because people tend to lose muscle and gain fat as they age, the BMI scale's accuracy tends to worsen as you age. Regardless, it's still the case that looking at your BMI alone may mask a trend toward normal weight obesity and cause you to underestimate your cardiovascular risks. About 30 million Americans may be considered normal weight obese and not know it. Fortunately, as with its role in targeting abdominal fat, exercise is one strategy that can help improve body composition and thus reduce the likelihood of normal weight obesity.

Putting it all together

Your BMI, fat distribution and body composition — as well as information about your diet, activity levels, and family and personal health history — will help you and your health care provider settle on a healthy weight target. Together, you can discuss any weight-related goals you might have, such as building muscle mass, improving your nutrition, losing fat or all the above.

It's important to note that some people are genetically predisposed to being overweight, and may be overweight despite being active and eating well. If this sounds familiar, make sure your practitioner is a trusted partner in your health. You should feel listened to and supported, no matter your weight.

And, if together you decide losing weight is your goal, you can discuss strategies to do it in a healthy way.

UNDERSTANDING YOUR ENERGY BALANCE

Weight gain and loss are dependent upon your energy balance — in other words, calories in versus calories expended. Calories from food provide the fuel you need to power your body's basic processes, such as breathing, circulating blood, digesting and performing physical activity, as well as regulating hormone levels and growing and repairing cells. The calories you need to maintain your current weight depend on a variety of factors, including your sex, age, body size and composition, and activity level.

If weight loss is the goal, it ultimately depends in part on tipping the balance of energy to burn more than you take in. You need to fuel your body with less food energy or increase the number of calories you burn, or both. The healthiest weight loss — and the type you're most likely to maintain — tends to be slow and steady. People sometimes lose weight faster in the first few weeks of a new regimen. However, long-term weight loss of about 1 or 2 pounds a week is considered a reasonable goal for most people.

In reality, though, weight loss is complex. As you lose weight, your body mass and composition change. Your body responds by undergoing a variety of hormonal changes that may make it more challenging to keep dropping pounds. And you also have the hormonal shifts of menopause to contend with. After you've lost weight, you tend to burn fewer calories through basic metabolic processes, and the calories you spend through exercise also decrease. What this all means is that the same food intake that originally gave you a negative energy balance may no longer be enough of a calorie deficit to continue losing weight.

This is a common experience — the dreaded weight-loss plateau — and it can be a frustrating time. Knowing in advance that it will likely happen may help you prepare for it. Take a look at your eating and exercise habits. Research has shown that plateaus often happen earlier than they would naturally because of slip-ups in sticking with your healthy routines. When you do reach a plateau, it's a good time to reassess your goals and remind yourself why you've committed to losing weight. In order to kick-start your weight loss, you might need to reduce your calorie intake further and rev up your workout routine. Exercise counteracts the decreased energy expenditure that occurs in response to the reduced calorie intake. Keep in mind that if you're strength training, increased muscle mass may mask fat loss if you're looking only at the number on the scale.

Weight loss is a journey that's best measured in years, not months. Keeping that in mind can help you set reasonable goals and prepare for the long haul and the inevitable bumps in the road.

FOUNDATIONS OF A HEALTHY DIET

As you go through menopause, mostly, the same old advice holds true: To feel your best and achieve a healthy weight, build from the right foundation.

A balanced approach

The foundation of healthy eating is a balanced diet based on vegetables, fruits, whole grains, lean proteins, healthy fats and limited sodium or added sugar. Fueling your body with a balanced diet like this can improve your health and help you reach your weight goals. It can also be satisfying, flexible and delicious — which makes it more likely you'll stick with it in the long run.

The Mayo Clinic Healthy Weight Pyramid can be a helpful tool as you seek to make healthy food choices. Vegetables and fruits form the base of the pyramid. The more fresh produce you eat, the better. These foods contain fiber, water and nutrients to fill you up and provide you with high-quality fuel. The serving recommendations for other food groups depend on your energy needs for your sex, age, body size and activity level. As you work your way up the pyramid, the less of each group you'll need as part of a balanced diet.

Is there a "menopause diet"?

No doubt you've seen various restrictive diets and weight loss methods touting extreme results. Some promote key nutrients to work with your metabolism for weight control during and after menopause. Others claim that the key to weight loss over 40 is intermittent fasting — alternating normal eating with periods of restricting calories. Different approaches involve eating no food or seriously restricting calories on certain days or during a window of time each day.

So, do any of these methods work? There is limited data from high-quality studies evaluating these specific plans. But in short, no

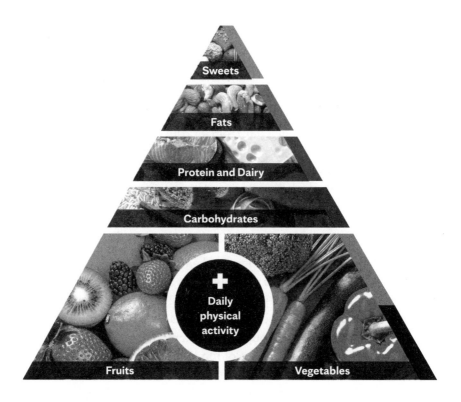

Mayo Clinic Healthy Weight Pyramid. See your health care provider before you begin any healthy-weight plan.

solid evidence shows that any specific diet is more effective than generally taking in fewer calories than you burn. The best "menopause diet" may be a take on a balanced diet that you can stick with long term. See what works for you. For example, some women find that eating fewer simple carbs, especially limiting alcohol, helps with weight control in midlife.

Focus on fiber

If you're eating from the base of the pyramid, you'll already be consuming foods that are low in energy density — that is, they have few calories for their volume. This means you can eat more of them, consume fewer calories and feel fuller. Water and fiber in food help contribute to low energy density, so most fruits and vegetables fall under this category.

Fiber is the part of plant-based foods that isn't absorbed by your body. It supports the health of your digestive tract and can reduce insulin resistance as well as the risk of high blood pressure, type 2 diabetes, stroke and heart disease. There's evidence that diets high in fiber are associated with lower body weight.

Unfortunately, most women don't get enough fiber. Try to eat at least 21 to 25 grams of fiber a day from a variety of foods. Fiber is found in fruits, vegetables, whole grains, beans, lentils, nuts and seeds. Eat your fruits and vegetables with their skins on to help increase your fiber intake, and drink plenty of water throughout the day to help fiber move through your digestive tract.

Portion distortion

A serving of food is a specific, measured amount of food. A portion is how much food we put on our plate and may contain many servings. An important part of weight loss or maintaining a healthy weight is eating moderate portion sizes. Large portions have become so prevalent that it seems normal to consume large amounts of food in a single meal. However, standard portions of food are often much more than your body needs. This distortion is reinforced by the size of our plates, serving utensils and meal packaging.

Visual cues can help you estimate serving sizes in your meals — see the table at right for some examples.

SIZING UP A SERVING

It's important to understand how much of a particular food makes up a serving. Many people envision servings to be larger than they are. These visual clues can help you sense how much to start with.

Vegetables	Visual cue
1 cup broccoli	1 closed fist
2 cups raw, leafy greens	2 closed fists

Fruits	Visual cue
½ cup sliced fruit	Tennis ball
1 small apple or medium orange	Tennis ball

Carbohydrates	Visual cue
½ cup pasta or dried cereal	Cupped handful
½ bagel	Front of a fist
1 slice whole-grain bread	DVD
½ medium baked potato	Tennis ball

Protein/Dairy	Visual cue
3 ounces of fish	Deck of cards
2-2½ ounces of meat	⅔ deck of cards
1½-2 ounces of hard cheese	⅓ deck of cards

Fats	Visual cue
1 teaspoon butter or margarine	Tip of thumb
1 tablespoon peanut butter	1 thumb

The data on drinks

It's easy to gulp down hundreds of extra calories in a matter of minutes, which is why high-calorie beverages can quickly sabotage your weight-loss goals. People who consume sugary drinks — including fruit juice with added sugar — are at an increased risk of weight gain.

Some evidence suggests that diet soda is no better if you're trying to lose weight. Studies have found that diet soda intake was associated with greater waist circumference and abdominal fat gain — even without a changing BMI. In one study, diet soda consumers had a gain in waist circumference that was three times greater than that of non-soda drinkers. This effect was exacerbated in individuals who were already overweight or obese.

Instead of sugary drinks, focus on getting lots of water. Try adding some lemon, cucumber or berries for some infused flavor without the calories, or try sparkling water if you need a bit of fizz. If high-calorie coffee drinks are your downfall, try a low-fat milk, such as 1% or skim, skip the whipped cream and try to find a satisfying, low-calorie alternative most of the time.

Alcohol is another source of concentrated calories. Alcohol has been associated with more fat being stored around the stomach area. If you drink, do so in moderation (up to one drink a day for women). However, even one drink every day may be too much if you're concerned about your weight.

EXERCISE AT MIDLIFE

The importance of exercise for menopausal women can't be overstated. At a time in life when your disease risk is often creeping up and you have a harder time managing your weight, exercise can be an invaluable tool in your toolbox.

The power of exercise

Exercise can play a unique role in combating two common trends experienced around menopause — loss of muscle mass and an expanding waistline. Exercise builds muscle, improving your body composition and making it less likely you'll fall into the category of normal

DIET VS. EXERCISE

So what's more important for maintaining or losing weight — diet or exercise? The answer is that they're equally important but for different reasons.

Exercise burns calories and is effective in preventing weight gain, even in individuals with a genetic predisposition to obesity. It also improves your body composition, targets visceral fat and has numerous health benefits. However, it's hard to lose weight through physical activity alone. Research indicates that diet is a more critical part of losing weight, at least in the initial stages, and that exercise has a greater impact on keeping the pounds off over time. A combined approach is likely the most effective way to maintain your healthy weight in the long term.

weight obesity. Greater muscle mass helps your body burn more calories at rest and during exercise. Some research shows that strength training can lead to a reduction in abdominal fat, even without a change in overall body weight or BMI. And you don't have to be a fitness addict to see benefits — high-intensity interval training (HIIT), a time-efficient approach, may help reduce visceral fat better than moderate- intensity exercise. After you've lost weight, exercise can specifically help prevent you from regaining belly fat.

Regardless of your BMI, exercise lowers the risk of death and reduces your risk of many conditions, such as osteoporosis and cardio-vascular disease, conveying important health benefits even while you may still be working on shedding pounds. Although it's hard to lose weight through physical activity alone, exercise does play an important role in preventing weight gain in the first place, as well as maintaining the weight loss achieved through calorie restriction.

By helping you maintain a healthy weight, exercise may help manage your menopausal symptoms. Regular exercise can improve sleep, lessen anxiety and stress, enhance sexual arousal and improve your overall quality of life. If you aren't used to exercising, it may initially be a trigger for hot flashes because it temporarily increases your core body temperature. If hot flashes are a problem, you may want to start slowly and pick up the pace as your fitness increases.

How much do you need?
U.S. guidelines recommend adults get at least 150 minutes of moderate-intensity aerobic exercise or 75 minutes of vigorous aerobic activity a week for health benefits and to maintain weight. This is equal to 30 minutes of moderate-intensity activity five days out of the week. Even greater health benefits will come from getting 300 minutes of moderate-intensity or 150 minutes of vigorous aerobic activity — and this higher amount is likely needed in order to lose weight and keep it off.

It's also important to include strength-training activities at least

EXERCISE FOR MULTIPLE BENEFITS

Exercise has many benefits in addition to helping you maintain a healthy weight. Exercise can:
- Build lean muscle mass, improving strength and increasing your metabolism.
- Reduce visceral fat.
- Slow the bone loss that comes with menopause and reduce the risk of falls and osteoporosis.
- Decrease insulin resistance and reduce your risk of various conditions, such as heart disease, type 2 diabetes, high blood pressure, and breast and colon cancers. Exercise can also function as a treatment for many of these same conditions.
- Stimulate your brain and perhaps even reduce the risk of cognitive decline and Alzheimer's disease.
- Boost your mood and combat depression.
- Enhance sexual arousal.
- Improve sleep and energy levels.

twice a week. This is especially true for menopausal women who are trying to prevent muscle loss and maintain bone strength. You can use weight machines, handheld weights, resistance bands or your own body weight. Consider finding a reputable personal trainer to get started with strength-training activities if you aren't familiar with them. Balance and flexibility exercises can round out your routine and help improve your stability and range of motion.

If you haven't exercised in a while, or if you have a health condition that prevents you from meeting these recommendations, talk to your health care provider before starting a new activity. Remember that something is always better than nothing! Make sure to keep your routine varied — an exercise plan pairing aerobic activity plus strength training tends to be the most effective for reducing body weight, waist circumference, overall fat mass and visceral fat.

CREATE LASTING CHANGE

Achieving and maintaining a healthy weight is no quick fix. It requires developing positive lifelong behaviors that will help you succeed — and strategies to continually reinforce these behaviors. This is why it's important to keep your motivation for change front and center in your mind. Whatever it is that you value — whether it's being able to live independently and travel long into your golden years or being a healthy role model for your kids and grandkids — this is the fuel for your commitment to lasting change.

Weight-loss success has more to do with sticking to a plan than choosing a specific diet. It will take commitment, planning and time to develop the weight-management strategies that will allow you to change existing habits. However, the return on investment in your health and quality of life can be tremendous. Here are some tips to help you get started.

Track your food and activity
There's solid evidence that keeping track of what you eat and how active you are can help with weight management. That's because we tend to underestimate the calories we consume and overestimate the

GET ON YOUR FEET

By now it's old news that sitting for long periods of time is linked with a number of health concerns, including obesity and metabolic syndrome — a cluster of conditions that includes increased blood pressure, high blood sugar, excess body fat around the waist and abnormal cholesterol levels. Too much sitting also seems to increase the risk of death from cardiovascular disease and cancer. And spending a few hours a week getting moderate or vigorous activity doesn't seem to significantly offset the risk.

But what if your job has you at a desk or behind the wheel for long periods? The solution seems to be less sitting and more moving overall. You might start by simply standing rather than sitting whenever you have the chance. For example:

- Stand while talking on the phone.
- If you work at a desk for long periods of time, try a standing desk — or improvise with a high table or counter.
- Go for a walk with a colleague rather than having a sit-down meeting.

The impact of movement — even leisurely movement — can be profound. For starters, you'll burn more calories. Even better, the muscle activity needed for standing and other movement seems to trigger important processes related to the breakdown of fats and sugars in the body. When you sit, these processes stall — and your health risks increase. When you're standing or actively moving, you kick the processes back into action.

amount of physical activity we do. Especially as you're establishing or adjusting habits, it's easy to misjudge. Tracking helps you remain aware, objective, accountable and goal-oriented as you consider your diet and activity each day.

There's no right or wrong way to keep food and activity records.

The following list includes common tracking tools. Don't be afraid to experiment as you choose one that's simple and convenient for you.

- **Apps.** Smartphone apps are a handy tool for many people, allowing you to enter food and activity throughout the day to track your calories. Some turn your phone into a pedometer or accelerometer to automatically track the duration and distance of an activity.
- **Wearable devices.** Trackers such as smartwaches can measure steps, distance, or calories burned. Some also monitor your sleep patterns.
- **Computer-based logs.** For some people, simple spreadsheets make the best logs. Different templates can be found online.
- **Paper workbooks or logs.** If you prefer pen and paper, a workbook or even a simple notebook may suit you best.

Set realistic goals

Set realistic goals so that you don't get discouraged, and remember that change takes perseverance and time. Unrealistic goals make it less likely that you'll adhere to your healthy behaviors.

- Goals will be most effective if they're aligned with your values. Remember that weight loss is a means to an end. Reflecting on your values and why you committed to losing weight in the first place can help renew your motivation and reinforce healthy behaviors when the going gets tough.
- Set intermediate goals that are SMART: specific, measurable, attainable, relevant and time limited. Instead of saying "I'm going to eat better," say "I'm going to eat one more serving of vegetables and fruit each day."
- Celebrate your milestones. Treat yourself to a weekend away or a massage. And keep revising your goals as needed.

Practice mindfulness

A holistic approach to weight loss engages the mind as well as the body. Mindfulness — the practice of being attuned to the present moment without judgment — may help you reinforce your positive behaviors.

- Tune in to your body and eat when you're hungry. Slow down and enjoy your food, paying attention to the physical sensations and

MEDICATIONS, SURGERY AND OTHER WEIGHT STRATEGIES

If you're having a hard time losing weight through diet and exercise, there are other options out there.

- **Prescription medications.** Used alongside diet changes and exercise, several drugs can help increase the amount of weight you lose. FDA-approved options for adults include orlistat (Xenical), phentermine combined with topiramate (Qsymia), naltrexone with bupropion (Contrave), liraglutide (Saxenda), and semaglutide (Wegovy). These generally work by reducing or regulating your appetite, making you feel full faster or preventing your body from absorbing fat. Semaglutide (Wegovy), a newer option, was originally approved to treat diabetes under the brand name Ozempic. It can lower blood sugar and blood pressure and may lead to significant weight loss, about 5% to 15% of total weight. Still, keep in mind that weight-loss drugs tend to have a number of adverse side effects, and they can be expensive. In addition, many people regain weight after stopping treatment.
- **Surgery.** When diet and exercise haven't worked, bariatric surgery may be an option. These procedures make changes to the digestive system to limit how much you can eat or absorb nutrients. Endoscopic weight loss surgery is a minimally invasive form in which a device is inserted down the throat to perform the procedure with no surgical incision.
- **Holistic and integrative therapies.** Despite a supplement market worth billions, dietary supplements and herbal remedies have little data supporting their safety and effectiveness for weight loss. Some studies have shown stress-relief practices combined with dietary counseling to help with weight loss.

There's no magic bullet when it comes to achieving a healthy weight. Still, these options — along with long-term healthy habits — may help with weight loss to reduce key health risks.

emotions you're feeling as you eat. This gives your body more time to signal that you're full. Eating while your mind is focused elsewhere may lead you to consume more calories, whereas chewing more times before swallowing may help reduce food intake. Stop eating when you're full. Take a pause before you reach for more. You might realize you don't need another serving after all. This more intuitive approach of noticing and following your body's internal cues has been shown to have positive impacts on healthy habits as well as body image.

- Part of weight loss is being able to make healthy decisions in spite of the forces working against you. An increased awareness of your behaviors may help you interrupt your default patterns and choose to engage in actions that are aligned with your goals and values. For example, sometimes you may experience hunger even when you don't physically need food. Being aware of this may help you choose whether to heed these cravings.

- Live life to the fullest now, even as you make a commitment to implement healthy changes. Don't wait for the weight to come off to engage in activities you enjoy.

Manage your triggers

Once you're aware of the cues that cause you to eat or avoid exercise, you may be able to circumvent them so that you don't have to rely on your willpower in the moment.

- If you eat when you're bored, try distracting yourself with an alternative activity, such as going for a brief walk. If you're always starving after work when you stop to get groceries, consider having a small snack before you leave the office so you're less tempted to buy unhealthy foods. Create a meal plan and shop for it on the weekend — filling your fridge with fruits and vegetables — so you don't have a "What are we having for dinner tonight?" moment that leads to less healthy choices. Cook healthy dishes on the weekend and freeze or save portions to have during the week.

- For many people, screen time is a trigger that can affect both diet and exercise, and excessive screen use is associated with an increased risk of obesity and type 2 diabetes. Consider setting daily time limits on your social media apps, or turn off autoplay on streaming services if you notice you're always getting sucked into the next episode instead of going for a walk. If you find yourself blankly munching food while scrolling or streaming video, you may want to limit screen time while eating to make sure you're mindfully enjoying each activity.

Get support

As you identify weight-related goals and strategies to meet them, lean on your health care provider as a source of information and support. You don't have to do it all alone.

- Enlist your partner, family or friends for support in achieving your weight goals. Let them know specific ways they can help — whether it's exercising with you or just sharing positive encouragement. Even a canine companion may be a source of motivation and help you stay committed to your regular walks.
- Consider signing up for a dedicated weight-loss program or a support group led by a professional.
- Remember that every woman goes through menopause. And though each person's experience is unique, many women are likely having the same symptoms and the same struggles with weight management as you are. Just knowing you're all in the same boat may help you keep some perspective as you go through this important and universal life transition.

A worthwhile commitment

This might all seem a bit daunting. You may be juggling a family, a career and an active social life — not to mention dealing with your menopause symptoms — and now you need to focus on your weight too? It's true that, like many worthwhile things, weight management is not necessarily easy. But making a deliberate choice to commit to your health and well-being at this critical time of life will likely pay off in how you feel while you're juggling everything else down the road. Approaching this self-care with a positive attitude can make a big difference in your experience.

17

Breast care

Perimenopause and menopause are associated with significant changes in your breasts. This transition marks a time when monitoring your breast health becomes more important.

In particular, in the years leading up to menopause, you and your health care provider will discuss breast cancer screening options. The American Cancer Society reports that a woman living in the U.S. has a 1 in 8 lifetime risk of being diagnosed with breast cancer.

But what are *your* risks of developing the disease? Is there anything you can do to reduce the risk? What screening options are best for you? This chapter will help you sort out these questions.

A LOOK INSIDE

Breasts are composed mainly of connective and fatty tissues. Suspended within the tissues of each breast is a network of milk-forming lobes.

Within each lobe are many smaller lobules, each of which ends in dozens of tiny bulbs that can produce milk. Thin tubes called *ducts* connect the bulbs, lobules and lobes to the nipple, which is surrounded by an area of dark skin called the *areola*. No muscles are in the breasts themselves, but the chest wall muscles covering your ribs lie underneath each breast.

Blood vessels and lymph vessels run throughout your breasts. Blood nourishes breast cells. Lymph vessels carry a clear fluid called *lymph*, which contains immune system cells and drains waste products from tissues. Lymph vessels lead to pea-size collections of tissue known as lymph nodes. Most of the lymph vessels in the breast lead to lymph nodes under the arm — axillary lymph nodes.

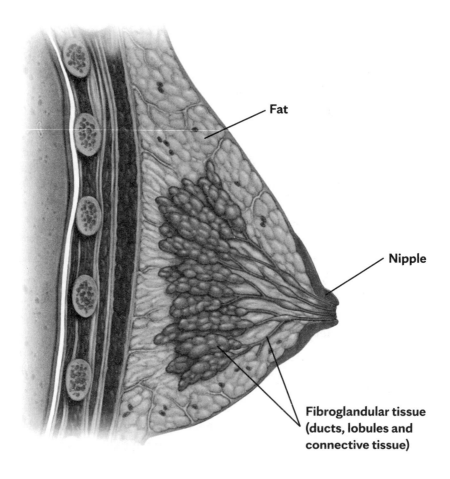

Fat

Nipple

Fibroglandular tissue
(ducts, lobules and
connective tissue)

Changes with menopause

The changes in your breasts during perimenopause and menopause are the result of hormonal changes that happen during this time. During perimenopause, you may notice at times that your breasts become more tender and swollen as estrogen levels fluctuate significantly. Later, as you approach menopause and estrogen levels decrease, the texture, shape and size of your breasts may also change.

You may notice a bumpy texture or lumpiness in your breasts, along with swelling, tenderness or pain. These are known as *fibrocystic changes*. While fibrocystic changes are common in menstruating women just before their periods, they can also happen in postmenopausal women taking hormone therapy. Hormone therapy may also make your breasts become denser than they would otherwise be.

What about cancer?

Cancer occurs when some cells begin growing abnormally. These cells divide more rapidly than healthy cells do and continue to accumulate, forming a lump or mass.

Breast cancer is the common term for a cancerous (malignant) tumor that starts in cells that line the ducts and lobules of the breast. If the cancer cells are confined to the ducts or lobules and haven't invaded surrounding tissue, the cancer is called *noninvasive*. Cancer that has spread through the walls of the ducts or lobules into connective or fatty tissue is referred to as *invasive*. Cancerous cells may spread (metastasize) through your breast to your lymph nodes or to other parts of your body.

The starting point matters. When abnormal cells are confined within the walls of the duct, this is known as ductal carcinoma in situ (DCIS). This condition may progress to invasive cancer over time and is therefore treated as breast cancer. Lobular carcinoma in situ (LCIS), in contrast, is not considered a breast cancer because the abnormal cells within the lobules don't usually progress to invasive cancer. However, women with LCIS are still at increased future risk of developing breast cancer.

Research shows that making healthy lifestyle changes can significantly reduce the risk of breast cancer, even in women at high risk. But if breast cancer does develop, finding it early is critical. With early detection, the disease is less likely to have spread or be fatal.

BREAST CANCER SCREENING

You shouldn't be worried if your health care provider has suggested that you begin breast cancer screening. The purpose of screening is to detect disease, such as cancer, in its earliest stages when it's the most responsive to treatment. Early detection of breast cancer reduces the need for aggressive treatment options and increases the chance of a cure.

There are a variety of breast cancer screening tests that may be used. The screening methods your health care provider recommends will be based on your breast cancer risk factors. For women at average risk, the screening technique that's universally recommended is mammography. Some organizations also recommend clinical breast exams.

Mammography

Mammography is an X-ray examination used to screen for breast cancer or to evaluate abnormalities noted on the breast examination. Low doses of radiation are used to create detailed images of the breasts. These images are captured on film or digitally stored on a computer. From these images, a radiologist can detect changes in breast tissue or evaluate areas of concern.

A screening mammogram is a breast X-ray that's done to detect breast cancer in a person with no breast symptoms or abnormality. A diagnostic mammogram is a breast X-ray used to investigate changes in the breast such as a lump, new differences in the size or shape of your breasts, nipple discharge or a thickening of a nipple, or change in the texture of the breast tissue. The diagnostic mammogram may involve more testing such as spot compression images taken to magnify an area of concern in your breast.

You may want to schedule your mammogram for the week after your period to minimize breast pain. When scheduling, you may be asked to provide your family history of breast disease. Be prepared to document who in your family has experienced breast disease and their age at the time of their diagnoses. You may also be asked about your personal history of breast issues, including previous biopsies, or any hormone therapy use. Your health care provider will use this information to assess your risk and settle on a screening strategy that is right for you.

On the day of the mammogram, you'll want to skip using deodorants, antiperspirants, powders, lotions or creams under your arms or on or near your breasts. These items sometimes contain metallic particles that could interfere with the quality of the images captured. Taking over-the-counter pain medication 1 to 2 hours prior to your appointment can help alleviate the discomfort.

During the mammogram you'll stand in front of the X-ray device. A technician will place each breast on a platform. Your breast will be compressed to help spread out the breast tissue, making it easier to examine. The compression also ensures that your breast remains still so the image is not blurred. The pressure may be uncomfortable. If you experience too much discomfort, tell the technician. You'll be asked to hold your breath for a few seconds while the image is taken. The entire examination usually takes less than 30 minutes.

Although mammography is the most widely used method for early breast cancer detection, not all cancers are found through mammography. You should never ignore a breast lump, nipple discharge or any other change in your breasts, even if your mammogram is normal.

BREAST SELF-AWARENESS

So far, research has failed to show that breast self-exams reduce breast cancer deaths. But that doesn't mean that you shouldn't check your breasts. Breast self-awareness is still important, and it's a two-part process. First, get familiar with your breasts — their appearance, texture and size — and take note when there are changes. Second, know how to respond to the changes that you observe in your breasts, seeking medical attention when warranted.

Premenopausal and perimenopausal women should remember that breast tissue changes in response to menstrual changes in your hormone levels. You may find that examining your breasts is more comfortable immediately after your period.

WHAT TO KNOW ABOUT BREAST DENSITY

Breast density is an important risk factor for breast cancer. Your risk of cancer is 4 to 6 times higher if you have dense breasts. Additionally, dense breasts can be challenging for traditional screening with mammography. Dense breast tissue has less fatty tissue and more fibroglandular tissue. On a mammogram image, fatty tissue appears dark and transparent.

Dense tissue, on the other hand, appears as patchy white areas. See examples below. Because cancers also look white on a mammogram, having dense breast tissue makes it more difficult to find breast disease through standard mammography.

Dense breasts are normal and are seen in about 40% to 50% of all women who have a mammogram. Some states require, by law, that you be notified if you have dense breast tissue. Your provider may recommend supplemental screening options if you have dense breasts. The decision on whether to do supplemental screening and which test to use will take into account your cancer risk and the risks versus benefits of screening. Insurance coverage of these options varies by state and insurer.

 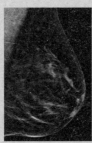 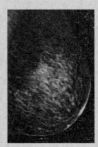 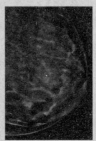

1. The breasts are almost entirely flat. **2.** There are scattered areas of fibroglandular density. **3.** The breasts are heterogeneously dense, which may obscure small masses. **4.** The breasts are extremely dense, which lowers the sensitivity of mammography.

Clinical breast exam

A clinical breast exam (CBE) may be performed by your health care provider during a regular checkup. If used, it's typically incorporated into your annual physical beginning in your 20s and repeated every 1 to 3 years.

During the CBE, your health care provider will visually inspect your breasts while you're in a seated or standing position. He or she will be looking for changes in the shape, size or appearance of your breasts.

As estrogen levels drop with menopause, there's a reduction in the glandular tissue of the breasts and an increase in fatty tissue. Breasts will often change shape as the breast tissue becomes less elastic. You may notice that your breasts sag more, have a noticeable elongated shape or flattened appearance, or that the position of your nipples relative to your breasts changes. It's important that you share with your health care provider any visual changes to your breasts that you've noticed so that he or she can assess those changes during your exam.

Your health care provider will also carefully feel (palpate) your breasts for any lumps or abnormalities. During this part of the physical exam, you'll be lying down. Your provider will make note of any changes to the texture or appearance of the skin of your breasts or nipples. He or she may also feel under each arm to figure out if you have enlarged lymph nodes.

It's important to remember that a lump does not necessarily indicate cancer. Normal breast tissue can feel lumpy, especially as breasts change in response to hormone fluctuations. Guide your health care provider to any abnormalities you may have noticed. Additionally, ask your provider to guide you to any lumps or changes in breast texture he or she identifies during your exam. This will help you become familiar with your breasts and recognize subtle changes. If a lump is found, more evaluation may be required.

Other screening methods

While mammography is the best screening option for most women, other techniques may be recommended if you are at high risk of breast cancer or have dense breasts. They include:

Breast tomosynthesis This procedure is sometimes referred to as *3D mammography* because it uses the same technology as digital mammography but takes multiple images of the entire breast to create a 3D image. This allows radiologists to see different layers of tissue within the breast and view details within the tissue at different angles. Breast tomosynthesis is most often used in combination with digital mammography and may reduce the number of false positive results from mammography alone. That can reduce the need for follow-up imaging.

Ultrasound This imaging method, also called *sonography*, uses sound waves to create an image of tissue. Breast ultrasound is most commonly used as a diagnostic tool to further evaluate abnormalities, such as a lump, that were identified on a mammogram or through a CBE. Ultrasound can be very useful in distinguishing a benign breast condition, such as a cyst, from a more suspicious mass that would require a biopsy.

Molecular breast imaging (MBI) This procedure, also known as a *nuclear medicine study*, uses tiny amounts of an intravenously injected radioactive tracer that's picked up mainly by tumor cells. The tracer is injected into a vein in your arm. A special camera detects the tracer in your breasts and produces images that identify areas where it has accumulated abnormally. Side effects are minimal. The radiation dose is very low, and the tracer usually leaves your body within a few hours. This test is used as a supplemental screening tool and is helpful for women with dense breasts.

Magnetic resonance imaging (MRI) MRI is a procedure that uses magnetic fields and radio waves, rather than radiation, to create a multidimensional image of the breasts. A contrast material, delivered into a vein through an IV, is used to enhance the appearance of tissues and blood vessels, which can help locate and identify tumors. Breast MRI is generally considered more sensitive than mammography and may be able to pick up some breast cancers that are not visible through mammography. It's not a perfect tool and can result in false positive test results, leading to the need for additional imaging with ultrasound and other tests. MRI is used as an additional screening tool in women at high risk of breast cancer who meet certain criteria.

Screening controversies and risks
Breast cancer death rates have dropped more than 40% since 1990. This decline has been attributed to earlier detection through screening

RED FLAGS: VISUAL BREAST CHANGES TO LOOK FOR

The following changes should be discussed with your health care provider.

- **Dimpling.** A puckering or retraction of the skin on the surface of the breast. The layer of skin on top of the breast may appear uneven and resemble cellulite or the texture of a golf ball.
- **Inflammation.** Localized swelling in the breast that may appear red and sore. This swelling happens quickly, within a day or two, and often looks like an infection of the breast. Your skin may be firm and warm to the touch. The inflammation may affect only one breast and could be accompanied by other symptoms such as a lump or changes in skin texture or appearance such as bruising or other discoloration of the skin.
- **Nipple retraction.** Some women are born with inverted nipples that appear indented into the breasts. New onset nipple retraction occurs when a woman whose nipples were previously raised above the surface of the breast experiences changes in the position or appearance of the nipple in relationship to the breast.
- **Nipple discharge.** Clear or bloody discharge that secretes either spontaneously from the nipple or as the result of lightly squeezing the nipple doesn't necessarily predict significant disease such as cancer but should always be evaluated.
- **Peau d'orange changes.** These are changes to the texture of the skin covering the breast, making the skin feel like and resemble an orange peel.
- **Rash on nipples.** May resemble eczema and leave the nipples looking red and scaly. Nipples may become itchier and more sensitive. Any rash on the nipple or the surrounding pigmented skin (areola) must be evaluated.

— specifically mammography — and more-effective treatment. You might wonder, then, how soon you should start screening for breast disease and how often to repeat screening. Unfortunately, there's not a clear answer to this question. In 2009, the U.S. Preventive Services Task Force (USPSTF) updated its position on breast cancer screening. It recommended that women wait until age 50 to begin regular screening mammography. USPSTF also recommended that screening mammography be done every two years rather than yearly. The task force cited evidence that early screening and more-frequent screening could lead to more false positives and unneeded testing, such as biopsies, which may outweigh the benefits.

For years, many medical organizations — including the American Cancer Society (ACS), American College of Radiology and Mayo Clinic — chose not to adopt the USPSTF recommendations and continued recommending screening with annual mammography beginning at age 40. However, in 2015, the ACS updated its breast cancer screening guidelines. The new guidelines shifted the recommended starting age for annual mammography for women at average risk from 40 to 45. In addition, the ACS recommended that women age 55 and older be screened every two years instead of every year and continue biennial screening as long as they're in good health and are expected to live at least 10 more years. The ACS also recommended that women ages 40 to 44 and over age 55 have the option of annual screening based on their personal preferences. Finally, the ACS chose to no longer recommend clinical breast exams for women of average risk at any age.

It's important to note that these guidelines are not intended for women with breast symptoms or changes or for those at high risk of breast cancer. Mayo Clinic recommends shared decision-making between women and their health care providers when considering the timing of screening.

In general, data shows that women between the ages of 50 and 74 experience the greatest benefits from screening. This is because your risk of breast cancer increases as you age. Mammograms are good at finding cancers early, before symptoms present and when treatment can be more effective and potentially less aggressive. In addition, the risks of mammography are greater for younger women. Studies have shown that women in their 40s who participate in regular

SCREENING GUIDELINES

The chart below provides a summary of the latest recommendations for breast cancer screening for women at average risk who have no symptoms.

Age	American Cancer Society recommendation	U.S. Preventative Services Task Force recommendation
20s and 30s	No routine screening	No routine screening
40 to 44	Individualized decision to begin mammogram every year	Individualized decision to begin mammogram every two years
45 to 49	Mammogram every year	Individualized decision to begin mammogram every two years
50 to 54	Mammogram every year	Mammogram every two years
55 to 74	Mammogram every two years (or yearly, if preferred)	Mammogram every two years
75 and older	Mammogram every two years (or yearly, if preferred), as long as the individual is in good health and has a life expectancy of 10 years or longer	No recommendation

screening mammograms are more likely to have false positive results, meaning the test identifies a concern that winds up not being cancer. False positive results lead to increased expense and anxiety for women as more tests are ordered. Mammography is much less effective at finding cancer in dense breast tissue than in fatty tissue. This may be a problem for younger women, who tend to have a greater amount of dense breast tissue. Mammography may also detect certain types of cancer that grow so slowly that they may never pose a threat.

Mammography is a useful screening tool, but deciding when to begin screening is a personal decision. Weigh your risk factors and discuss with your health care provider which screening methods are best for you.

RISK ASSESSMENT

Many women want to understand what their chances are of developing breast cancer and if there's anything they can do to reduce their risk. Understanding your personal risk can help you and your health care provider make decisions about how often you should be screened, what screening methods should be used and what types of risk-reduction strategies you should consider.

Estimating breast cancer risk is difficult because researchers don't fully understand how certain risk factors affect breast health in individual women. Researchers can't say for certain why one woman develops breast cancer and why another woman does not.

Cancer begins when there is a change (mutation) in a cell that causes it to grow out of control. The mutation may be inherited — passed down from a parent to a child — or it may occur spontaneously in response to aging or environmental factors or without a known cause. Many women diagnosed with cancer are surprised because they don't have a family history of cancer. The truth is, most cancer is not hereditary. In fact, only 5% to 10% of breast cancers are the result of inherited genetic mutations. In addition, having a genetic mutation doesn't mean that you will develop cancer, just that you are more likely to develop cancer when combined with other factors.

Common risk factors

There are risk factors for breast cancer that you can control and others that you cannot. Here's a look at some of them:

- **Sex.** Both women and men have breast tissue. However, breast cancer is 100 times more common in women than men. This is because women have more breast cells than men do and those cells are constantly exposed to higher levels of the hormone estrogen, which stimulates breast growth.
- **Age.** You're more likely to get breast cancer as you get older.
- **Family history.** Having one female first-degree relative — such as a mother, sister or daughter — who has been diagnosed with breast cancer increases your own risk. The age of your first-degree relative at the time of her diagnosis is also important. In general, your risk of breast cancer increases with the number of first- and second-degree relatives who have been diagnosed with breast cancer and increases further still the younger those relatives were at the time of their diagnoses. While family history is a very significant risk factor for breast cancer, 85% of women with breast cancer do not have a family history of the disease.
- **Genetic mutations.** Certain inherited changes in your genes (mutations) increase the risk of breast cancer. The most common mutations are found on two specific genes: BRCA1 and BRCA2. These mutations can be inherited from a parent of either sex. There are other gene mutations that can lead to inherited breast cancer risk, but they are much less common and don't increase your overall risk as much as a BRCA mutation.
- **Breast density.** Your breast cancer risk increases with your level of breast density. In fact, breast cancer risk for women with dense breast tissue is 4 to 6 times higher than for women with nondense breasts. Dense breasts also impact the effectiveness of a mammogram, as cancers may be missed.
- **Radiation therapy.** Women who, as children or young adults, were treated with chest radiation for another cancer such as lymphoma have increased risk.
- **Previous history of breast cancer.** If you've survived breast cancer, you are at greater risk of another breast cancer diagnosis.
- **Menstrual history.** The ages at which you start and end menstruation

influence your risk of breast cancer. Women who began menstruating before the age of 12 or finish menstruating after the age of 55 have increased risk. The increased risk may be related to a longer duration of hormone exposure through a greater number of menstrual cycles.

- **Race and ethnicity.** There are certain groups that are more likely to develop breast cancer or be diagnosed with more-aggressive forms of breast cancer. Black women, compared to white women, have lower rates of breast cancer, but they're more likely to be

ARE YOU AT HIGH RISK?

Women with average risk have:
- No personal history of breast cancer
- No previous history of certain types of benign breast disease, including atypical hyperplasia or lobular carcinoma in situ
- No family history of breast cancer in a first-degree relative of either sex (parent, sibling or child) or family history of ovarian cancer in a first-degree female relative
- No previous chest radiation therapy

Women at increased or high risk may have (any or all):
- A personal history or family history of breast cancer
- A past diagnosis of proliferative benign breast disease such as atypical hyperplasia or lobular carcinoma in situ
- Dense breast tissue
- A history of chest radiation while a child or young adult, such as the radiation used to treat lymphoma

Women at very high risk have:
- Genetic testing results that indicate a BRCA1 or BRCA2 mutation or other genetic predisposition to breast cancer, or a family history of those mutations and no previous testing

diagnosed before age 40 with cancers that are fast growing and more difficult to treat. Hispanic women also have a lower diagnosis rate than white women. BRCA1 and BRCA2 mutations are more common in women of Ashkenazi Jewish ancestry.

Risk factors that you can control are more aptly described as lifestyle factors. These will be covered in more detail later on in this chapter.

Risk models

Researchers have developed computer models to predict or estimate a woman's risk of breast cancer. These models are based on data collected from many women in clinical studies. While each model has limitations, these tools can help you and your health care provider make decisions about screening, testing and other options that may reduce risk and protect breast health. Here are a few of the most common models:

The Breast Cancer Risk Assessment Tool, which is based on the Gail model, is one of the most widely used and studied tools. This model estimates the likelihood that a woman with certain risk factors will develop invasive breast cancer. Eight questions look at a person's history of previous breast cancer, current age, age at first period, age at first live birth, number of first-degree relatives (mother, sister or daughter) with breast cancer, number of previous biopsies, race and known BRCA1 or BRCA2 genetic mutations. This model can make predictions for white, Black, Hispanic and Asian and Pacific Islander women in the United States, but it isn't very exact in predicting an individual's risk.

Other models are similar but look at various factors. The Claus model captures more details about first- and second-degree relatives' history of cancer. This model is used to look at the breast cancer risk for a woman with a documented family history of breast cancer. The Tyrer-Cuzick model, used in the IBIS prediction tool, estimates the likelihood that a woman carries the BRCA1 or BRCA2 gene mutations, as well as the risk of developing breast cancer. It takes into account factors such as body mass index (BMI), previous benign breast disease and age at menopause, in addition to a detailed family history of breast cancer. The BWHS (Black Women's Health Study) Breast Cancer Risk Calculator is a model developed for U.S. Black women, based solely on data from that group.

It's important to remember that all the breast cancer risk assessment models give risk estimates only. Even women with low risk can develop breast cancer, so talk with your practitioner about the steps for screening and prevention that make sense for you.

Genetic screening

If you're considering having genetic screening, you may still have mixed feelings about it. Maybe you worry about living with the knowledge that comes from the results. You may be unsure about how and when to talk to others about it. The decision to go ahead with genetic screening is best made with the support of a genetic counselor who will walk you through the process, help you understand the benefits and limitations, and work with you to understand the results of your tests.

The role of a genetic counselor is to help you identify whether there is a pattern of cancer that runs through your family and to discuss the benefits and limitations of specific tests, the cost and insurance coverage information, and the people in your family who would benefit the most from being tested. The counselor can then guide you through the process once you've made the decision that is best for you. Genetic counselors will never push you to undergo testing, nor will they tell you what you should or shouldn't do.

If you decide to go ahead with genetic testing, the test itself is relatively simple. A blood or saliva sample will be sent to a specialized lab for analysis. Depending on the complexity of the tests ordered, your results should be available in 2 to 4 weeks. Only a small percentage of individuals will test positive for a genetic mutation. Your genetic counselor will help you understand your results and identify appropriate options for reducing your risk of breast cancer going forward.

REDUCING YOUR CANCER RISK

What can you do to prevent breast cancer? While we have some strategies that can reduce the risk of breast cancer, and research holds promise for developing better risk-reduction strategies, there's currently no guaranteed way to prevent the disease. For all women, irrespective of risk factors, a change in certain lifestyle habits may lower their risk to some degree. Women at high risk of breast cancer have other options to consider, as well.

Lifestyle

For most of us, the power of making healthy lifestyle choices and the impact of those choices on our health isn't a mystery. We know that maintaining a healthy weight, exercising regularly, eating a low-fat diet with diverse and healthy food choices, and limiting alcohol consumption are all important to our overall health. Often, the challenge is in establishing these habits. These specific steps can support better breast health and limit your risk of developing breast cancer:

Maintain a healthy weight. There's little doubt about the connection between obesity and an increased risk of breast cancer after menopause. Excess body fat leads to higher levels of estrogen, which in turn increases the risk of breast cancer. Excess weight increases your risk of other cancers too, including cancers of the kidney, colon, liver, pancreas, stomach, ovary, uterine lining, esophagus and thyroid.

Limit alcohol. Drinking alcohol increases the risk of breast cancer both before and after menopause. Research now shows that even one drink or less a day is linked with a higher breast cancer risk. The risk increases with the amount of alcohol consumed.

Choose a healthy diet. Women who eat a Mediterranean diet may have a reduced risk of breast cancer. This healthy dietary pattern includes a variety of fiber-rich whole plant foods, including fruits, vegetables, whole grains, legumes, nuts and seeds. It limits red meat and processed meat, refined grains, and added sugars, including fruit juice.

Exercise regularly. Aim for at least 30 minutes of exercise on most days of the week. In addition, aim to move more and sit less.

Assess hormone therapy

As you learned in Chapter 6, combination hormone therapy may increase the risk of breast cancer (although by less than other risk factors such as obesity or consuming more than one alcoholic drink a day). This doesn't mean you should avoid hormones — the increased risk may be acceptable to find symptom relief. But this is why it's important to talk to your health care provider about the benefits and risks.

WHAT ABOUT BREAST PAIN?

Nearly all women will experience breast pain (mastalgia) at some point in their lives. Breast pain can occur in one or both breasts and may include tenderness, aching, burning, tightness, soreness or a dull heaviness. Sometimes the pain will be focused more on the side of the breast. It's also common to experience pain in the armpit or on the front of the breast, centered around the nipple.

Pain that occurs around your menstrual cycle, lasting several days and then resolving, is called *cyclic mastalgia*. As your menstrual cycle becomes less regular, it may be difficult to distinguish cyclical from noncyclical breast pain. Noncyclical mastalgia is breast pain that cannot be associated with the hormone changes that accompany your menstrual cycle. Post-menopausal women are more likely to experience noncyclical breast pain. This pain may be centered more in the chest wall.

It's very rare for breast pain to signal something more concerning such as breast cancer. Talk to your health care provider about any breast pain that doesn't go away after one or two menstrual cycles, or pain that persists after menopause. There are treatment options that may help. In addition, your health care provider may want to review your medications to see if your breast pain could be a side effect of a specific drug. Caffeine in beverages or diet may also contribute to breast pain. Even a simple issue such as an improperly fitting bra could be the culprit.

Risk-reducing medications

If you've discovered that you're at high risk of developing breast cancer, you may want to consider this option. Chemoprevention — risk reduction using one of several medications — is best suited for women who meet any of the following criteria:

- Have received a risk model score greater than the general population

- Have had a recent biopsy that identified a high-risk condition such as lobular carcinoma in situ or atypical hyperplasia
- Are at least 35 years old and have a strong family history of cancer
- Have certain gene mutations, such BRCA2

However, there are often side effects to risk-reducing medications that may make the benefit not worth the risk for you. In addition, using the drug doesn't guarantee that you'll never develop breast cancer. You'll still need to keep up with regular breast screening.

Here's a look at some of the drugs used for chemoprevention:

Tamoxifen This drug is within a class of drugs called *selective estrogen receptor modulators* (SERMs) — drugs that change how estrogen interacts with breast cells by blocking estrogen from signaling cell growth in breast cells. Tamoxifen is one of the most studied SERMs used today. It's used both to treat estrogen-sensitive breast cancer and reduce the risk of recurrence. Tamoxifen is frequently given as a pill that you take once a day, typically for five years. The effects of tamoxifen on cancer prevention may continue for 10 years or longer after the medication has been stopped.

Women under the age of 50 without a BRCA1 mutation will experience the greatest preventive benefits from tamoxifen. Side effects include hot flashes, blood clots and increased risk of stroke and cataracts. While tamoxifen blocks the effects of estrogen in breast tissue, it mimics the effects of estrogen on uterine tissue, slightly increasing the risk of uterine (endometrial) cancers. Antidepressants known as selective serotonin reuptake inhibitors (SSRIs) may interact with tamoxifen and impact its effectiveness. Tamoxifen can be used by both premenopausal and postmenopausal women.

Raloxifene Raloxifene (Evista) is another frequently prescribed SERM used as a risk-reducing medication for invasive breast cancer. Like tamoxifen, it increases the risk of blood clots. But raloxifene does not affect the risk of endometrial cancer because it does not simulate the effect of estrogen on the uterus. While tamoxifen is more effective, raloxifene may be a better choice if you are postmenopausal and haven't had a hysterectomy. Raloxifene also helps preserve bone mass. However, it may cause hot flashes.

Aromatase inhibitors (AIs) The drugs in this class — including

PERSONAL STORY: JAMIE | AGE 47

" In 2013, my sister passed away after a 9-year battle with ovarian cancer. She was positive for a BRCA1 gene variant, and she had me promise I would get genetic testing. Almost a year later, I found the courage. When my results were positive, all I could think about was everything my sister went through, and *will that be my story too?* It's an understatement to say I was scared about my future as a woman, and as a mom.

At age 39, I had surgery to remove my uterus and ovaries and reduce my cancer risk.

The surgery itself was easy to recover from. But in the days after, due to the immediate hormonal imbalance, my mind was cloudy, I couldn't sleep and the hot flashes were unbearable. I couldn't control my emotions. I just wanted to stay in bed and cry. Headaches consumed my life, and my libido was at zero, so my relationship took a beating as well. After several months, and multiple doctor appointments to find the right dose of hormones, there was finally a light at the end of the tunnel. I slowly started getting my drive back, my energy increased, the headaches subsided and my sleep improved. I regained my confidence, which also helped me focus.

At the time, it was difficult to figure out if all my symptoms were related to my surgery or grief around losing my sister and, only a few months prior, my mom to lung cancer. The weight I felt was heavy. And when I started to feel better emotionally, mentally I was still struggling with the loneliness of losing two of the most important women in my life. My health care team worked together to meet with me and find the right medication combination that was safe for me, being a BRCA1 carrier. I'm very thankful for their trusted partnership in trying different approaches to care for my emotional, mental and physical well-being.

anastrozole (Arimidex), exemestane (Aromasin) and letrozole (Femara) — reduce the amount of estrogen in your body, depriving breast cancer cells of the fuel they need to grow. They are used to treat cancer that is hormone receptor positive in women who are postmenopausal. Some women may choose to use AIs to reduce the risk of breast cancer, although the drugs aren't currently FDA approved for this use. Although AIs aren't associated with an increased risk of blood clots or uterine cancer, they're newer medications and not much is yet known about long-term health risks. They do increase the risk of osteoporosis and may cause side effects such as hot flashes and vaginal dryness.

Risk-reducing surgery
Women at high risk of breast cancer also have surgical options for reducing their risk. While very effective at lowering risk, surgery has significant drawbacks. The decision should be made with your health care team and based on a thorough understanding of all options.

Preventive mastectomy Removal of both breasts (bilateral mastectomy) is an option for women at very high risk, such as BRCA1 and BRCA2 mutation carriers or women with a strong family history that suggests a gene mutation. Women with BRCA1 or BRCA2 mutations have a lifetime risk of breast cancer of 40% to 85%.

Prophylactic bilateral salpingo-oophorectomy This procedure — which involves the removal of both ovaries and fallopian tubes — is generally offered to women with BRCA1 or BRCA2 mutations who are at elevated risk of ovarian cancer in addition to elevated breast cancer risk. When performed before menopause, the risk of breast cancer is also reduced.

18

Strong bones

Whether you're approaching menopause or have already transitioned beyond it, you may be concerned about your bone health. Maybe you've heard that menopause comes with significant bone loss. Or perhaps you know some women in your life who are dealing with osteoporosis, a condition that causes bones to become brittle, weak and more prone to breaks. While some bone loss is inevitable as you age, weak bones and osteoporosis are not. There are proven steps you can take to protect the health of your bones and keep them strong.

YOUR CHANGING BONES

Bones are living, growing tissues that are continually changing. Throughout life, old bone is broken down and removed, and new bone is formed. When you're young, your body makes new bone faster than it breaks down old bone, and your bone mass increases. Most people reach their peak bone mass by their early 30s. As you age, you lose more bone mass than is created.

Around the time of menopause, the speed at which you lose bone mass increases. A big reason for this change is a decline in estrogen, a hormone that plays an important role in building and maintaining bone. It's estimated that women lose bone mass most rapidly beginning the year or two before menopause and continuing for 5 to 10 years after menopause. From that point on, bone loss continues but at a slower rate.

A loss of bone mass increases your risk of osteoporosis, which in turn increases your risk of fractures. Postmenopausal women are especially susceptible to fractures of the hip, wrist and spine. Worldwide, an

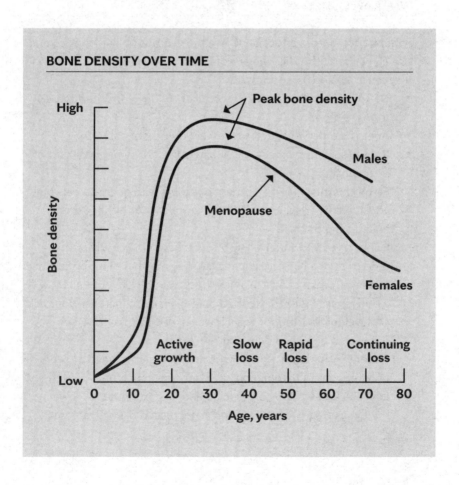

BONE DENSITY OVER TIME

estimated 1 in 3 women over the age of 50 will break a bone because of osteoporosis.

Because osteoporosis doesn't cause obvious symptoms, it's often called a silent disease. Many women don't know they're at risk until a bone is broken. A loss in height or a stooped posture can also be a sign of osteoporosis because these changes may be due to fractures in the bones of the spine (vertebrae). Fortunately, protecting your bones and preventing osteoporosis is easier than you think — and it's never too late to start.

WHAT AFFECTS BONE HEALTH?

A number of factors affect bone health — some you can control, and some you can't. The following risk factors may increase the likelihood that you'll develop osteoporosis:

- **Gender.** Women are much more likely to develop osteoporosis than are men.
- **Age.** The older you get, the greater your risk of osteoporosis.
- **Race.** You're at greatest risk of osteoporosis if you're white or of Asian descent.
- **Family history.** Having a parent or sibling with osteoporosis puts you at greater risk, especially if your mother or father experienced a hip fracture.
- **Body frame and weight.** People who have small body frames tend to have a higher risk because they may have less bone mass to draw from as they age. A low body weight for your height, with a body mass index (BMI) of 20 or less, can also increase your risk of developing osteoporosis. However, obesity may also be harmful to bone health in different ways.
- **Sedentary lifestyle.** People who are more active have a lower risk of osteoporosis than people who don't get much physical activity.
- **Low calcium intake.** Low calcium intake contributes to lower bone mass, early bone loss and an increased risk of fractures.

EVALUATING YOUR RISK

It's a good idea to take stock of your bone health in the early post-menopausal years, even if you aren't concerned about bone loss. Research shows that women, especially older women, often underestimate their risk of fractures owing to bone loss. In one study, more than 50% of patients with a moderate risk for developing fractures believed their risks were significantly lower. That number jumped to over 80% among patients at high risk of bone fractures.

- **Tobacco and alcohol use.** Research suggests that tobacco use contributes to weak bones. Similarly, regularly having more than two alcoholic drinks a day may increase your risk of osteoporosis.
- **Hormone levels.** An absence of menstruation (amenorrhea) for prolonged periods before menopause can increase the risk of osteoporosis. So can entering menopause before the age of 45. Having an overactive thyroid gland or using too much thyroid hormone for an underactive thyroid can also harm bone health.
- **Medical conditions.** Diabetes, other endocrine disorders and gastrointestinal disorders can increase the risk of low bone mass.
- **Weight loss.** Losing extra pounds through surgery, medication or lifestyle changes may lead to lower bone mass.
- **Eating disorders.** People who have anorexia or diet excessively are at risk of bone loss.
- **Certain medications.** Long-term use of steroid medications, such as prednisone, cortisone, prednisolone and dexamethasone, are damaging to bone. Other drugs that may increase the risk of osteoporosis include aromatase inhibitors to treat breast cancer, selective serotonin reuptake inhibitors, methotrexate, some anti-seizure medications, proton pump inhibitors and excessive amounts of aluminum-containing antacids.

One way to get a better sense of your bone health is to take advantage of the Fracture Risk Assessment Tool (FRAX). FRAX is a simple questionnaire that can estimate your risk of a bone fracture in the next 10 years. It was developed using data from several multithousand patient studies performed in different parts of the world.

FRAX is intended for postmenopausal women and men ages 40 to 90 who are not currently taking medications for osteoporosis. It's available free and online to anyone and takes into account age, sex, race, prior broken bones, family history of hip fracture, tobacco use, steroid medication use and medical conditions known to affect bone health. One way to access the tool is at the FRAX calculator online (frax.shef.ac.uk/FRAX). Once you're there, select the "Calculation Tool" tab, choose your country of origin, and enter your personal information.

Based on your answers to the FRAX questionnaire, an algorithm will calculate your chances of having any major fracture due to osteoporosis, as well as specific chances of a hip fracture, in the next 10 years. While this estimate is very generalized, it can help you and your health care provider decide when you might need further testing for osteoporosis.

FRAX can also be useful if your provider has already screened you for bone loss and found that you have low bone mass — reduced bone density that increases your risk of developing osteoporosis. FRAX results can help you and your care team decide if and when to start preventive therapy.

Keep in mind that FRAX isn't a perfect predictor, and it can't determine whether you have osteoporosis. It's also not intended for people currently taking medication to treat osteoporosis. If you use the FRAX calculator, it's best to discuss the results with your health care practitioner, who can make recommendations for you based on a more thorough understanding of your particular medical history, lifestyle and circumstances.

GETTING YOUR BONES TESTED

The gold standard for assessing your risk of fracture due to bone loss is bone density testing, a fast and painless process. Bone density testing is the most accurate way to find out whether you have osteoporosis or

WHAT'S THE DIFFERENCE BETWEEN OSTEOPOROSIS AND LOW BONE MASS?

Osteoporosis and low bone mass, also called osteopenia, are both conditions relating to bone density. Having osteoporosis means that your bones are significantly weakened, increasing your risk of developing bone fractures.

If you have low bone mass, your bone density is lower than normal but not low enough to be diagnosed as osteoporosis. Having low bone mass increases your risk of osteoporosis and bone fractures, but it doesn't mean you'll end up developing the disease. The lifestyle habits described in this chapter can help prevent low bone mass from progressing to osteoporosis.

low bone mass. When done repeatedly over time, bone density tests can also track the rate at which you're losing bone density. If you're already being treated for osteoporosis, the test can track how well your bones are responding to the treatment.

A bone density test measures the mineral content of your bones. The greater the mineral content, the denser and stronger your bones are. The most commonly used and most exact bone density test is the dual energy X-ray absorptiometry (DXA) test. It's also known as *DEXA*. This noninvasive test uses low levels of X-rays. Hip and spine density is measured using a central DXA machine. For a DXA scan, you lie on a padded table as a scanner passes over your lower spine or hip. This scan is the best way to diagnose osteoporosis and predict your risk of fractures. In some instances, a peripheral DXA (pDXA) test may be used to screen for osteoporosis. The pDXA uses a smaller, portable machine to scan your wrist, fingers or heel.

Once the DXA scan measures how dense your bones are, the measurement from the scan is converted to a T-score. A T-score reflects how your bone density compares to the average peak bone density of a healthy young adult of the same sex. The typical reference database for comparison is white men or women. So a T-score value of 0 means that your bone density is equal to the average bone density of a healthy, white young adult. The following T-score classifications have been established by the World Health Organization:

Normal	T-score above -1
Low bone mass (osteopenia)	T-score between -1 and -2.5
Osteoporosis	T-score of -2.5 or lower
Severe osteoporosis	T-score of -2.5 or lower with skeletal fracture

Your test results will also include a Z-score. While your T-score compares your bone density to a young adult's, the Z-score compares it with the average bone density for someone of your age, sex and ethnicity. A low Z-score can help flag whether something other than aging or menopause may be contributing to bone loss.

When should you be tested?

It's recommended that all women have a bone density screening by age 65. Testing is also recommended if you're transitioning into menopause or are in the early years of postmenopause and have other risk factors for osteoporosis (such as those on pages 310–311). If you've been taking medications that are known to cause bone loss, such as glucocorticoids, it's also recommended that you be tested.

How often should you be tested?

Your health care practitioner will recommend how often you undergo bone density testing based on your T-score and other factors. If the test shows that you don't need to be treated for osteoporosis, you likely won't need to be tested again for another 2 to 5 years or more. If you're already taking medication to treat osteoporosis, it's recommended that you be tested again a year or two after you begin treatment to determine whether the treatment is working.

Other tests for bone loss

To get a better sense of your current bone health, your practitioner may suggest gathering additional information about your bone strength with DXA or computerized tomography (CT). For example, if you have a DXA bone density test, it may include a trabecular bone score (TBS). This analysis looks at the structure, rather than the density, of your bone on a DXA image of your lower (lumbar) spine. Together with a bone density measurement, TBS can provide a fuller understanding of your bone quality and fracture risk.

PREVENTING BONE LOSS

Your current bone health has a lot to do with the strength of your bones in your late teens and early 20s. Adults who attained a high bone mass by their early 20s, when bones often reach their peak density, are at a lower risk of low bone density later in life.

That doesn't mean midlife is too late to take action. While it's normal to continue losing some bone mass as you age, there are steps you can take to slow that process and prevent osteoporosis. Even if you've been diagnosed with osteoporosis, it's important to do all you can throughout your life to improve your bone health.

Good nutrition

Eating a balanced diet of nutritious foods is important in maintaining an appropriate weight, which helps maintain healthy bones. In particular, the mineral calcium, along with vitamin D, is needed for healthy bones. Getting the recommended amounts of calcium and vitamin D is important throughout the rest of your life.

Calcium About 50% to 70% of bone tissue is made of calcium, the mineral that gives bones their hardness and strength. Getting enough calcium each day can help keep your bones strong, reduce bone loss and lower your risk of fractures. If you're a woman age 50 or younger, you need 1,000 milligrams (mg) of calcium a day. This daily amount increases to 1,200 mg when you're over the age of 50.

It's best to get your calcium from what you eat and drink. Dairy products, dark green leafy vegetables, and calcium-fortified fruit juices

GETTING ENOUGH CALCIUM IN YOUR DIET

Getting calcium in the foods you eat may be easier than you think. Here are just a few examples of calcium-rich foods:

Food source	Amount of calcium in milligrams (mg)
8 ounces plain, low-fat yogurt	450 mg
8 ounces fortified almond milk	449 mg
8 ounces fortified oat milk	350 mg
1 cup frozen chopped collard greens, boiled	325 mg
1.5 ounces cheddar cheese	307 mg
8 ounces fat-free milk	300 mg
½ cup firm tofu	250 mg
6 ounces calcium-fortified orange juice	263 mg
Calcium-fortified cereals	100–1,000 mg
1 cup fresh kale, cooked	175 mg
1 cup ice cream	170 mg
1 cup white beans	155 mg
1 cup pinto beans	80 mg
1 cup bok choy, cooked	185 mg
5 dried figs	70 mg

and soy beverages contain good amounts of calcium. For example, an 8-ounce glass of milk or calcium-fortified soy milk contains about 300 mg of calcium. Green vegetables such as broccoli, spinach or kale provide about 75 to 240 mg of calcium in a 1-cup serving when fresh or steamed.

You may need to take a calcium supplement if you're not getting enough calcium in your diet. Supplements are absorbed well and they are typically inexpensive. If you have or have had kidney stones or high blood calcium, talk to your doctor before taking calcium supplements. Taking more than 1,200 mg a day has not been shown to improve bone strength and may increase the likelihood of developing kidney stones, particularly in people who have a family history of developing them. Too much calcium taken in supplements may also be linked to heart problems. Establish a habit of taking the supplement at the same time each day, such as at bedtime or with a meal.

Vitamin D Vitamin D is an important nutrient for bone health. It allows your body to absorb calcium by enabling it to leave your intestine and enter your bloodstream. It also works in the kidneys to help your body absorb calcium that would otherwise be excreted. In combination with calcium, vitamin D can help slow bone loss and prevent osteoporosis. The recommended daily allowance for vitamin D is 15 micrograms (mcg), or 600 international units (IU) a day, for adults up to age 70. When you turn 71, the recommendation increases to 20 mcg (800 IU) a day.

Your body naturally produces vitamin D when your skin is exposed to direct sunlight. The amount your skin produces depends on the intensity of sunlight, the amount of skin exposed, your age and the pigment of the skin. Older skin and brown and Black skin will produce less vitamin D from the same exposure, compared with a young, white person's skin. Keep in mind that exposing your skin to sunlight increases your risk of skin cancer. For that reason, it's a good idea to wear protective clothing and use sunscreen if you're out in the sun for more than a few minutes.

If you tend to avoid the sun, or if you have Black or brown skin, you may need to get more vitamin D in other ways. Most dairy or plant-based milk is fortified with about 3 mcg (120 IU) of vitamin D a cup, although other dairy products usually aren't fortified. Many cereals are also fortified with vitamin D. Other good food sources include fatty fish such as trout, salmon and tuna. Most multivitamins also contain vitamin D. Be aware, though, that taking too much vitamin D can lead to high levels of calcium in the blood, which can increase your risk of kidney stones. The safe upper limit of vitamin D for adults is 100 mcg (4,000 IU) a day.

Exercise

Staying physically active is another way to help prevent bone loss. Exercise protects bone density and may even help to modestly increase it. Physical activity also improves posture, balance, strength and agility, all of which can prevent falls and reduce your risk of breaking a bone. What's more, exercise can help prevent disease, reduce stress, increase your energy levels and improve your overall sense of well-being.

The two types of physical activity that will most benefit your bones are weight-bearing and strength-training exercises. Being active in these ways throughout your life helps to build stronger bones, but it's never too late to start.

Weight-bearing exercise Weight-bearing activities involve doing aerobic exercise on your feet, with your bones supporting your weight. Examples include walking, running, dancing, tennis, elliptical training and stair climbing. Along with strengthening your bones, these activities can boost your heart health. It's worth noting that not all aerobic exercises strengthen bones. Swimming and cycling, for example, are good for your overall health but aren't weight-bearing exercises.

The general recommendation for adults is to get at least 150 minutes of aerobic exercise a week. That amounts to about 30 minutes on most days. You don't have to do all 30 minutes at once, though.

Strength training Strength training includes the use of free weights, weight machines, your body weight, resistance bands or water exercises to strengthen your muscles and bones. Strength training can also work directly on your bones to slow mineral loss. Aim to do strengthening exercises 2 to 3 days a week. If this seems daunting, consider focusing on one area of the body each day.

Keep in mind that the best weight-bearing and strength-training exercises for your bones are the ones you enjoy doing. You'll be less likely to stick with an activity if it feels like a chore.

If you haven't exercised much and you want to get started, it's a good idea to talk with your health care practitioner before you begin. Also consult your doctor if you've been diagnosed with osteoporosis or low bone mass, since certain activities may increase your risk of fractures.

Other lifestyle choices

Eating well and exercising are the best ways to protect the health of your bones, but other factors may also come into play. Here are some more steps you can take:

Avoid cigarette smoking and vaping. Smoking speeds up bone loss and increases the chance that you'll experience a fracture. Heavy smokers are also more likely to experience early menopause. And recent research shows that vaping may have a harmful effect on bone health too. On the other hand, quitting smoking has been shown to improve bone strength.

Avoid excessive alcohol. Research suggests that drinking moderate amounts of alcohol may strengthen bones. But having more than two alcoholic drinks a day may negatively affect your bone density. Being under the influence also increases your risk of falling.

Prevent falls. To lower your risk of falling and breaking a bone, wear shoes that offer good support and have nonslip soles. Clear your floors of clutter and check your house for electrical cords, area rugs and slippery surfaces that might cause you to fall. Keep rooms and stairwells brightly lit, and use nonslip mats in the bathtub and on shower floors.

MEDICATIONS FOR BONE LOSS

If you are postmenopausal and have been diagnosed with osteoporosis, or if you have a history of broken hip bones or fractured vertebrae, your health care practitioner may prescribe medication to strengthen your bones in order to reduce your risk of breaks. You might also receive treatment if you have low bone mass and are at a high risk of developing a fracture in the next 10 years.

When considering medication options, your practitioner will take into account your overall health, the severity of your bone loss and drugs you may be taking for other health conditions.

Bisphosphonates

Bisphosphonates are commonly prescribed for postmenopausal women with osteoporosis or with an increased risk of fracture. These drugs work by slowing the rate at which your body breaks down old bone. They have relatively few side effects. Bisphosphonates prescribed to strengthen bones include alendronate (Fosamax, Binosto), risedronate (Actonel, Atelvia), ibandronate (Boniva) and zoledronic acid (Reclast). They're taken in pill form on an empty stomach daily, weekly or monthly, or intravenously once a year.

The length of treatment with bisphosphonates should be discussed with a doctor. Using them for more than five years has been linked to a rare type of fracture in the thighbone (femur) and, in rare cases, osteonecrosis of the jaw, in which a section of jawbone deteriorates.

Estrogen

Hormone therapy containing estrogen can help maintain bone density, especially when started soon after menopause. It is approved in the U.S. for preventing osteoporosis after menopause, even in women without other hormone-related symptoms. For more information on hormone therapy and the related risks, see Chapter 6.

Raloxifene and conjugated estrogens-bazedoxifene

Raloxifene (Evista) is a type of selective estrogen receptor modulator (SERM). It slows bone loss in postmenopausal women by mimicking estrogen's beneficial effects on bone density. It is approved both for preventing and treating osteoporosis, and it may also reduce the risk of breast cancer. Raloxifene comes in a daily tablet. Its side effects include hot flashes, leg cramps, blood clots, swelling and flu-like symptoms.

A newer medication (Duavee) pairs a SERM (bazedoxifene) with estrogen. It offers the benefits of each drug. Conjugated estrogens help maintain bone density, while bazedoxifene helps protect the uterine lining from the effects of estrogen alone. The combination drug is approved for prevention of osteoporosis and is taken as a daily pill.

Denosumab

Denosumab (Prolia) also treats osteoporosis by slowing the rate of bone loss. It's delivered with a shot under the skin every six months. The most common side effects are back and muscle pain, high cholesterol, and an inflamed bladder. Denosumab may also lower your calcium levels or cause skin rashes. If you have a weakened immune system, you may have a higher risk of developing serious infections, especially skin infections.

Before you stop taking denosumab, it's important to talk with your practitioner about how to prevent bone loss, which may mean taking a different medication.

Teriparatide and abaloparatide

Teriparatide (Forteo) is a type of synthetic parathyroid hormone. Rather than slowing the loss of old bone, it helps build new bone. You take it by injection, using a pre-loaded pen. Side effects include leg cramps, upset stomach and dizziness. Abaloparatide (Tymlos) is another drug similar to parathyroid hormone. For most people, it's not recommended that you take these drugs for more than two years.

After stopping teriparatide or abaloparatide, you'll need to take a medication that slows bone loss to protect the bone you've built up.

Romosozumab

Romosozumab (Evenity) is the first drug to work by both slowing bone loss and promoting new bone growth. It's given as an injection every month at your doctor's office and is limited to one year of treatment. After that, you'll need to switch to a medication that slows bone loss. Romosozumab may increase the risk of heart attack or stroke and isn't recommended for anyone at high risk of these conditions.

PROTECTING YOUR BONES FOR LIFE

Although low bone density impacts many older women, you can take steps at any age to reduce your risks and prevent or control osteoporosis. Getting enough calcium, vitamin D and regular exercise can make a real difference. If medication is needed, the good news is that a growing number of options are available. Research continues to offer hope for new ways to diagnose, treat and prevent bone loss.

19

Heart health

It's a fact: About 1 in 3 women dies of heart disease. Every year, heart disease is the No. 1 killer of both men and women in the U.S. While the rates vary somewhat among racial and ethnic groups, heart health is a leading health concern in each group. And your chances of developing heart disease increase as you age — particularly once you've gone through menopause.

That may seem like sobering news. But knowledge is power, and the information in this chapter can help you take charge of your heart health. By making healthy choices today, you can significantly reduce your risk of heart disease in the future.

MENOPAUSE AND HEART DISEASE

Before menopause, women are less likely to have heart disease than are men of the same age. But once you enter menopause, your risk of heart disease increases significantly. Menopause itself doesn't cause heart disease, but declining levels of estrogen may play a role. Estrogen is thought to have a protective effect on a woman's blood vessels.

Aging also may have a significant impact on the health of your blood vessels. As you age, your arteries become less flexible. Stiff arteries are not as effective at maintaining a healthy blood flow, so your heart has to work harder to pump blood throughout your body. After menopause you're also more likely to develop conditions that increase your risk of heart disease, including high cholesterol, high blood pressure and weight gain.

Going through menopause early has an even greater effect on your chances of developing heart disease. If you've experienced menopause between the ages of 40 and 45, your risk of heart disease doubles compared with that of women your age who haven't yet gone through menopause.

All of this news might be unsettling, but you can do a lot to reduce your risk of heart disease. Many of the most significant risk factors are ones you can control. That's true at any age, regardless of when you experience menopause. Knowing about these risks — and dealing with them in a proactive way — can make all the difference.

STRAIGHT TALK ABOUT HEART DISEASE

The term *heart disease* is often used interchangeably with the term *coronary artery disease. Coronary artery disease* generally refers to problems caused by narrowed, blocked or stiffened arteries. Atherosclerosis is a particular condition that happens when there's a buildup of fatty plaques in your arteries. Atherosclerosis can lead to chest pain (angina), a heart attack or stroke. Other heart conditions, such as those that affect your heart's muscle, valves or rhythm, are also considered forms of heart disease.

KNOWING YOUR RISKS

According to the American Heart Association, nearly half of U.S. women over age 20 have some form of heart disease. You're more likely to face many of the risk factors for heart disease in your post-menopausal years, but you can take steps to reduce these risks.

High cholesterol

Cholesterol is a fat found in the bloodstream and in all your body's cells. Cholesterol comes from two sources. It's produced in your body,

---

RED FLAGS: SIGNS AND SYMPTOMS OF HEART DISEASE IN WOMEN

Did you know that heart disease symptoms in women can be different from those in men? That knowledge has improved the diagnosis and treatment of heart disease in women and has empowered them to seek help sooner rather than later.

For many women, the first symptom of heart disease is a heart attack. The most common heart attack symptom in both men and women is some type of pain or discomfort in the chest. But in women, chest pain isn't always severe or the most notice-able symptom. You may experience:

- Pressure, tightness or fullness or even pain in the chest
- Neck, jaw, shoulder, upper back or abdominal discomfort
- Shortness of breath
- Right arm pain
- Upset stomach or vomiting
- Sweating
- Lightheadedness or dizziness
- Unusual fatigue

If you experience these symptoms or think you're having a heart attack, call for emergency medical help immediately.

---

mostly in the liver, and it's found in foods that come from animals, such as meats, poultry, fish, seafood and dairy products.

Cholesterol often gets a bad rap, but your body uses it positively to build cells and certain hormones. Cholesterol becomes a problem and a major risk factor for heart disease when there's too much of it in your blood. Cholesterol can build up in your arteries, increasing the risk of a blood clot forming and blocking blood flow to critical organs such as the brain (stroke) and the heart (heart attack).

Cholesterol is carried through your blood, attached to proteins. This combination of proteins and cholesterol is called a *lipoprotein*. You may have heard of the different types of cholesterol, which are based on what type of cholesterol the lipoprotein carries.

Low-density lipoprotein (LDL) This is often referred to as "bad" cholesterol. The levels of LDL in your blood tend to increase once you reach menopause. Too much LDL cholesterol can lead to a buildup of plaque in the arteries (atherosclerosis), increasing your risk of heart attack or stroke.

High-density lipoprotein (HDL) HDL is known as "good" cholesterol because a high level of HDL protects against heart attacks, while a low HDL level is linked to a greater risk of heart attacks. Some experts believe HDL removes excess cholesterol from arteries and carries it back to the liver to be broken down and removed from your body. Estrogen raises HDL levels, which may be why women tend to have higher levels of HDL than men do. When you reach menopause, HDL levels tend to decline. However, having high HDL doesn't mean that you're not at risk of ever having a heart attack or stroke. In fact, new evidence suggests that HDL may become less protective in women after menopause

Triglycerides Cholesterol that's produced in the liver is released into the bloodstream to supply body tissues with a type of fat called *triglycerides*. Triglycerides are stored in your fat cells and released for energy between meals. They are what's measured in the lipid panel when your cholesterol is checked. Having high triglycerides results in a greater risk of heart disease in women than in men.

You're more likely to have high cholesterol if it runs in your family. Being overweight, eating a diet high in saturated and trans fats, and leading a sedentary lifestyle also increase your risk. The American

HEART PROBLEMS THAT ARE MORE COMMON IN WOMEN

Women are much more likely than men to have certain heart problems. The good news is that these conditions are treatable.

Spontaneous coronary artery dissection (SCAD)
SCAD is an emergency condition that occurs when a tear forms in a blood vessel in the heart, like wallpaper that starts to peel away. This can slow or block blood flow to the heart, causing a heart attack, heart rhythm problems (arrythmias) or death. SCAD most commonly affects women, and it may occur during pregnancy or soon after giving birth. Other risk factors include fibromuscular dysplasia, hormone use, connective tissue disease and high blood pressure.

Heart failure with preserved ejection fraction (HFpEF)
Nearly half of all people with heart failure have normal pumping function, called *preserved ejection fraction (EF)*. With HFpEF, the walls of the heart become stiff, and taking in enough blood to maintain a healthy output puts stress on the heart. This form of heart failure is twice as common in women as in men. It is associated with systemic inflammation and seems to be influenced by traditional risk factors for heart failure, including obesity, diabetes, high blood pressure and smoking.

Heart Association recommends having your cholesterol levels checked every 4 to 6 years, starting at age 20. More-frequent screenings are recommended starting in midlife. Your health care provider also may suggest testing more often if you have risk factors for heart disease.

Blood pressure
High blood pressure (hypertension) is another condition that increases your risk of developing heart disease. Hypertension is when the pressure in your blood vessels is too high. Over time, this pressure can

Coronary microvascular disease

Coronary microvascular disease is sometimes called *small vessel disease*. It develops when the small arteries in your heart become narrowed so that they don't expand properly when you're active. This inability to expand is called *endothelial dysfunction*, and it increases your risk of heart attack. Small vessel disease can be treated with changes in lifestyle and medication. Warning signs of the disease are similar to those of a heart attack. They include chest pain or discomfort; upper body discomfort in the arms, back, neck, jaw or stomach; shortness of breath; and sleep problems or fatigue.

Broken heart syndrome

Broken heart syndrome is sometimes called *takotsubo cardiomyopathy, apical ballooning syndrome* or *stress cardiomyopathy*. This condition is often brought on by stressful situations. It involves a disruption of your heart's normal pumping function, which may be a reaction to a surge of stress hormones. With broken heart syndrome, you may have sudden chest pain or shortness of breath and think you're having a heart attack. Medications are used to treat the weakened heart muscle, and the reduction in heart pumping function usually resolves within days or weeks.

damage your arteries, leading to an increased risk of serious conditions such as heart attack, heart failure or stroke.

Blood pressure is determined by the amount of blood your heart pumps and the amount of resistance to blood flow in your arteries. The more blood your heart pumps and the narrower your arteries, the higher your blood pressure. Before menopause, your chances of having high blood pressure are lower than those of men your age. But after menopause, you're more likely to develop high blood pressure compared with your male peers, especially once you've turned 65. This can be true even if you've had normal blood pressure throughout your life. Changes in your body after menopause, including increased weight and possibly lower estrogen levels, contribute to higher blood pressure.

Your chances of having high blood pressure are also higher if the condition runs in your family or if you're Black. Your lifestyle can play a role too. You're more likely to develop high blood pressure if you smoke, get little activity, eat a diet high in fats, sugars and salt or are overweight.

Diabetes

Diabetes is also strongly linked to heart disease, and your chances of developing it increase as you age. Having diabetes doubles your risk of

KNOW YOUR BLOOD PRESSURE NUMBERS

You can have hypertension for years without any symptoms. That's why it's so important to have your blood pressure checked regularly. If you discover you have high blood pressure, you can work with your health care provider to control it.

Your category	Systolic (mm Hg) (top number)	Diastolic (mm Hg) (bottom number)
Normal	Less than 120	Less than 80
Elevated	120 to 129	Less than 80
Hypertension Stage 1 Stage 2	 130 to 139 140 or higher	 80 to 89 90 or higher
Hypertensive crisis (seek emergency care immediately)	Higher than 180	Higher than 120

Source: American Heart Association

having a heart attack or stroke. If you have diabetes, you're also more likely to have other risk factors that increase your risk of heart disease, such as high blood pressure, high cholesterol and obesity.

The term *diabetes* refers to a group of diseases that affect the way your body uses blood sugar, also called *glucose*. The most common forms of diabetes are type 1 and type 2. Type 1 diabetes most often develops in children and young adults. Type 2 diabetes develops more commonly in midlife and beyond and is associated with increased body weight. If you have diabetes, it means your body can't produce enough insulin or it can't use insulin properly. When that happens, the glucose in your bloodstream is unable to enter your cells, which results

A blood pressure reading contains a top number and a bottom number. The top number is the systolic measurement. Your systolic reading tells you the pressure in your arteries during a heartbeat, when your heart is pushing blood through your arteries. The bottom number is the diastolic measurement. This number represents the pressure in your arteries when your heart is at rest between heartbeats. Your systolic number will be higher than your diastolic number.

Keep in mind that one high reading isn't enough for your provider to determine that you have high blood pressure. High blood pressure is diagnosed when you've had several high readings over a period of time. There's no cure for high blood pressure, but the healthy lifestyle habits discussed later in this chapter can help you prevent or manage the condition. Your health care provider may also prescribe medication to lower your blood pressure if you have stage 1 or stage 2 hypertension. If you're concerned about your blood pressure, make an appointment to discuss it with your provider.

in a potentially dangerous buildup of glucose in your bloodstream.

Because symptoms of type 2 diabetes can be mild or nonexistent, it's common to be unaware that you have the condition. The American Diabetes Association recommends being screened regularly if you are 45 or older. If the results of your test are normal, you should get retested every three years. If the test indicates that your blood sugar levels are higher than normal, your doctor will likely want to test you on a yearly basis.

Your risk of developing type 2 diabetes increases if the disease runs in your family. Being overweight or obese, not getting enough exercise, and eating an unhealthy diet also increase your chances of diabetes. Managing these risks with a healthy lifestyle will not only help you prevent or manage diabetes but also lower your risk of heart disease.

Because diabetes increases the risk of heart attack or stroke, additional preventive steps are now recommended for people with type 2 diabetes who have heart disease or are at high risk of it.

Your family history

Many of the conditions that increase your risk of heart disease run in families. The same is true for heart disease itself, especially if a close relative developed heart disease at a young age.

As you reach menopause, it's a good idea to gather information about your family's medical history and share it with your health care provider. Make sure your practitioner knows about parents, siblings and grandparents who've had heart disease. It's also important to note the age at which any of those close relatives had a first heart attack. In addition, tell your practitioner about any other conditions that increase your own risk, including high cholesterol, high blood pressure and diabetes. If heart disease does run in your family, it's more important than ever to protect your heart health by making good choices and controlling the risk factors that you can.

Risk factors specific to women

Certain factors that are known to increase the risk for heart disease are specific to women. These include menopause, especially early or premature menopause, depression, rheumatologic disease and having high blood pressure or diabetes during pregnancy. Radiation to the left chest as part of lymphoma or breast cancer treatment, as well as certain types of chemotherapy, may also affect the risk of future heart disease.

However, the current risk calculators for heart disease do not take all these novel risk factors into consideration. Because of this, they may underestimate the overall risk in women. Talk with your health care practitioner to get a full picture of your risk.

HEART PROTECTION STRATEGIES

You may not be able to change your age or your family history, but there's a lot you can do to prevent heart disease. Taking charge of your heart health now will help you enjoy the years to come.

Aspirin and heart disease

You may have heard that an aspirin a day keeps heart disease at bay. That's because aspirin can reduce the chance of a blood clot developing in your arteries. If your arteries are narrowed, a blood clot can prevent blood flow to your heart or brain and cause a heart attack or stroke. But aspirin can have serious side effects, including internal bleeding.

A series of recent trials have led to updated guidelines from the U.S. Preventive Services Task Force and the American Heart Association for taking aspirin preventively. Across these studies, aspirin showed no clear benefit for people over the age of 60 with risk factors for heart disease. Gastrointestinal bleeding was also more common. For people in younger age groups, low-dose aspirin slightly reduced the risk of heart failure, but also slightly increased the risk of internal bleeding. Based on these findings, the U.S. Preventive Services Task Force and the American Heart Association do not recommend taking a daily dose of aspirin to prevent heart attack for people over 60 without existing heart disease. However, for women ages 40 to 59 who have an increased risk of heart disease, daily aspirin may be considered. Women ages 60 to 69 who have diabetes and a higher risk of heart disease also may want to make an individualized decision with their practitioner.

Guidelines are evolving as more research is done. The bottom line is that you should have a discussion with your health care provider before taking a daily dose of aspirin. Your medical history and any medications you're taking will be factors in deciding whether using aspirin to prevent heart disease is a good option for you. Of course, if you have already had a heart attack, a daily baby aspirin is recommended for life, unless you have significant reasons for not taking it.

Statins

If you have high cholesterol, it's smart to be proactive when it comes to heart disease. Changes in your diet and exercise routine may be enough to get your cholesterol levels under control. If not, your health care provider may suggest that you take a statin.

DIAGNOSING HEART DISEASE IN WOMEN

For decades, the stress test — in particular the exercise stress test — has been the gold standard for noninvasive testing of heart disease. It usually involves walking on a treadmill or riding a stationary bike while your heart rate, heart rhythm and blood pressure are monitored.

The stress test can be an effective way to find heart disease in both men and women, but some women may also benefit from more testing. That's because women are more likely than men to develop small vessel disease, which is not as easily identified using a stress test. Unlike atherosclerosis, which blocks blood flow to the heart and major arteries, small vessel disease results from damage to small arteries or the inner lining of the main arteries leading to the heart. Research has shown that this condition can increase the risk of serious heart disease.

For this reason, imaging techniques — such as magnetic resonance imaging (MRI), positron emission tomography (PET), echocardiography or specialized vascular tests to evaluate the health of the lining of the blood vessels (endothelial testing) — may be recommended in addition to a stress test for women with symptoms of heart disease.

Statins are drugs that work by blocking a substance your body needs to make cholesterol. Statins may also help your body reabsorb cholesterol that has built up in plaques on your artery walls, preventing further blockage in your blood vessels and lowering your risk of heart attacks. Statins include medications such as atorvastatin (Lipitor), fluvastatin (Lescol XL), lovastatin (Altoprev), pitavastatin (Livalo), pravastatin (Pravachol), rosuvastatin (Crestor) and simvastatin (Zocor). Lower cost generic versions of many statin medications are available.

Statins and women To date, most studies have focused on the ability of statins to help prevent heart disease in men. It's not as clear whether statins produce a similar benefit for women. Recent research has raised the possibility that statins may not lower women's risk of developing heart disease, although more research is needed. However, it has been clearly shown that in women who've had a heart attack, statins prevent recurrent heart attack and prolong survival just as well as in men, if not better.

In the past, risk assessment tools didn't factor sex differences into the equation. However, current guidelines do consider that women's risk may differ from men's. The latest risk calculator, developed from guidelines by the American College of Cardiology (ACC) and American Heart Association (AHA), helps to predict your 10-year and lifetime risks of developing heart disease by taking into account several risk factors, such as blood pressure, cholesterol levels, and whether you smoke. A high 10-year risk score is one factor health care providers use to decide whether to prescribe a statin.

Current recommendations for taking statins In the past, a person's LDL cholesterol level was used to guide the use of statins. Newer recommendations are based primarily on the 10-year risk of heart disease, along with other factors. Current evidence supports prescribing statins to help lower LDL and overall heart disease risk in four main groups of women who are most likely to benefit:

- Those who already have heart disease. If you've had a heart attack, stroke caused by blockages in a blood vessel, ministroke (transient ischemic attack), peripheral artery disease, or prior surgery to open or replace coronary arteries, a statin is recommended.
- Those who have very high LDL cholesterol. If your LDL cholesterol reading is 190 mg/dL or higher, statins are recommended.

- Those who have diabetes. If you are between the ages of 40 and 75 and you have diabetes, regardless of your risk of cardiovascular disease, you may want to consider taking statins.
- Those who have a higher 10-year risk of heart attack. From age 40 to 75, if your 10-year risk of a heart attack is 7.5% or higher, especially if you have other risk factors such as premature menopause or a history of preeclampsia, your doctor may prescribe a statin.

Side effects of statins The most common side effect is mild muscle pain. Very rarely, statins can cause rhabdomyolysis, a serious condition that can lead to severe muscle pain or damage to your kidneys. Rhabdomyolysis can develop when you take statins in combination with certain drugs or if you take a high dose of statins. Statins are also associated with a slightly increased risk of diabetes and liver damage.

If you're concerned about your cholesterol levels, talk to your provider about your total risk of heart disease and discuss how your sex and lifestyle play a role in your decision about taking medication for high cholesterol.

HORMONE THERAPY AND PREVENTION OF HEART DISEASE

Hormone therapy isn't recommended for prevention of heart disease. And if you've already developed heart disease, hormone therapy may not be right for you. But studies have shown that using hormone therapy to treat symptoms early in menopause, in healthy women without heart disease risk factors, may reduce the risk of developing heart disease. As discussed in Chapter 6, the timing hypothesis suggests that taking estrogen therapy within 10 years of menopause and before age 60 may reduce your risk of heart disease, among other benefits. On the other hand, taking estrogen after age 60, when some atherosclerosis is likely already present, is believed to have a harmful effect.

A HEART-HEALTHY LIFESTYLE

So far the focus of this chapter has been on medical conditions that can affect your heart health. But your lifestyle can have a huge impact on your chances of developing heart disease.

Believe it or not, about 80% of cardiovascular diseases can be prevented through a combination of healthy lifestyle habits. These habits include not smoking, eating a healthy diet, exercising and maintaining a healthy weight. Many of these habits can also prevent conditions that increase your risk of heart disease, including diabetes, high cholesterol and high blood pressure. By leading a healthy lifestyle, you'll be improving your overall health, longevity and well-being.

Avoid tobacco

Smoking or using tobacco of any kind is one of the most significant risk factors for developing heart disease, particularly in women. Chemicals in tobacco can damage your heart and blood vessels. Using tobacco may also increase your risk of blood clots and lower your levels of HDL (the "good") cholesterol. Carbon monoxide in cigarette smoke replaces some of the oxygen in your blood. This increases your blood pressure and heart rate by forcing your heart to work harder to supply enough oxygen.

When it comes to heart disease prevention, no amount of smoking is safe. But, the more you smoke, the greater your risk. Even so-called social smoking — smoking only while at a bar or restaurant with friends — is dangerous and increases the risk of heart disease. So does exposure to secondhand smoke.

The good news is quitting smoking can rapidly reduce your risk. And it's never too late to quit. Women who quit smoking between the ages of 45 and 54 gain an average of six years of life compared with women who continue to smoke. Quitting smoking can also lower your risks of other diseases linked to tobacco use, such as lung cancer.

Quitting strategies If you smoke, quitting may seem like an impossible mountain to climb. You'll improve your chances of success if you get the right support. That support can come from family, friends, your health care provider, a counselor, a support group or a telephone quit line. Support can also come from using a medication for smoking cessation. Seeking out smoke-free restaurants, bars and workplaces can also make a big difference. The more committed you are to sticking with a plan, the more likely it is that you'll be able to kick the habit.

Eat a heart-healthy diet

One of the best things you can do to protect your heart is to eat a healthy diet. Depending on your eating habits, that may mean fine-tuning your diet or making more significant changes. Taking on a new eating plan may seem daunting, but it's well worth the effort. A healthy diet can help you prevent not only heart disease but factors linked to heart disease risk, such as diabetes, high cholesterol and weight gain.

Eating well isn't just about how many calories you consume. Heart-healthy diets such as Dietary Approaches to Stop Hypertension (DASH), the Mediterranean diet and the Mayo Clinic Diet focus on enjoying a variety of foods that meet your body's needs. Following are some tips to consider when it comes to eating for your heart health.

Eat more vegetables and fruits. Vegetables and fruits are good sources of vitamins and minerals. They are also low in calories and rich in dietary fiber and contain substances found in plants that may help prevent cardiovascular disease. Eating more fruits and vegetables may help you eat less high-fat foods, such as meat, cheese and snack foods.

Choose whole grains. Whole grains are good sources of fiber and other nutrients that play a role in regulating blood pressure and heart health. You can increase the amount of whole grains in your diet by making simple substitutions for refined grain products. Or be adventuresome and try a new whole grain, such as farro, quinoa or barley.

Eat healthy fats. Limiting how much saturated fat you eat and avoiding trans fat in processed foods is an important step to reduce your blood cholesterol and lower your risk of heart disease. The best way to reduce saturated fat in your diet is to limit the amount of butter and other solid fats you add to food. Instead, choose monounsaturated fats, such as olive oil or canola oil. Polyunsaturated fats, found in certain fish, avocados, nuts and seeds, are also good choices for heart health.

Choose low-fat protein sources. Lean meat, poultry, fish, low-fat dairy products, eggs and legumes are some of your best sources of protein. But be careful to choose lower fat options, such as skim milk rather than whole milk and skinless chicken breasts rather than fried chicken with the skin on. Fish is another good alternative to high-fat meats. And certain types of fatty fish are rich in omega-3 fatty acids, which can lower triglycerides in your blood.

Avoid excess salt. Sodium is an essential mineral that your body needs to perform a variety of functions. The amount of sodium most adults need is very low (less than 500 mg daily) compared with the average intake in the U.S. (over 3,200 mg daily). Lowering how much salt you consume in the foods you eat can lower your blood pressure and reduce your risk of heart disease, while consuming too much salt can raise your blood pressure. The American Heart Association recommends consuming less than 1,500 mg of sodium a day, but even reducing your sodium intake to 2,400 mg a day can have a positive effect on your blood pressure and heart health.

Limit sugary drinks and foods. Too much sugar in your diet can increase your likelihood of developing heart disease. The American Heart Association recommends that women consume no more than 6 teaspoons or 100 calories of sugar a day. A can of soda contains 8.75 teaspoons or 140 calories of sugar. Drinking fewer sweetened beverages — or cutting them out altogether — is a great way to reduce the amount of sugar you consume. Also beware of foods packed with added sugar, such as bakery goods, breakfast cereal, candy and some yeast breads.

Get moving
When it comes to your heart, healthy eating and exercise go hand in hand. While being inactive can increase your risk of heart disease as much as smoking can, physical activity not only reduces your risk but can also help you maintain a healthy weight and prevent high blood pressure, high cholesterol and diabetes. Exercising regularly will also strengthen your muscles and bones, raise your energy levels and boost your self-confidence. The American Heart Association recommends you get at least 150 minutes of moderate exercise, 75 minutes of vigorous exercise or a combination of both each week. Aim for at least 30 minutes of aerobic activity most days of the week. Shorter bursts of three 10-minute exercise sessions throughout the day can offer the same health benefits.

Running, swimming, bicycling and active sports such as tennis are all forms of heart-healthy aerobic exercise. So are daily activities such as gardening, housekeeping, taking the stairs and walking the dog. You don't have to exercise strenuously to achieve benefits, but you can see bigger benefits by increasing the intensity, duration and frequency of your workouts. The most important thing is to avoid being inactive, so choose the activities that are most enjoyable to you.

If you haven't been exercising much, take things slowly at first. For example, start by walking for 5 to 10 minutes most days and gradually work your way up to 30 minutes or more. If you have any concerns about starting a new exercise program, talk with your health care provider.

Maintain a healthy weight

Maintaining a healthy weight is an important part of reducing your chances of developing heart disease. But the hormonal changes of menopause might make you more likely to gain weight, especially around your stomach area. Muscle mass also tends to diminish with age, while fat increases.

Even a small weight loss can be beneficial. A good goal if you're overweight is to aim to lose 5% to 10% of your body weight over a period of six months. For example, if you weigh 150 pounds, that's 7 to 15 pounds. Reducing your weight by that much can help decrease your blood pressure, lower your cholesterol level and reduce your risk of diabetes. Even a lasting weight loss of 3% to 5% can have a positive impact on your heart health.

See Chapter 16 for specific strategies on maintaining a healthy weight in menopause and beyond.

A healthy heart for life

Now is a good time to change many of your risk factors for heart disease. Seek out the support of friends and family members who might also benefit from taking on healthier habits. Reward yourself for accomplishments, and don't be discouraged by bumps in the road. By sticking with these healthy habits, you'll be going a long way toward protecting your heart.

20

Brain changes
with aging

Ask any group of women who are going through menopause whether the transition has affected their brains and the answer is likely to be an emphatic yes. Some complain of the inability to remember familiar names or common words, others of a lack of focus or concentration, and still others of forgetting where they put things. Now where did those keys go again?

We know that estrogen does indeed have an influence on key aspects of brain processing and metabolism. In fact, recent research has shed new light on the complex question of how estrogen and other hormones affect the brain. A variety of studies have tried to tease out the link between the hormonal fluctuations of menopause, the cognitive symptoms that commonly occur during this period, and brain health and dementia in the longer term. While scientists have made some exciting discoveries in this area, there is still much to learn about how the brain changes during and after the menopause transition — and why.

Part of the difficulty is that menopause isn't just an isolated event. It happens in the broader context of aging, which brings multiple changes. Many of the physical symptoms that are common during menopause — irregular periods, hot flashes, mood swings and disrupted sleep — can have an effect on your ability to think and remember. As a result, there almost certainly are multiple factors at play.

In fact, a recent study confirmed that not only are age and menopause both factors in brain health, but they interact. Researchers looked at biomarkers in the brain for dementia, seen on an MRI. In midlife women, age, sex and menopause factors interacted in predicting the total brain volume and other measurements of brain matter.

Although there's still much to be discovered, this chapter will try to help you understand what's going on with your brain at this stage in your life. It will also delve into what you can do to protect your most valuable asset — your brain.

CHANGES THAT OCCUR WITH AGING

Many of your body's cells are constantly replacing themselves throughout your life. In contrast, most of the brain nerve cells (neurons) you have in adulthood are what you'll have to work with for the duration. Neurons are capable of living for up to 100 years or longer, but they're not automatically replaced when they die or get damaged. Thus, their number declines as you get older.

But neurons don't just sit there. They're abuzz with signals and messages (electric impulses) to each other, lighting up paths of communication across the brain that make today's complex transmission of wireless data look like child's play. Each neuron is designed to collect and process messages and then relay the information to other neurons. Neuronal communication regulates actions you consciously think about, such as writing an email or talking with a friend, along with actions you don't think about, such as breathing, experiencing pain or blinking dust from your eye.

Collectively, your neurons are also a repository for instincts, memories, intellectual analyses and creative thoughts. Together, they organize and shape your emotions and guide your actions and reactions.

To stay healthy, neurons are constantly maintaining and repairing themselves. As you age, however, some of these maintenance and repair processes may start to malfunction or get out of sync. Also, trauma or disease can irreparably damage neurons.

After about the fifth or sixth decade of life, the brain typically undergoes changes that include:

- A loss of neurons, especially in certain areas of the brain such as the prefrontal cortex — an area at the front of the brain — and the hippocampus, a small portion found deep inside toward the center of the brain. Both of these areas are important to cognitive skills such as learning, remembering, planning and decision-making. Losing neurons means the volume of your brain shrinks (atrophies) slightly.
- Disruption of communication between neurons due to loss or damage.
- Diminished coordination between brain regions.
- Reduced blood flow in the brain due to narrower arteries and fewer new blood vessels.
- Accumulation of debris inside and around neurons.
- Increased damage from free radicals — molecules that are unstable and hyperreactive.
- Increased inflammation.

For most women, these changes mean becoming a little more forgetful — experiencing momentary lapses often brought on by inattention or distraction. It may be a bit harder to recall information "on the spot," for example, such as rattling off the date of a best friend's birthday or the title of a book you finished recently. And distant memories that you don't call upon often may fade even further.

You might catch yourself being more absent-minded. You become so preoccupied with one thought that you overlook everything else. Or you're doing too many things at once and forget some of them.

In addition to memory, other cognitive functions become vulnerable, such as your brain's processing speed. Your brain may require more time to solve complex problems or assess visually challenging input, compared with people in their 30s and 40s.

Your brain may also need more time to make sense of new or

unfamiliar information, or you might need more details or instruction to master a new skill.

This doesn't mean that you're not as smart as you once were or that you can no longer think for yourself. It just means you might take a little longer to figure out an answer or grasp concepts that are new to you. In fact, when given enough time, older adults deliver solutions to problems that are just as accurate and effective as those of younger adults.

On the other hand, many important cognitive functions are hardly affected at all by the normal aging process. Generally, your ability to focus, concentrate and create aren't diminished by time. Your ability to correctly choose your words and access a rich vocabulary actually improve over the years.

And don't forget the benefits that age can bring, such as wisdom and experience. In your 50s and 60s and beyond, you have much more knowledge and insight to draw upon than in previous decades.

HORMONES AND THE BRAIN

You're aware by now how influential estrogen can be. It affects organs and systems throughout your body, and it plays an important role in your brain health.

Biologic studies have pinpointed cells throughout the brain that contain estrogen receptors. Circulating estrogen binds to these special molecules that function as a gateway for estrogen to exert its influence on targeted brain cells. Research suggests that estrogen may have protective effects on neurons and cognitive function by:

- Increasing the production of acetylcholine, which regulates learning and memory
- Enhancing the glutamate neurotransmitter system, a communication route involved in long-term potentiation — how you learn new things
- Regulating genes that influence how neurons survive, differentiate, regenerate and adapt
- Buffering neurons from overstimulation by neurotransmitters and protecting them from harmful free radicals

RED FLAGS: WHEN IS FORGETFULNESS A PROBLEM?

Occasional forgetfulness is typical of normal aging, so don't stress out too much about forgetting an appointment or misplacing a set of keys. On the other hand, forgetfulness caused by disease may begin suddenly and it becomes progressively worse. Early signs of cognitive impairment are often noticed by others and may include:

- Asking the same questions repeatedly without remembering the answer
- Stopping in the midst of a conversation without remembering what the discussion was about
- Mixing words up — saying *bed* instead of *table*, for example
- Taking longer to complete familiar tasks, such as putting on makeup or brushing teeth
- Placing items in inappropriate places, such as putting the mail in the freezer
- Getting lost while walking or driving in familiar places
- Making rash decisions, such as about personal safety or money
- Undergoing sudden changes in mood or behavior for no clear reason
- Experiencing increasing difficulty following directions

Studies of progesterone, the female hormone that has the job of counterbalancing the effects of estrogen, are fewer, but they also indicate a protective effect of progesterone on neurons.

Women and cognitive decline
Alzheimer's disease is a progressive degeneration of the brain that involves an overwhelming loss of neurons and the connections between them. It's one of the most common illnesses of old age, and one of the most devastating.

Yet despite the protective nature of female hormones toward the brain, Alzheimer's affects many more women than men. According to the Alzheimer's Association, women make up nearly two-thirds of American seniors living with Alzheimer's. In addition, at age 65, women have a 1 in 5 chance of developing Alzheimer's over the remainder of their lives, compared to men, who have a 1 in 10 chance.

Why is this? One obvious reason is that women generally live longer than men, which increases their overall chances of developing Alzheimer's. But there are likely other sex differences at play too, and scientists are only beginning to uncover what some of these might be.

Interestingly, mild cognitive impairment (MCI), a stage that often precedes Alzheimer's disease, is more prevalent in men than women. This may be in part because women generally perform better on verbal memory tests, masking early impairment. Women with MCI are typically diagnosed later, with more symptoms. And they appear to decline at a faster rate than men, descending more abruptly into dementia. It's possible that men may experience cognitive decline earlier in life but at a more gradual pace, whereas women may rapidly move from normal cognition to dementia at a later age.

Estrogen plays a role in brain health, but exactly how is uncertain. It's tempting to draw a neat line between estrogen decline during the menopause transition and increased risk of cognitive impairment. In animal studies, for example, abrupt withdrawal of estrogen results in increased cellular stress and faulty memory. On the flip side, clinical trials of younger women who take estrogen after a hysterectomy show improved verbal memory.

As with most diseases, Alzheimer's most likely results from a complex interplay between genetics, environment and other individual characteristics including sex, metabolism and lifestyle choices. Investigators are working to tease out what these various factors may be, as well as how the choices we make may affect the outcome.

An example of this interplay can be found in a study that focused on the links between telomeres, APOE e4 status, menopause and hormone therapy.

Telomeres are the protective endcaps on every chromosome. They're often likened to the plastic ends on a shoelace that help keep the shoelace from unraveling. In the same way, telomeres keep the

DNA within a chromosome from unraveling or becoming damaged. Telomere length is often used as a measure of cellular aging. Longer telomeres are associated with greater health and longer life spans. Although women and men have similar telomere length at birth, by adulthood women generally have longer telomeres, possibly due to the beneficial effects of circulating estrogen.

APOE e4 is a genetic variant that increases the risk of Alzheimer's disease. Researchers theorized that the healthy middle-aged women participating in their study who had the APOE e4 genetic variant would display shorter telomeres at the end of a two-year period than women who didn't have this variant. They also speculated that hormone therapy, initiated at the start of the menopause transition, would protect against telomere shortening.

Study results showed that the odds of telomere shortening over the two-year period were more than six times greater in APOE e4 carriers compared to noncarriers. In other words, cells appeared to age a lot faster in women with the APOE e4 variant.

Hormone therapy was a game changer for the APOE e4 carriers, however. APOE e4 carriers who were on hormone therapy showed little to no decline in telomere length. But for noncarriers, hormone therapy had little protective effect on cell aging. In fact, noncarriers who went off hormone therapy experienced increased telomere length.

These results need to be explored and validated by more research. But they suggest that disease — and the medicine needed to effectively treat it — is much more individualized than previously thought.

Hormone therapy and the brain
If estrogen is an important factor in brain health, it would seem to make sense that replacing hormones when they're low — such as around menopause and after — would improve cognitive function and even help prevent dementia. But evidence from clinical trials so far has been mixed and inconsistent, and in some instances, hormone therapy has had harmful effects.

In the early 2000s, investigators published results based on several large, long-term, rigorous clinical trials on women's health. One of the largest was the Women's Health Initiative (WHI). An offshoot of this study, the Women's Health Initiative Memory Study (WHIMS) followed over 4,500 women between the ages of 65 and 79 for about four years to see what effects hormone therapy might have on cognitive health, the general assumption being one of benefit. On the contrary, the WHIMS trial found that use of hormone therapy in older women didn't improve cognition at all. In fact, use of conjugated estrogens (CEE) plus progesterone doubled the risk of dementia. The use of estrogen alone did not significantly increase the risk, but it had no benefit.

Another offshoot study of the Women's Health Initiative, the WHI Study of Cognitive Aging (WHISCA), enrolling women 66 years and older, found neither benefit nor persistent harm on cognitive health in older women using hormone therapy.

Other smaller studies have found similar results. The Heart and Estrogen-Progestin Replacement Study (HERS), which looked into the long-term effects of hormone therapy on cognition and heart health, found that among older postmenopausal women, hormone therapy for four years didn't result in any improvement on cognitive tests.

The publication of this data swung opinion against using hormone therapy for preventing cognitive decline. Without stronger scientific evidence of a protective benefit, hormone therapy isn't recommended at any age for preventing or treating Alzheimer's or other dementias.

However, that isn't the end of the story. Research continues to investigate speculations that timing, dose, route of administration and the specific hormone therapy regimen used may play an important role in the balance of benefits and risks.

In fact, additional follow-up from the WHI suggest that the long-term effects of hormone therapy on cognition may be more promising. Eighteen years of WHI follow-up data showed that women who had taken conjugated estrogens actually had lower rates of death from Alzheimer's. However, the same wasn't true for women who had been assigned to estrogen plus progesterone.

All in the timing?

As far as we know, the risks of hormone therapy use in healthy women ages 50 to 59 remain very low. On the other hand, greater risks are associated with starting hormone therapy in your 60s or 70s.

As researchers continue to explore the connection between hormone therapy and cognition, a lot of current research revolves around the idea that there's a critical window in which hormone therapy can have positive effects. This is called the timing hypothesis. Another theory is that estrogen therapy can help protect cognition when used in someone with healthy neurons. But if the brain is already diseased, the effect is likely to be neutral or harmful.

Observational studies suggest that hormone therapy used in women who more recently transitioned to menopause decreases the risk of Alzheimer's disease, whereas hormone therapy used in later years — especially a combined estrogen and progestin formulation — increases the risk. Additionally, brain imaging studies of women who use hormone therapy early on in menopause have shown enhanced function of the hippocampus and prefrontal cortex, areas of the brain important for memory and thinking.

Other recent studies have yielded different results. The Kronos Early Estrogen Prevention Study (KEEPS) involved about 700 women who enrolled within three years of their final menstrual period — a substantially younger group than the preceding WHIMS and other studies. An offshoot of the study, KEEPS Cognitive and Affective Study (KEEPSCog), evaluated the cognitive effects of hormone therapy in these women over a period of four years. Results showed that hormone therapy was neither helpful nor harmful to learning or memory. However, one type of hormone therapy, conjugated equine estrogens (CEE) taken orally, did improve mood symptoms such as depression and anxiety. The same effect wasn't found with transdermal estradiol.

One study specifically compared the effects of hormone therapy early in menopause with later use to test the timing hypothesis. In the Early Versus Late Intervention Trial with Estradiol (ELITE), women who had entered menopause less than six years or more than 10 years earlier received either hormone therapy (oral estradiol plus a vaginal progesterone gel) or a placebo. Researchers tested the women's verbal memory, executive function and cognition after about 2.5 years and about 5 years. But in fact, the study found that estrogen therapy made no significant difference in the scores in either group. It neither helped nor harmed the cognitive abilities tested.

It's important to keep in mind, however, that for women who experience premature menopause, hormone therapy has important proven benefits. Refer back to Chapter 4 for more details.

KEEPING YOUR BRAIN HEALTHY

Rest assured that menopause is no guarantee of mental decline. Long-term observational studies of women going through menopause

MEMORY BOOSTERS

Habit-based (procedural) memory is used to store skills developed by repetition and practice — like riding a bike. It stays with you all your life.

You can capitalize on procedural memory skills to sharpen everyday memory skills and speed up information processing. This in turn allows you to take full advantage of other invaluable skills, such as insight and experience, which can be acquired only over time. Here's how:

Keep a calendar
Like most women these days, you're probably bombarded with lots of information coming from all directions — names, numbers, passwords, to-do lists. Trying to track too many tedious details can actually make you more prone to memory lapses.

Instead, create an effective calendar and organization system to help you keep extraneous information readily available and yet free up brain space for more important tasks. Use tools that can help you organize and remember appointments and other info — from paper calendars to notebooks to apps. The most important thing is to pick one and use it regularly, to the point where it becomes a habit — this is how procedural memory can make up for faulty recent memory.

It also helps to categorize the information you're trying to remember. Instead of one big long list, create separate sections for scheduled events, tasks that need to get done and static information such as phone numbers, addresses and other contact information.

Organize the clutter
Keeping your environment clutter-free and relatively organized can

are generally encouraging. For example, the brain fog that's common in perimenopause is typically not enough to make you score poorly on a memory test. In addition, these menopause-related difficulties are usually temporary and have little long-term effect on your brain health.

help minimize distractions and improve memory. For example, make a habit of always returning keys and handbags to a designated place. This makes it simple to find them next time.

Putting correspondence in order can help you stay on top of the endless stream of mail and paper that enters the home. It can also prevent unpaid bills and missed appointments. One method is to create different folders or places for: information that requires a response or action, such as bills or invitations; information that you'll need to consult occasionally, such as bank statements or insurance policies; and information to read at your leisure, such as magazines and catalogs.

Focus your attention
Attention is an important part of memory processing. It takes concentration to input information into your brain so that it can be stored and retrieved properly. Slow down and focus on the task at hand. Use your senses — sight, hearing, taste, touch and smell — to tune in to the present. Minimize distractions in order to give your undivided attention to a person or project.

Use memory tricks
Memory tricks are creative techniques that prompt you to manipulate new information in a way that helps you recall it later. For example, repeating information out loud or associating mental images with names or facts can help you remember. Breaking up information into chunks is useful too. Instead of remembering a grocery list of seven random items, think of the list as four vegetables and three fruits.

Scientists are just beginning to uncover factors that may help people protect their minds into their later years. One thing that's becoming clear is that permanent, age-related changes to the brain begin much earlier than once believed and can eventually accumulate enough damage to cause severe loss of memory and thinking skills. What this also means, however, is that there most likely are measures you can take in midlife to preserve and enrich your brain health.

So far, three steps are known to have a real impact on preserving brain health: protecting your heart health, staying active and building up a strong mental reserve.

Protect your heart

Mounting evidence indicates that what's good for your heart is good for your brain too. As one of the largest and busiest organs in your body, the brain has a vast network of blood vessels that feed it the oxygen and nutrients necessary to operate successfully. As such, the brain also relies heavily on the heart's capacity to pump out the optimal amount of blood it needs.

Over time, the brain's vascular system begins to resemble that of the rest of the aging body — arteries in the brain become more narrow and less elastic, some become clogged with fatty deposits (a condition known as *atherosclerosis*), and the growth of new capillaries (offshoots from the main arteries) slows down.

At the same time, the heart may not pump with its previous efficiency. As a result, the brain may receive less blood, and the blood that does arrive may not flow through the brain as well as it once did. This wear and tear on the brain's vascular system can result in microscopic injuries, inflammation and oxidative stress. In addition, other conditions such as high blood pressure, atherosclerosis or diabetes can further worsen these effects on the brain's vascular system.

It's possible that a faulty, aging vascular system may create a brain environment that makes it easier for nerve cells and communication pathways to be damaged. Various studies have linked cardiovascular risk factors in midlife — such as high blood pressure, high cholesterol and obesity — to later cognitive impairment and dementia.

Alzheimer's disease and cerebrovascular disease — such as strokes or ministrokes, which themselves can cause brain injury and dementia

— also frequently occur together. In fact, it's often difficult to separate one from the other.

The good news is that keeping your heart and blood vessels healthy will aid in keeping your brain supplied with the right amount of blood. It will also help keep blood flowing freely through your brain. Chapter 19 outlines specific strategies to increase your heart health.

Keep moving

Physical activity can have additional brain benefits too. Exercise seems to help the brain not only by keeping your blood flowing but also by directly supporting the health of brain cells.

Animal and human studies indicate that aerobic exercise increases the release of a substance called *brain-derived neurotrophic factor* (BDNF). BDNF promotes neuron survival and growth, enhances the formation of connections between neurons, supports new blood vessel formation and encourages the generation of new neurons in the hippocampus, the key memory center of the brain.

Clinical studies also suggest that exercise inhibits some Alzheimer's-like changes in the brain. Several studies in mice and in humans show an association between long-term exercise and lower levels of amyloid plaques — abnormal structures in the brain that are a characteristic feature of Alzheimer's disease.

Evidence suggests that, in the short term, aerobic exercise improves various measures in cognitive testing, including memory, attention, processing speed, and judgment and decision-making. Exercise may also enhance the connectivity and activation of neurons.

In the long term, regular physical activity can reduce your risk of dementia. An analysis of multiple studies found that adults who routinely engaged in physical activities, sports or regular exercise during midlife had a significantly lower risk of dementia years later. Likewise, the risk of mild cognitive impairment, often considered a precursor to Alzheimer's disease, was reduced in women who reported exercising earlier in life. One study connected a program of regular walking with increased volume in the hippocampus, thus potentially countering age-related loss of brain volume and associated memory impairment.

Most studies have focused on aerobic exercise — the kind that increases your heart rate and breathing — but it's possible that strength training and resistance exercise may help as well.

Keep in mind, also, that exercise doesn't have to mean hours at the gym. Put on your sneakers and walk. Doing yardwork, dancing, cleaning (dancing while cleaning!), or hiking all count, too. Aim for 30 minutes a day, most days of the week.

More research is needed to know to what degree adding physical activity improves memory or slows the progression of cognitive decline. Nonetheless, evidence so far strongly suggests that regular exercise is important to stay mentally fit.

Build up your reserve

There's another factor that may play an important role in preserving your brain health. It involves the concept of cognitive reserve — essentially your brain's ability to adapt to age- or disease-related changes by

CROSS-TRAIN YOUR BRAIN

Just as you can exercise your body to gain physical strength, you can also exercise your brain to increase intellectual capacity. Early research suggests that brain-training programs may improve your memory, mental processing speed and ability to perform everyday activities.

There's a wide range of available online brain-training programs, computer software programs and smartphone apps with scientific merits. These programs run you through various exercises, often on a timer, that gradually ramp up the level of difficulty so that your brain is continually stretched and challenged.

Of course, you can achieve much the same effect on your own by doing increasingly harder number games or crafts, for example. The key is to practice, practice, practice. Challenge yourself and target a range of skills — do jigsaw puzzles to sharpen spatial relationship skills, and play speed-based card games with a partner to increase mental processing speed.

drawing on existing neuronal networks or generating new neuronal connections where old ones may fail.

Your cognitive reserve relates to brain networks set up by factors such as brain size and neuron count, natural intelligence, life experience, education and occupation. The greater your reserve, the more leeway your brain has when asked to perform certain tasks. This implies that you may be able to prevent or compensate for cognitive decline by strengthening nerve networks and even building new ones through intellectual and social stimulation.

Most studies show a link between having an active social and intellectual life throughout the adult years and a decreased risk of cognitive impairment in later years. A study by Mayo Clinic researchers offers a good example. The investigators found that intellectually stimulating activities such as using a computer, playing games, reading books and engaging in crafts — including knitting, woodworking and other types of handiwork — were associated with a 30% to 50% decrease in the chances of developing mild cognitive impairment.

As with physical exercise, some activities seem to offer more of a cognitive workout than others. Find what you enjoy. The important part may be choosing activities that absorb your mind, draw you in and engage your thought processes.

It may also be that engaging in intellectually and socially stimulating activities helps reduce stress. For example, playing a game with another person usually involves a deliberate effort to pay attention to what you're doing. People who are working on a craft often find themselves becoming completely immersed in it.

This is similar in some ways to meditative techniques that focus on becoming fully aware of the here and now. Such techniques tend to produce a relaxation response — sort of the opposite of the body's fight-or-flight response to stress. The relaxation response decreases your blood pressure, heart rate and breathing rate. It increases concentration, immersion in the moment, and feelings of contentment and well-being. It may also help buffer areas of the brain from stress-related changes, thus preserving neurons and their connections.

Finally, participating in enjoyable leisure activities, especially social ones, can help prevent depression and loneliness, both of which have been associated with poor cognitive health.

21

Caring for your hair, eyes, ears, teeth, skin and joints

There's no question you've earned your stripes in the years leading up to menopause. You may just not have realized the stripes would appear as crow's-feet.

Chapter 2 outlined many of the common body changes that happen with menopause. Now it's time to look at what you can do to keep your body in its best operating shape throughout this next season of your life.

Earlier chapters have touched on important steps for overall health — a nutritious diet, regular exercise, stress management and ample sleep. In this chapter, you'll learn about specific tips to care for the areas commonly affected by menopause, from your hair to your joints. With some maintenance efforts, some common menopausal changes may be preventable. And those that do occur can be minimized and managed.

With a bit of care, you might even find yourself healthier than ever in the years after menopause.

CARE FOR CHANGING HAIR

Your hair may have been your greatest fashion asset in your teens and 20s. But as you age, your glands produce less oil, leaving hair drier and less shiny. And other hair is cropping up in the most unexpected — and annoying — of places. New facial hair growth is especially common after menopause. Can anything be done about it? Absolutely.

Avoiding damage

Hair damage happens when the protective fat (lipid) layer that makes hair shiny and pliable —already in shorter supply with age — is destroyed. This gives hair a dried out, dull and frizzy appearance and also makes hair more brittle and prone to breakage. To keep hair healthy, avoid damage caused by:

Chemical products Frequent coloring, relaxing or perms can damage your hair. A natural color and style involving minimal chemicals is optimal. Short of that, try to space colorings as far apart as possible. Avoid care involving coloring and a perm or relaxer at the same sitting.

Heat Too much heat can damage hair. Try letting your hair air-dry or going with your natural level of curliness. Or use a hair dryer or curling iron on a low setting. With hair straighteners, place a moist cloth over the hot plates so that they don't directly touch the hair.

Rough handling Straight, wavy or loosely curled hair breaks more easily when wet. Be gentle when towel-drying. Let hair become mostly dry before gently combing it with a wide-toothed comb. For those with tightly curled hair, combing hair while damp is preferred. Comb only as little as needed to style your hair.

Tight hairstyles Avoid the prolonged wearing of hairstyles such as ponytails, cornrows or braids.

Improper shampooing Massage shampoo into your scalp with your fingertips and rinse it away. After shampooing, use a conditioner on your hair if it tends to be dry or tangle easily.

Thinning hair solutions

If your hair seems to be pulling a disappearing act, you can once again thank the change in hormones — along with natural aging and, probably, genetics. Still, there are options to explore:

Treat your hair gently. Take extra care to prevent damage.

Eat a nutritionally balanced diet. Poor nutrition can increase your risk of hair loss. Be sure you're getting a good mix of fruits, vegetables and sources of protein. Certain supplements may help by adding key nutrients for hair growth. Several proprietary supplements, such as the brands Viviscal and Nutrafol, have been shown to help fight hair loss.

See your health care provider. While menopause is often a common culprit for hair loss, it's not always the cause. Be sure to rule out any underlying health conditions before you explore treatments.

Consider minoxidil (Rogaine). Minoxidil is an over-the-counter liquid or foam that you rub into your scalp twice a day to grow hair and to prevent further hair loss. The effect peaks at 16 weeks, and you need to keep applying the medication to retain benefits. Side effects may include scalp irritation, facial hair growth, and rapid heart rate (tachycardia). For women who can't tolerate topical minoxidil, a low-dose pill may be available with a prescription.

MEDICATIONS FOR UNWANTED HAIR

Medications usually take several months before you see a significant difference in hair growth. Medications may include:

Oral contraceptives Birth control pills or other hormonal contraceptives, which contain estrogen and a progestin, treat hair growth by decreasing androgens in a few different ways. Possible side effects include dizziness, upset stomach, headache and stomach upset.

Anti-androgens These drugs block sex hormones from attaching to their receptors in your body. The most commonly used anti-androgen for hair growth is spironolactone (Aldactone).

Topical cream Eflornithine (Vaniqa) is a prescription cream specifically for excessive facial hair in women. It's applied directly to the affected area of your face and helps slow new hair growth but doesn't get rid of existing hair.

Dealing with unwanted hair

Self-care measures to combat rogue body hair include:

Bleaching Instead of removing the hair, you may want to opt for using bleach to make it less visible. Bleach may cause skin irritation for some women, so be sure to test on a small area first.

Plucking The trusty tweezers. While plucking is a good method to remove a few stray hairs, it's not very practical for removing large areas of hair.

Shaving Shaving is quick and inexpensive, but it needs to be repeated regularly since it removes the hair only down to the surface of your skin.

Depilatory products These products are generally available as gels, lotions and creams that you spread on your skin. Chemical depilatories work by breaking down the protein structure of the hair shaft. It's a good idea to test a small patch of the product before applying on a larger area.

Wax Waxing involves applying warm wax on your skin where the unwanted hair grows. Once the wax hardens, it's pulled back from your skin against the direction of hair growth, removing hair. Waxing removes hair from a large area quickly, but it may sting temporarily and sometimes causes skin irritation and redness.

Laser hair removal During this procedure, a laser beam passes through the skin to an individual hair follicle. The intense heat of the laser damages the follicle, which inhibits future hair growth. However, it doesn't guarantee permanent hair removal. It typically takes multiple treatments, and periodic maintenance treatments might be needed as well. Laser hair removal is most effective for people who have light skin and dark hair.

Electrolysis This treatment involves inserting a tiny needle into each hair follicle. The needle emits a pulse of electric current to damage and eventually destroy the follicle. Electrolysis is an effective hair removal procedure, but it can be painful. A numbing cream spread on your skin before treatment may reduce this discomfort.

SAVOR YOUR SKIN

However young you may feel in spirit, your skin may be starting to tell a different story. As you age, your skin becomes drier and more lax and wrinkled — you'll likely lose about 30% of the collagen in your skin in the first five years after menopause. And you may start to notice more spots and growths too.

You may not be able to change all your spots — or wrinkles. But proactive skin care can help keep your skin youthful and healthy.

Practice sun protection

Start with skin care rule No. 1 — protect yourself from the sun.

Avoid the sun during peak hours. Generally this is between 10 a.m. and 2 p.m., regardless of season. These are prime hours for exposure to skin-damaging ultraviolet (UV) radiation from the sun, even on overcast days.

Wear protective clothing. This includes pants, shirts with long sleeves, wide-brimmed hats and sunglasses. Consider investing in sun-protective clothing or using an umbrella for shade. Laundry additives are also available that give clothing an added layer of ultraviolet protection.

Don't neglect sunscreen. Apply generously and reapply regularly — generally every two hours, or even more often if you're swimming or perspiring. Use enough sunscreen to fully cover all bare skin, including your neck, face, ears, tops of your feet, back and legs.

Skip the tanning beds. All UV radiation damages your skin. In fact, tanning beds emit UVA rays, which might increase the risk of melanoma, the deadliest form of skin cancer.

Don't smoke

Smoking makes your skin look older and contributes to wrinkles. Smoking narrows the tiny blood vessels in the outermost layers of your skin, which decreases blood flow. This depletes the skin of oxygen and nutrients that are important to skin health. Smoking also damages collagen and elastin — the fibers that give your skin strength and elasticity.

If you smoke, the best way to protect your skin is to quit. Ask your health care provider for tips or treatments that can help.

Eat a healthy diet

A healthy diet can help you look and feel your best. Eat plenty of fruits, vegetables, whole grains and lean proteins, and drink enough water.

CHOOSING A GOOD SUNSCREEN

No matter what stage of life you're in, using sunscreen can help prevent age-related skin changes and skin cancer. Choose a broad-spectrum sunscreen with a sun protection factor (SPF) of at least 30.

A broad-spectrum, or full-spectrum, sunscreen is designed to protect you from two types of ultraviolet light that can harm your skin — UVA and UVB. SPF is a measure of how well a sunscreen deflects UVB rays. But you also want protection against UVA. UVA rays may increase the risk of melanoma, the deadliest form of skin cancer.

Some research suggests that a diet rich in vitamin C and low in unhealthy fats and refined carbohydrates might promote younger looking skin.

Manage stress

Uncontrolled stress can make your skin more sensitive and trigger pimple breakouts and other skin problems. To encourage healthy skin, take steps to manage your stress and make time to do things you enjoy.

Treat your skin well

Daily cleansing and shaving can take a toll on your skin. To keep it gentle, limit your bathing time, as long showers and hot water remove precious oils from your skin. Wash with a mild cleanser. Apply shaving cream, lotion or gel before shaving to protect and lubricate your skin, and shave in the direction the hair grows. After washing, use a moisturizer with ingredients that both hydrate and hold water in the skin.

Conquer adult acne

It's not only a teenage problem. Why are you suddenly getting acne again in midlife? The shift in hormone levels with the transition to menopause may kick off a new period of acne problems. Wash your face

A GUIDE TO ANTI-WRINKLE PRODUCTS AND TREATMENTS

Many creams, lotions and other products promise to reduce wrinkles and prevent or reverse damage caused by the sun. Do they work? That often depends on the specific ingredients and how long you use them, but they may have modest benefits.

The Food and Drug Administration (FDA) classifies nonprescription creams and lotions as cosmetics, which are defined as having no medical value. These products are regulated less strictly than medications, and they don't undergo the same testing for safety and effectiveness that prescription creams do. When deciding whether to use a cream, consider the cost, ingredients and potential side effects (such as skin irritation).

Common anti-wrinkle ingredients

The effectiveness of over-the-counter anti-wrinkle creams depends in part on the active ingredients. Here are some common ingredients that may modestly improve the appearance of wrinkles.

- **Retinol.** Retinol is a vitamin A compound and an antioxidant. Antioxidants are substances that neutralize free radicals — unstable oxygen molecules that break down skin cells and cause wrinkles.
- **Vitamin C.** Another potent antioxidant, vitamin C may help protect skin from sun damage.
- **Hydroxy acids.** Alpha hydroxy acids, beta hydroxy acids and poly hydroxy acids are exfoliants. Exfoliants remove the top layer of old, dead skin to stimulate the growth of smooth, evenly pigmented new skin.
- **Coenzyme Q10.** This ingredient may help reduce fine lines around the eyes and protect the skin from sun damage.
- **Tea extracts.** Green, black and oolong teas contain compounds with antioxidant and anti-inflammatory properties.
- **Grapeseed extract.** This extract has anti-inflammatory and antioxidant properties. It also promotes wound healing.

- **Niacinamide.** A potent antioxidant, this substance is related to vitamin B-3 (niacin). It helps reduce water loss in the skin and may improve skin elasticity.

Dermatology treatments

If you're looking for a face-lift in a bottle, you probably won't find it in over-the-counter creams. To explore more intensive treatments that can give more dramatic results, you may want to visit a dermatologist. This specialist can help you create a personalized skin care plan by assessing your skin type, evaluating your skin's condition and recommending products or treatments that are likely to help you achieve your desired results.

A variety of medical treatments are available to reduce wrinkles. Here are some options your dermatologist may offer.

- **Prescription creams.** These may include more-potent active ingredients, compared with nonprescription creams.
- **Botulinum toxin (Botox) injections.** Botox shots use a toxin to block certain chemical signals from nerves that cause muscles to contract. Botox can be used to relax the facial muscles that cause frown lines and other facial wrinkles.
- **Chemical peel.** This skin-resurfacing technique uses a chemical solution to remove the top layers of skin so that smoother skin will grow back. It can help treat wrinkles, discolored skin or scars. The skin heals in days to weeks.
- **Dermabrasion.** A rapidly rotating device removes the outer layer of skin. This may improve the look of acne scars, age spots and wrinkles. Healing may take weeks to months.
- **Facial fillers.** Substances injected into the skin can smooth wrinkles and make them less noticeable.
- **Laser resurfacing.** This procedure directs an intense beam of light at your skin to stimulate growth of new cells and collagen. It may lessen the appearance of lines, scars and redness.

and pimple-prone areas with a gentle cleanser twice a day — but not more, to avoid irritation. Use an acne cream or gel to help dry excess oil. Look for products containing benzoyl peroxide or salicylic acid as the active ingredient. Choose oil-free cosmetics, sunscreens and moisturizers that won't clog pores (noncomedogenic), and remove any makeup before going to bed. Also, it's a good idea to throw out old makeup and regularly clean your cosmetic brushes and applicators with soapy water.

THE EYES HAVE IT

The eyes are said to be the window to the soul. Keep those windows functioning their best with a little self-care.

Help for dry eyes

As mentioned in Chapter 2, dry eyes are an especially common problem around the time of menopause. But you can take steps to stay comfortable and prevent complications such as infection or damage to the surface of the eyes.

If you experience dry eyes, pay attention to the situations that are most likely to cause your symptoms. For instance:

Avoid air blowing in your eyes. Try to direct hair dryers, car heaters, air conditioners or fans away from your eyes.

Add moisture to the air. A humidifier can add moisture to dry indoor air.

Consider wearing wraparound sunglasses or other protective eyewear. Safety shields can be added to the tops and sides of eyeglasses to block wind and dry air.

Take eye breaks during long tasks. If you're reading, working on a computer or doing another task that requires visual concentration, take periodic eye breaks. Try the 20-20-20 rule: Every 20 minutes, look at something 20 feet away for at least 20 seconds.

Be aware of your environment. The air at high altitudes, in desert areas and in airplanes can be extremely dry. When spending time in such an environment, it may be helpful to frequently close your eyes for a few minutes at a time to minimize evaporation of your tears.

Position your computer screen below eye level. If your computer screen is above eye level, you'll open your eyes wider to view the screen. Position your computer screen below eye level so that you won't open your eyes as wide. This may help slow the evaporation of your tears between blinks.

Stop smoking and avoid smoke. If you smoke, ask your health care provider for help devising a quitting strategy that's most likely to work for you. Smoke can worsen dry-eye symptoms.

Use artificial tears regularly. If you have chronic dry eyes, use eye drops to keep them lubricated even when your eyes feel fine. In addition, there are gels, gel inserts and ointments available over the counter. See the sidebar below for tips on choosing the right product for you.

Everyday eye care
Your overall eye health is important at any age. As you enter into a stage where eye concerns become more common, here are tips for maintaining optimal vision:

Have regular eye exams. Eye exams can help detect eye problems at their earliest stages. As a general rule, have a comprehensive eye exam every four years beginning at age 40 and every two years from age 65. You may need more-frequent screening if you're at high risk of eye disease or if you have corrected vision.

Know your family's eye health history. Some eye diseases, such as glaucoma, tend to run in families.

Quit smoking. Smoking puts you at risk of common eye conditions

CHOOSING A DRY-EYE PRODUCT

When you're choosing eye drops off the shelf to treat dry eyes, it's best to avoid drops that are formulated to reduce redness. Prolonged use can cause irritation. If you've tried more than one eye drop product and are still not finding any relief, ask your health care provider about prescription medications and procedures that may be effective in your case.

such as macular degeneration and cataracts. Ask your health care provider for suggestions about how to stop smoking. Medications, counseling and other strategies are available to help you.

Reduce alcohol use. Excessive alcohol use can increase the risk of some eye problems.

Wear sunglasses. Ultraviolet light from the sun may contribute to the development of cataracts. Wear sunglasses that block ultraviolet B (UVB) rays when you're outdoors.

Manage other health problems. Follow your treatment plan if you have diabetes or other conditions that can increase your risk of eye disease.

Maintain a healthy weight. Being overweight increases your risk of developing diabetes, high blood pressure and cardiovascular diseases. Each of these conditions can damage the small, delicate vessels found in the eye and potentially lead to vision loss.

Choose a healthy diet that includes plenty of fruits and vegetables. Adding a variety of colorful fruits and vegetables to your diet ensures that you're getting ample vitamins and nutrients. Fruits and vegetables have many antioxidants, which help maintain the health of your eyes. Aim to include foods that contain beta carotene, lutein, zeaxanthin, and vitamins C and E. Zinc and omega-3 fatty acids are also important.

SLOWING HEARING CHANGES

Hearing loss that happens gradually as you age is common. In fact, it's estimated that about 25% of people in the U.S. between the ages of 55 and 64 have some degree of hearing loss. After age 65, that number creeps closer to 50%.

You can't reverse most types of hearing loss. But try not to speed up the process by putting yourself at risk from chronic noise exposure.

Protect your ears
Here are steps you can take to prevent noise-induced hearing loss and avoid worsening age-related hearing loss:

Wear earplugs or earmuffs. If you have to shout to be heard by someone an arm's length away, you're being exposed to too much noise. In such situations, wear protective earplugs or specially designed earmuffs that meet federal safety standards. This guideline applies at work and at home.

Manage recreational risks. Activities such as riding a motorcycle or snowmobile, attending a concert, or firing a gun can damage your hearing. Wear hearing protection to blunt the noise. When using headphones or earbuds, turning down the volume and setting volume limits on your devices can help you avoid damage.

Keep the noise down at home. It's easy to overlook the daily racket. To reduce noise, control the volume on the TV and stereo, don't run multiple appliances at the same time, and when possible, purchase quieter appliances.

Have your hearing tested. If you work in a noisy environment, have regular hearing tests. Testing can detect hearing loss early so that you can take steps to prevent further damage.

SHOWCASE YOUR SMILE

One of the best weapons you can have in your menopause arsenal is your smile. Are you keeping it healthy?

Brushing 101

Keeping the area where your teeth meet your gums clean can prevent gum disease, while keeping your teeth surfaces clean can help you stave off cavities. Consider these brushing basics:

Brush your teeth at least twice a day. When you brush, don't rush. Take enough time to do a thorough job.

Use the proper equipment. Use a fluoride toothpaste and a soft-bristled toothbrush that fits your mouth comfortably. Consider using an electric or battery-operated toothbrush, which can reduce plaque and a mild form of gum disease (gingivitis) more effectively than manual brushing.

Practice good technique. Hold your toothbrush at a slight angle — aiming the bristles toward the area where your tooth meets your gum. Gently brush with short back-and-forth motions. Remember to brush the outside, inside and chewing surfaces of your teeth, as well as your tongue.

Keep your equipment clean. Always rinse your toothbrush with water after brushing. Store your toothbrush in an upright position if possible and allow it to air-dry until using it again. Don't routinely cover toothbrushes or store them in closed containers, which can encourage the growth of bacteria.

Know when to replace your toothbrush. Invest in a new toothbrush or a replacement head for your electric or battery-operated toothbrush every 3 to 4 months — or sooner if the bristles become frayed.

HANDLING HEADACHES

During perimenopause, when estrogen levels are swinging wildly as menstrual cycles become more erratic, migraines often get worse. Other menopausal symptoms — such as disrupted sleep, mood swings and hot flashes — may also contribute to headaches, including migraines, tension-type and chronic daily headaches.

For women with migraine, the good news is that once your final period occurs and estrogen levels smooth out, migraines often improve. The exception is for women who have migraine with aura, who may not experience the same type of relief with menopause. The arrival of menopause also doesn't seem to "cure" tension-type and chronic daily headaches.

If you experience a new headache — of any kind — during perimenopause or any other time, tell your health care provider. Together you can exclude other causes for headache as well as find the right type of relief.

Does hormone therapy help or hinder?

In some women, hormone therapy can worsen migraines, while in others it may ease them. It's important to talk to your health care provider about your individual circumstances and any kind of headache you have. Easing other symptoms of menopause may help with headaches.

Don't pass on the floss

You can't reach the tight spaces between your teeth and under the gumline with a toothbrush. That's why daily flossing is important. When you floss:

Don't skimp. Break off about 18 inches of floss. Wind most of it around the middle finger on one hand and the rest around the middle finger on the other hand. Grip the floss tightly between your thumbs and forefingers.

In general, experts recommend avoiding hormonal fluctuations if possible. In the time leading up to menopause, this might mean taking a hormonal contraceptive in a continuous rather than a cyclical regimen or including a shortened hormone-free period.

Finding relief

Treatment for headaches during menopause is really no different than at other times. If you have migraine, you'll want to avoid migraine triggers and take quick-relief medications — such as ibuprofen, acetaminophen-caffeine combinations or a prescription medication such as a triptan — as soon as you feel one coming on. In addition, your health care provider may have you on a preventive medication to decrease recurrences. Work with your provider to find an option that works well for you.

For tension-type headaches, nonprescription pain relievers such as nonsteroidal anti-inflammatory drugs are often effective. Keep in mind that overuse of pain relievers — more than twice a week, for example — can result in the development of chronic daily headaches. You might also consider nondrug therapies, which can be helpful. These might include stress management, relaxation therapy, acupuncture or biofeedback.

Be gentle. Guide the floss between your teeth using a rubbing motion. Don't snap the floss into your gums. When the floss reaches your gumline, curve it against one tooth.

Do one tooth at a time. Slide the floss into the space between your gum and tooth. Use the floss to gently rub the side of the tooth in an up-and-down motion. Unwind fresh floss as you go around your mouth.

Keep it up. If you find it hard to handle floss, use an interdental cleaner — such as a special wooden or plastic pick, stick or brush designed to clean between the teeth.

See your dentist

To prevent gum disease and other oral health problems, schedule dental cleanings and exams at least once or twice a year.

DON'T NEGLECT YOUR JOINTS

Your joints undergo a certain amount of wear and tear as you age. In addition — surprise, surprise — the shift in hormone levels at menopause seems to affect the joints too. At the cellular level, estrogen has a protective effect on joint tissues, though its role in joint health and the development of arthritis isn't fully understood. Large studies such as the WHI have shown that women using hormone therapy experience less joint pain and stiffness, compared with women taking a placebo. More research is needed to explore this connection.

Protecting your joints is one of the most effective ways to avoid or ease pain and prevent further joint damage. Follow the principles below to protect your joints from unnecessary strain.

Recognize and acknowledge your pain

Learn to recognize the difference between general discomfort from a joint condition such as arthritis and pain from overuse of a joint. Then change your activity level or how you do a task to avoid excessive pain.

Pain that lasts more than an hour after an activity or exercise indicates the activity was too stressful. If you experience pain after an activity, consider the following factors, which may have contributed to the pain:

- What were you doing that involved the use of the painful joints?
- What position were you in?
- How long were you involved in the activity?
- Was the task too heavy or forceful?

The next time you're involved in the same activity, try changing one of these variables, and keep changing them (one at a time) until you learn what and how much your joint can handle without causing pain.

Practice correct body mechanics
Consider these ergonomic tips to protect your joints:
- When sitting, the proper height for a work surface is 2 inches below your bent elbow. Make sure you have good back and foot support when you sit. Your forearms and upper legs should be parallel with the floor.
- If you type at a computer or other keyboard for long periods and your chair doesn't have arms, consider using wrist or forearm supports.
- Increase the height of your chair seat to decrease the stress on your hips and knees as you get up and down.
- When standing, the height of your work surface should enable you to work comfortably without stooping or reaching.
- To pick up items from the floor, stoop by bending your knees and hips. Or sit in a chair and then bend over.
- Carry heavy objects close to your chest, supported by your forearms.
- Maintain good posture. Poor posture causes uneven weight distribution and may strain your ligaments and muscles.

Give it a rest
Your joints need breaks just like the rest of you. Alternate light and moderate activities throughout the day. Work at a steady and deliberate pace — don't rush! Try to rest before you become fatigued or sore.

Reduce excess body weight
Carrying extra body weight contributes to joint problems in several ways. It puts added stress on weight-bearing joints, such as your hips

and knees. In addition, fat tissue produces proteins that may cause harmful inflammation in and around your joints, which may lead to osteoarthritis.

Remain active

In addition to helping you feel good and control your weight, exercise can help strengthen muscles that support your joints, reduce joint pain and help you maintain your mobility — when it's done right.

The main precaution to take is to protect your joints from further damage. Listen to your body — don't force a motion if you feel pain, and cut back on the intensity if your muscles ache long after the activity is over.

Low-impact activities such as cycling, swimming and moderate strength training place less stress on your joints. Follow these tips:

- Start easy and increase intensity gradually.
- Warm any bothersome joints with a heat source before exercise and apply ice to them after.
- Make stretching part of your routine to maintain flexibility. The key is to stretch gently, as the chance of tearing a tendon — the fibrous tissue that attaches muscle to bone — increases with age.
- Cross-train by alternating between a variety of flexibility, strengthening and aerobic exercises throughout the week.
- Use appropriate equipment, such as proper footwear or a well-adjusted bicycle.

22

Preventive care and screenings

You may be dreading that first colonoscopy that was put on your schedule for next month — they're going to do what, exactly? While the procedure itself may be less than appealing, it might help to look at this important screening exam as an opportunity to invest in your health.

As you approach menopause and move into a new stage in life, make prevention a priority. Rather than focusing only on treating illnesses as they pop up, prevention means taking steps in your daily life and with your routine health care to prevent these concerns in the first place, as well as to catch and treat important diseases and conditions at an early, more manageable stage.

Two important pillars of prevention are to eat a healthy diet and exercise regularly. Additionally, prevention involves staying on top of routine screening tests and recommended vaccinations, which are the focus of this chapter. These are key to catching any health problems early and avoiding complications.

RECOMMENDED SCREENINGS

Here's a look at routine screening tests that are recommended for women as they enter into midlife and beyond. Keep in mind that the recommended screening schedules are for women at average risk — if you're at increased risk of a particular condition, your health care provider will work with you to come up with a screening schedule that's appropriate for you.

Blood pressure measurement
This test — using an inflatable cuff around your arm — measures the peak pressure your heart generates when pumping blood through your arteries (systolic pressure) and the amount of pressure in your arteries when your heart is at rest between beats (diastolic pressure).

What's the test for? This test is used to detect high blood pressure. If you have high blood pressure, the longer it goes undetected and untreated, the higher your risk of a number of health problems, including heart attack, stroke, heart failure, kidney damage and eye damage.

MULTI-CANCER EARLY DETECTION TESTS

The cancer screening tests that are currently recommended cover five common cancers. A new type of screening technology, using a simple blood test, may be able to greatly expand the number of cancers caught early. A multi-cancer early detection (MCED) test, such as the Galleri test, is a blood test that looks for evidence of many types of cancer at the same time. While it does not diagnose cancer, it can identify where in the body a cancer signal is detected, to guide follow-up testing. This broader early detection has life-saving potential. The technology is still very new, though. For now, MCED testing is not widely available or recommended, and it shouldn't replace any routine screenings.

When and how often should you have it done? Have your blood pressure checked at least every two years. However, you'll likely have it checked every time you see a health care provider. If your blood pressure is elevated, your provider may recommend more-frequent monitoring. Testing is especially important if you are Black, overweight or inactive, or have a family history of high blood pressure (hypertension). These factors increase your risk of high blood pressure.

What do the numbers mean? An ideal or normal blood pressure for an adult of any age is 119 millimeters of mercury (mm Hg) over 79 mm Hg or lower. This is commonly written as 119/79 mm Hg. See page 328 for the table of blood pressure categories and ranges.

Breast cancer screening
Two tests — a clinical breast exam and mammogram — are typically done in conjunction with one another. A clinical breast exam (CBE) is a physical check of your breasts and underarms that's often part of a routine physical. With a mammogram, images are taken of your breast tissue while your breasts are compressed between X-ray plates.

What's the test for? CBEs and mammograms aim to detect cancer and precancerous changes in the breasts. With a CBE, your health care provider examines your breasts looking for lumps, color changes, skin irregularities and changes in your nipples. He or she then feels for enlarged lymph nodes under your arms. A mammogram can help point out small breast lumps and calcifications — often the first indication of early-stage breast cancer — that are too small to be detected on a physical exam.

When and how often should you have it? Based on current research, there's uncertainty around the benefits of CBEs and whether or when to recommend them. For this reason, your practitioner may offer the exam as part of shared decision-making. Before age 40, women may be offered a CBE at least every three years. For women age 40 and older, the exam may be offered every year. Having regular breast exams is particularly important if you have a family history of breast cancer or other factors that put you at increased risk of breast cancer.

As outlined in Chapter 17, there's been disagreement in recent years over the best screening schedule for mammograms. At Mayo Clinic, the current practice is to offer an annual screening mammogram beginning at age 40. Talk with your health care practitioner about a schedule that's right for you. Chapter 17 also outlines other breast imaging methods that may be used.

Cervical cancer screening

With a Pap test, your health care provider inserts a plastic or metal speculum into your vagina to view the cervix. Then, using a spatula and a soft brush, he or she gently obtains scrapings from the cervix, places the sample in a bottle and sends it to a laboratory for analysis. This test is often accompanied by a human papillomavirus (HPV) screening, which involves the same process and can be done at the same time. Or an HPV test may be done on its own.

What's the test for? The Pap test detects cancer and precancerous changes in the cervix. HPV screening is done to check for the presence of a high-risk strain of HPV. Almost all cervical cancers are linked to infection with a high-risk strain of this sexually transmitted virus.

When and how often should you have it? Multiple guidelines exist. For women ages 21 to 29, a Pap test is recommended every three years. Women ages 30 to 65 should have co-testing — HPV testing in addition to the Pap — every five years. Alternately, an HPV test may be done on its own every five years in women ages 25 to 65.

For women who've had a total hysterectomy — which includes removal of the cervix — for a noncancerous condition, these routine tests aren't necessary. They're also not necessary if you're age 65 or older, you've had normal Pap and HPV test results over the past 10 years, and you aren't at high risk of developing cervical cancer. When in doubt, ask your health care practitioner what's appropriate for you.

Regular cervical cancer screening is especially important if you've had a sexually transmitted infection or multiple sex partners, or if you have a history of cervical, vaginal or vulvar cancer. You're also at increased risk of cervical cancer and should be screened regularly if your immune system is suppressed (including infection with HIV) or you were exposed to the synthetic hormone diethylstilbestrol (DES) in utero. Smoking increases your risk too.

Although there's no known cure for HPV infection, the cervical changes that result from it can be treated. Fortunately, for most women, HPV infection clears on its own within 1 to 2 years.

Cholesterol test

A blood cholesterol test is actually made up of several blood tests. It measures total cholesterol in your blood, as well as levels of low-density lipoprotein (LDL), or "bad," cholesterol, high-density lipoprotein (HDL), or "good," cholesterol and other blood fats called *triglycerides*.

What's the test for? Cholesterol tests measure the levels of cholesterol and triglycerides (lipids) in your blood. Undesirable lipid levels raise your risk of heart attack and stroke. Problems happen when your LDL cholesterol contributes to fatty deposits (plaques) developing on your artery walls or when your HDL cholesterol carries away too little LDL cholesterol from the arteries.

When and how often should you have it? Have a cholesterol evaluation at least every five years if the levels are within normal ranges. If the readings are abnormal, have your cholesterol checked more often. Cholesterol testing is especially important if you have a family history of high cholesterol or heart disease, are overweight, are physically inactive or have diabetes. These factors put you at increased risk of developing high cholesterol and heart disease.

What do the numbers mean? The National Cholesterol Education Program has established guidelines to help determine which numbers are acceptable and which carry increased risk. However, desirable ranges vary, depending on your individual health conditions, habits and family history. Talk with your health care provider about your cholesterol levels and any steps you can take to keep them in a healthy range. General guidelines are given in the table on page 376.

Colorectal cancer screening

For this screening exam, a variety of tests may be used.

- *Colonoscopy.* With this exam, a long, flexible tube (colonoscope) is inserted into the rectum, which allows the health care provider to examine the entire length of your colon. This is considered the gold standard for colon cancer screening.
- *Virtual colonoscopy.* For this exam, computerized tomography (CT) produces cross-sectional images of your abdominal organs.
- *Flexible sigmoidoscopy.* Similar to a colonoscopy, a thin tube is inserted into your rectum. However, this test evaluates only the lower part of the colon (sigmoid colon).

BASIC CHOLESTEROL GUIDELINES

While individual cholesterol goals may vary, here's a breakdown of general cholesterol guidelines.

Total cholesterol	
Below 200 milligrams per deciliter (mg/dL)	Desirable
200-239 mg/dL	Borderline high
240 mg/dL and above	High
LDL cholesterol	
Below 100 mg/dL	Optimal
100-129 mg/dL	Near optimal
130-159 mg/dL	Borderline high
160-189 mg/dL	High
190 mg/dL and above	Very high
HDL cholesterol	
Below 50 mg/dL (for women)	Poor
50-59 mg/dL	Better
60 mg/dL and above	Best
Triglycerides	
Below 150 mg/dL	Desirable
150-199 mg/dL	Borderline high
200-499 mg/dL	High
500 mg/dL and above	Very high

Based on NCEP Expert Panel. Third report of the National Cholesterol Education Program (NCEP) Expert Panel on Detection, Evaluation, and Treatment of High Blood Cholesterol in Adults (Adult Treatment Panel III) final report. Circulation. 2002; 106:3143.

- *Barium enema.* For this test, an X-ray is taken of your colon after you have an enema with a white, chalky substance that outlines the colon (barium X-ray).
- *Fecal occult blood test or fecal immunochemical test.* With these tests, a stool sample is tested in a lab for hidden (occult) blood.
- *Stool DNA test (Cologuard).* This test uses a stool sample to look for DNA changes in cells that might indicate the presence of colon cancer or precancerous conditions. It also looks for signs of blood in your stool.

What's the test for? Colorectal exams detect cancer and precancerous growths (polyps) on the colon's inside wall that could become cancerous. While a colorectal cancer screening may seem embarrassing or uncomfortable, this screening could save your life by detecting precancerous polyps, which can be removed.

When and how often should you have it? If you're at average risk of developing colorectal cancer, have a screening test every 3 to 10 years, beginning at age 45. The frequency of screening will depend on the type of test you have. If you have a personal or family history of colorectal cancer or polyps, you will require more-frequent screening.

Talk with your health care practitioner about which screening approach and frequency are best for you. If you're at increased risk of developing colorectal cancer, you may decide to begin screenings at an earlier age and schedule them more frequently.

Dental checkup

In a dental checkup, your dentist examines your teeth and checks your tongue, lips, mouth and soft tissues.

What's the test for? A dental exam is done to detect tooth decay, problems such as tooth grinding and diseases such as gum (periodontal) disease. Your dentist also looks for sores and other abnormalities in your mouth that could indicate cancer.

When and how often should you have it? Have a dental checkup every six months to one year, or as your dentist recommends. Regular dental checkups are especially important if your drinking water doesn't contain fluoride or if you use tobacco, regularly drink alcoholic or high-sugar beverages, or eat foods that are high in sugar.

DIABETES SCREENING NUMBERS

	Blood sugar level	A1C
Normal	70 to 99 milligrams per deciliter (mg/dL)	Below 5.7%
Prediabetes*	100 to 125 mg/dL	5.7% to 6.4%
Diabetes	126 mg/dL or higher on two separate tests	6.5% or higher on two separate tests

*Prediabetes means that your blood sugar level is higher than normal, but it's not yet high enough to be classified as type 2 diabetes. Still, without intervention, prediabetes is likely to become type 2 diabetes in 10 years or less.

Diabetes screening

Two blood tests are commonly used to screen for diabetes. A fasting blood sugar test measures the level of sugar (glucose) in your blood after an eight-hour fast. An A1C test measures your average glucose level over the last two or three months by measuring what percentage of your hemoglobin — a protein in red blood cells that carries oxygen — is coated with sugar.

What's the test for? Diabetes screening can detect high (elevated) glucose levels, which can damage your heart and circulatory system.

When and how often should you have it? Have a baseline screening by age 45. If your results are normal, have your blood sugar rechecked every three years. If you have a family history of diabetes or other risk factors for the disease, such as obesity, your health care provider may recommend that you be tested at a younger age and more frequently. Screening is also recommended if you have signs and symptoms of diabetes, such as excessive thirst, frequent urination, unexplained weight loss, fatigue, or slow-healing cuts or bruises.

What do the numbers mean? A normal blood glucose level for an adult of any age is 70 to 99 milligrams per deciliter (mg/dL). If your blood sugar is between 100 and 125 mg/dL, you're considered to have prediabetes. Prediabetes is a medical condition that puts you at a higher risk of developing diabetes in the future. If your blood sugar is equal to or greater than 126 mg/dL on two separate tests, you'll be diagnosed with diabetes. For someone who doesn't have diabetes, a normal A1C level is below 5.7%, while an A1C between 5.7% and 6.4% indicates prediabetes. An A1C of 6.5% or higher on two separate tests indicates that you have diabetes.

Eye exam

During an eye exam, you read eye charts and have your pupils dilated with eye drops. Your health care provider also views the inside of your eye with an instrument called an *ophthalmoscope* and checks the pressure inside your eye with tonometry, a painless procedure.

What's the test for? An eye exam allows your ophthalmologist or optometrist to check your vision and figure out whether you may be at risk of developing vision problems.

When and how often should you have it? If you wear glasses or contact lenses, have your eyes checked once a year. If you don't wear corrective lenses and have no risk factors for eye disease, have your eyes checked every 2 to 4 years until age 65. After age 65, it's best to have an exam every year or two.

Hearing test

During a hearing test, a hearing specialist (audiologist) or other health care provider checks how well you recognize speech and sounds at various volumes and frequencies.

What's the test for? These screenings check for hearing loss, which becomes more common with increased age.

When and how often should you have it? Have your hearing checked every 10 years until age 50. Starting at age 50, have it checked every three years. Hearing tests are especially important if you've been exposed to loud noises through your job or recreational activities, have had frequent ear infections, or are older than age 60. These factors increase your risk of hearing loss.

Osteoporosis screening

Bone density is measured by way of a specialized X-ray scan of a few bones — usually in the hip and spine.

What's the test for? Bone density tests detect osteoporosis — a disease most common to women that involves gradual loss of bone mass, making your bones more fragile and likely to fracture. Osteoporosis most often increases the risk of fractures of the hip, spine and wrist. There are several different types of scans available. They include dual energy X-ray absorptiometry (DXA) and computerized tomography (CT). These tests are described in detail in Chapter 18.

When and how often should you have it? Women should have a baseline exam at age 65. However, if you have a family history of osteoporosis or other risk factors, earlier testing is a good idea. Risk factors for osteoporosis include early menopause, frequent or extended use of certain medications, including steroids, smoking, excessive alcohol consumption, low body weight, rheumatoid arthritis and a history of fractures.

What do the numbers mean? The T-score is a number that describes how much your bone density varies from what's considered "normal." Normal is based on the typical bone mass of white women in their 30s — the period of life when bone mass is at its peak. Peak bone mass varies from one person to another and is influenced by many factors, including genes, sex and race. People who are white or of Asian descent generally have lower bone density than do Black people and Hispanic people.

Normal	T-score above -1
Low bone mass (osteopenia)	T-score between -1 and -2.5
Osteoporosis	T-score of -2.5 or lower
Severe osteoporosis	T-score of -2.5 or lower with skeletal fracture

Sexually transmitted infection screening

Sexually transmitted infections (STIs), such as chlamydia and gonorrhea, are not just a problem for young adults. Anytime you have a new sexual partner, you're at risk of an STI. And often, these infections don't show symptoms to alert you in the early stages.

What's the test for? These tests determine the presence of STIs, which are generally acquired by sexual contact. The organisms that cause these infections may pass from person to person in blood, semen, or vaginal and other body fluids. Apart from HPV screening — which is discussed with cervical cancer screening — STI screening is not routine for women in midlife. But if you're engaging in unprotected sex or you have multiple partners, screening is important.

When and how often should you have it? Before having intercourse with a new partner, and after exposure to a new partner, be sure you've both been tested for STIs. It's recommended that you get screened for HIV and for hepatitis C at least once during your lifetime. Testing again may be appropriate if you engage in behaviors that increase your risk, such as having unprotected sex and having sexual contact with multiple partners.

Skin examination

In this exam, your health care provider inspects your skin from head to toe, looking for moles and spots that are irregularly shaped, have varied colors, are asymmetrical, are greater than the size of a pencil eraser, bleed or have changed since the previous visit.

What's the test for? Skin exams check for signs of skin cancer or other skin changes that may put you at increased risk of skin cancer.

When and how often should you have it? Consider having a full-body skin exam yearly once you turn 50. Regular screening for skin cancer is especially important if you have many moles, fair skin, sun-damaged skin or a family history of skin cancer or if you had two or more blistering sunburns in childhood or adolescence. These factors put you at increased risk of developing skin cancer. It's also important to check your own skin for changes, preferably once a month.

PREVENTIVE SCREENING EXAMS FOR WOMEN

This schedule of recommended screenings can help you stay on top of your health for the long run. These recommendations are based on

Type of screening	Ages 50-59	Ages 60-69
Blood pressure	At least every 2 years	At least every 2 years
Breast cancer	Every 1-2 years	Every 1-2 years
Cervical cancer	Every 3-5 years	Every 3-5 years; ask health care provider after age 65
Cholesterol	At least every 5 years	At least every 5 years
Colorectal cancer	Every 3-10 years (depends on test) starting at age 45	Every 3-10 years (depends on test)
Diabetes	Every 3 years	Every 3 years
Eye health	Every 2-4 years; yearly if you wear glasses or contacts	Until age 65, every 2-4 years; beginning at age 65, every 1-2 years; yearly if you wear glasses
Hearing	Every 3 years	Every 3 years
Osteoporosis	Ask health care provider	Baseline by age 65
Sexually transmitted infections	Every year if at increased risk; at least one lifetime HIV screening	Every year if at increased risk; at least one lifetime HIV screening
Skin	Ask health care provider	Ask health care provider

average risk and normal results on prior testing. Talk with your health care practitioner to tailor it for you.

Ages 70-79	Ages 80 and older
At least every 2 years	At least every 2 years
Every 1-2 years	Ask health care provider
Ask health care provider	Ask health care provider
At least every 5 years	At least every 5 years
Every 3-10 years (depends on test). Ask health care provider after age 75	Ask health care provider
Every 3 years	Every 3 years
Every 1-2 years; yearly if you wear glasses	Every 1-2 years; yearly if you wear glasses
Every 3 years	Every 3 years
Ask health care provider	Ask health care provider
Every year if at increased risk; at least one lifetime HIV screening	Every year if at increased risk; at least one lifetime HIV screening
Ask health care provider	Ask health care provider

RECOMMENDED VACCINATIONS

One of the best ways to prevent many diseases is to make sure you've received all the recommended vaccinations. Vaccines work by stimulating your body's natural defense mechanisms to resist infectious disease, destroying the disease-causing microbes before you become sick. Most vaccinations are given in childhood. But there are some vaccines that are recommended specifically for adults or may be recommended regularly throughout life. Or it may be that you didn't receive a vaccination in childhood that, if given now, could still be of benefit.

When in doubt, follow your health care provider's advice on which vaccinations to receive and when. He or she may recommend additional vaccinations depending on your occupation, hobbies or travel plans.

Chickenpox (varicella)

This viral disease spreads easily from person to person. Chickenpox is much more serious in adults than in children.

When you're at increased risk You're a health care worker without immunity or an adult who has never been exposed to the disease or never been vaccinated.

Doses for adults A two-dose series is given 4 to 8 weeks apart. Avoid this if you have weakened immunity or cancer of the lymph nodes or bone marrow or if you've had a serious allergic reaction to gelatin or the antibiotic neomycin.

COVID-19

This contagious respiratory disease is caused by the virus SARS-CoV-2. Infection can lead to mild to serious illness and can be fatal. The virus usually spreads between people in close contact by way of droplets that are released when someone breathes, coughs, sneezes, talks or sings.

When you're at increased risk Serious illness from COVID-19 is more common among people who are older or have asthma, heart disease, diabetes, obesity, stroke or dementia, kidney or liver disease, cancer, or other conditions. Anyone with a weakened immune system also has a higher risk.

Doses for adults A two-dose series, given 3 to 8 weeks apart, is most common for adults and children age 5 and older. A booster dose can be given at least two months after the primary series is complete. Additional boosters may be recommended. Talk with your practitioner about vaccine doses if you have a weakened immune system.

Hepatitis A
This viral infection of the liver is transmitted primarily through contaminated food or water or close personal contact.

When you're at increased risk You're traveling to a country without clean water or proper sewage, you have chronic liver disease or a blood-clotting disorder, or you use illegal drugs.

Doses for adults A two-dose series is given with at least six months between doses. Avoid this vaccination if you're hypersensitive to alum or 2-phenoxyethanol, a preservative.

Hepatitis B
This viral infection of the liver is often transmitted through contaminated blood, sexual contact or prenatal exposure.

When you're at increased risk Your occupation puts you at risk of exposure to blood and body fluids, you have chronic liver disease, you're on dialysis or have received blood products, or you're sexually active with multiple partners.

Doses for adults A three-dose series is given during a six-month period to prevent the disease. Avoid this if you're allergic to baker's yeast.

Influenza (flu)
The flu is a respiratory disease that spreads from person to person when you inhale infected droplets in the air.

When you're at increased risk You are age 50 or older, have a chronic disease or a weakened immune system, work in health care or have close contact with people who are at high risk of the disease.

Doses for adults One dose every year is recommended for all adults. The vaccine is typically available as an injection or as a nasal spray. If you're age 65 or older, consider receiving the high-dose version of the vaccine. Talk to your health care provider if you're allergic to eggs or if you've had a previous reaction to a flu shot —

some preparations may be available that are less likely to cause an allergic reaction.

Measles, mumps and rubella

These are viral diseases that spread from person to person when infected droplets in the air are inhaled.

When you're at increased risk You were born after 1956 and don't have proof of previous vaccination or immunity.

Doses for adults One or two doses are given. Avoid this if you received blood products in the past 11 months, have weakened immunity or are allergic to the antibiotic neomycin.

Meningococcal disease

This is a disease caused by the bacteria that can cause meningitis, which is an inflammation of the membranes surrounding the brain and spinal cord.

When you're at increased risk You have a compromised immune system or you travel to certain foreign countries.

Doses for adults A single dose can prevent bacterial meningitis.

Pneumonia

Pneumonia is an infection of the lungs and can have various causes, such as bacteria or viruses.

When you're at increased risk You're age 65 or older, you have a medical condition that increases your risk, such as chronic lung, liver or kidney disease, or you have a missing or damaged spleen.

Doses for adults There are currently two types of pneumococcal vaccines, which are recommended for all adults age 65 or older, with at least one year between the two doses. They may also be recommended for adults under age 65 with certain risk factors.

Tetanus and diphtheria (may include pertussis)

Tetanus is a bacterial infection that develops in deep wounds. Diphtheria is a bacterial infection contracted when you inhale infected droplets. Whooping cough (pertussis) causes upper respiratory symptoms and a hacking cough.

When you're at increased risk You experienced a deep or dirty cut or wound. For pertussis, you're at risk if you haven't received a previous pertussis vaccination — especially if you have close contact with an infant, for whom pertussis is particularly risky.

Doses for adults An initial tetanus and diphtheria (Td) series is given with a booster every 10 years. If your most recent booster was more than five years ago, get a booster within 48 hours after sustaining a wound. Tetanus, diphtheria and pertussis (Tdap) is also given as an initial three-dose series if you didn't finish the Td series as a child, and a Tdap booster is given during pregnancy to help protect the baby from whooping cough in the first months of life. Otherwise, get one dose of Tdap when you're due for a booster, followed by a Td booster every 10 years.

Shingles

Shingles is a viral infection that causes a painful rash. It's caused by varicella-zoster — the same virus that causes chickenpox.

When you're at increased risk You're older than age 50 and you have had chickenpox.

Doses for adults Two doses of the Shingrix vaccine, given 2 to 6 months apart, are generally recommended for adults age 50 or older. It doesn't matter if you've previously had shingles or chickenpox or if you received a dose of Zostavax, an earlier vaccine that's no longer available in the United States. The vaccine also is recommended for anyone over age 19 with a weakened immune system.

PARTNER WITH YOUR PRACTITIONER

Keep in mind that the recommendations in this chapter are general guidelines. For example, if you're planning to travel internationally, you'll want to make sure you're up to date on routine vaccinations. Also, depending on your destination, length of stay and medical history, you may need additional vaccines. Check the Centers for Disease Control and Prevention (CDC) recommendations for your destination.

Talk with your health care provider about your individual risks and preferences for care. Developing a healthy partnership with your provider — one where you can candidly discuss your risks, concerns, dreams, goals and symptoms — is a key step in maintaining good health.

Index

I